Oxidative Stress and Cardiac Failure

Edited by

Marrick L. Kukin, MD

Associate Professor of Medicine
Mount Sinai School of Medicine
Director, Heart Failure Program
The Zena and Michael A. Wiener Cardiovascular Institute
Mount Sinai Medical Center
New York, New York

Valentin Fuster, MD, PhD

Richard Gorlin, MD/Heart Research Foundation Professor of Cardiology
Mount Sinai School of Medicine
Director, The Zena and Michael A. Wiener Cardiovascular Institute
Mount Sinai Medical Center
New York, New York

Futura Publishing
Company, Inc.
Armonk, NY

Library of Congress Cataloging-in-Publications Data

Oxidative stress and cardiac failure / edited by Marrick L. Kukin,
Valentin Fuster.
     p. ; cm.
Includes bibliographical references and index.
   ISBN 0-87993-709-2 (alk. paper)
   1. Heart failure—Pathophysiology. 2. Stress (Physiology) 3. Free radicals (Chemistry)—Pathophysiology. 4. Active oxygen—Pathophysiology.
   [DNLM: 1. Heart Failure, Congestive—physiopathology. 2. Free Radicals. 3. Oxidative Stress—physiology. WG 370 O98 2002] I. Kukin, Marrick L. II. Fuster, Valentin.
   RC682.9 .O96 2002
   616.1′2907—dc21

                                       2002011514

Copyright ©2003
Futura Publishing Company, Inc.

Published by
Futura Publishing Company
135 Bedford Road
Armonk, NY 10504
www.futuraco.com

LC#: 2002011514
ISBN#: 0–87993–709-2

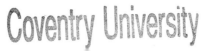

Dedication

This book is dedicated to my parents, Ira and Doris, my wife, Phyllis, and my children, Sarah, William, and Dana. Their collective and individual support, encouragement, understanding, and love helped me reach this point in my cardiology career where I could attempt to undertake the humbling and daunting task of editing a book.

MK

Acknowledgments

I am indebted and appreciative to my friends and colleagues who so generously provided their time and expertise in their respective chapter contributions. Their seminal contributions to the field of heart failure and oxidative stress have defined and advanced this field of study, which has thereby reached a time point that allowed me to prepare this book.

Mr. Steven Korn of Futura Publishing has been a steady source of encouragement, advice, and help. His initial note to me over 2 years ago after a review article that I had written started this endeavor.

Finally, I am most appreciative of the time, effort, advice, mentoring, and friendship of my co-editor and Division Chief, Valentin Fuster.

Foreword

Heart failure was viewed not too many years ago as a complication of primary damage to the heart muscle. Its progression was assumed to represent the consequence of further myocardial damage from the primary disease. Dysfunction of the heart muscle was presumed to be the cause of symptoms and of shortened life expectancy. Treatment therefore was obligatorily aimed at pharmacological support of the failing muscle and at reversing the disease that was at the root of the myocardial contractile deficiency.

How far we have come! A focus on contractile dysfunction has been replaced by a recognition that structural remodeling changes affecting the wall and chamber of the left ventricle are the primary determinants of the poor prognosis. And the dysfunction that contributes to symptoms may be as much a consequence of this remodeling process than of the primary disease process itself.

This focus on myocardial and interstitial structure has led to the recognition that the primary disease process, important as it is, may not be the critical determinant of progression of the disease. Instead, focus has been shifted to the neurohormonal, cellular, and molecular factors that may directly influence the myocyte, the fibroblast, and their structural organization. The number of these systems that appear to be activated in heart failure and contributing to the structural remodeling is now overwhelming. Inhibition of some of these systems has been associated with slowing of disease progression, thus supporting the hypothesis that these systems are contributing directly to the poor outcome in clinical heart failure.

But are these diverse mechanisms exerting their adverse effects through different pathways? Or might there be a common pathway for muscle dysfunction, cellular growth and remodeling, and myocyte death? This text, edited by Marrick Kukin and Valentin Fuster, proposes that oxidative stress may be the common pathway. Most of the putative adverse mechanisms may be associated with generation of reactive oxygen species and most of the effective therapies appear to attenuate oxidative stress. Still to be confirmed is whether antioxidants themselves exert a favorable effect. Disappointment from early clinical trials can certainly be attributed to ineffective agents given in the wrong doses.

The provocative chapters contributed by acknowledged experts in this field provide a persuasive argument for raising the profile of oxidative stress as an important and perhaps critical contributor to the adverse consequences of heart failure. As in all areas of physiology, separation of primary contributors from epiphenomena is challenging. Future research will reveal the importance of this hypothesis, but the present volume should serve in the meantime as a rich source of supportive data.

Jay N. Cohn, MD
Professor of Medicine
University of Minnesota Medical School

Introduction

Free radicals and oxidative stress in biological systems have been considered modulators and mediators of numerous disease states. The regulation of these systems appears to be essential for a biological homeostasis. Over the past 15 years, there has been increasing evidence that free radicals and oxidative stress play a significant role in the pathogenesis of heart failure.

This book should appeal to clinical and basic science investigators as well as to the practicing cardiologist. Depending on one's background and interest, different chapters will be read in great detail or skimmed. In an effort to provide a 'road map,' the following is an outline of highlights of the various chapters to help the reader navigate the book. Each chapter also emphasizes not only what is currently known, but also future directions in research in the respective areas.

Heart failure is a syndrome that encompasses a spectrum of disease states from asymptomatic left ventricular dysfunction to New York Heart Association class IV symptoms with congestion. In fact, the acronym CHF has dual meaning in many situations, with the C often being used interchangeably between chronic and congestive heart failure. In this book, when CHF is used, it is intended to mean congestive heart failure, and in the other instances the word chronic is spelled out. The distinction is important, as patients may have the symptoms of low-output chronic heart failure such as fatigue and dyspnea without congestive symptoms.

This book has been divided into three sections. The first part is current concepts in heart failure. Chapter 1, by Drs. Tang and Francis, provides an excellent and in-depth review of the definition of heart failure, including systolic and diastolic dysfunction and the epidemiology and natural history of the disease. The authors examine how differing databases can provide different information and insights into the natural history information. The detailed tables are extremely helpful in amplifying the information in the text. As a syndrome rather than a specific disease, heart failure has an enormous heterogeneity of presentation and natural history in patients. This is followed by a chapter on the pathophysiology of heart failure by Drs. Tsvetkova and Bristow. The authors present an excellent discussion of the intrinsic and modulatable categories of left ventricular contractile dysfunction.

The second part of this book details the pathophysiology of free radicals and oxidative stress with emphasis on the clinical and laboratory evidence. It starts with a comprehensive overview of the chemistry of oxygen free radicals and reactive oxygen species in biological systems by Drs. Zweier and Villamena. Using detailed chemical equations and illustrations, they demonstrate the cascade and amplification of these reactions, emphasizing the effects of unregulated oxygen free radicals to impact myocardial dysfunction. In addition, they review some of the techniques available to measure and quantify free radical activity.

In chapter 4, Drs. Wong, Struthers, and Belch review and expand upon the seminal contribution to the field of free radicals and heart failure, with Professors Belch's initial observations in 1991 of increased oxidative stress in heart failure patients. The evidence of oxidative stress in heart failure is clearly and cogently presented with the impact of how free radicals affect the course and pathophysiology of heart failure.

The next three chapters in this section provide the experimental evidence and translational understanding of oxidative stress beginning with animal models detailed by Drs. Sabbah and Tanhehco. They provide an excellent review of the relationship between apoptosis (programmed cell death) and progression of heart failure while exploring the possibility that oxidative stress is a mechanism that increases apoptosis.

This is followed by an outstanding chapter by Drs. Shawky, Khaper, and Liu that bridges bench to bedside by detailing free radicals, iron, and cytokines. These authors review a model of iron overload that causes diastolic heart failure, which has been found to be directly attributable to free radical excess, and a model of systolic dysfunction following cardiac injury that involves cytokine/free radical excess, which leads to progressive remodeling and cell deaths.

The section concludes with chapter 7 by Drs. Siwik, Pimentel, Xiao, Singh, Sawyer, and Colucci, focusing on complementary mechanisms leading to oxidative stress in the myocardium—adrenergic and mechanical factors. In this excellent chapter, which is a superb model of translational research, the authors cite relevant experiments demonstrating that reactive oxygen species act as intracellular signaling molecules in cardiac myocytes and fibroblasts and may thus play a central role in determining the myocardial response to extracellular remodeling stimuli such as mechanical strain and neurohormones.

The third section enters the clinical realm by focusing on therapeutic pathways and modulation of oxidative stress. It is divided by pharmacological or biological targets. Each of the chapters is based on a current effective therapy for heart failure. A careful reading of this section will form the underpinning of current pharmacological therapies for heart failure. Within the framework of this book, there is an emphasis on developing the current knowledge associating these effective therapies with their effect on reducing oxidative stress as a potential causative mechanism of their benefits. There are three chapters on neurohormonal antagonists that have shown evidence of reducing oxidative stress: β-blockers, angiotensin-converting enzyme (ACE) inhibitors, and angiotensin II receptor blockers.

Chapter 8 reviews the major mortality studies of β-blockers in heart failure and then explores the data of β-blockers and oxidative stress, with both carvedilol and metoprolol. Reduction of oxidative stress by β-blockers may be an important mechanism of action of this crucial therapy in chronic heart failure. The next chapter, by Drs. Singh and Abraham, focuses on ACE inhibitors and their crucial role in treating heart failure and their impact on oxidative stress. They elegantly review the laboratory, animal, and human evidence for ACE inhibitors in reducing oxidative stress as a mechanism of its beneficial effects.

In chapter 10, Drs. Berry and McMurray provide an excellent review of the data on angiotensin II receptor blockers and oxidative stress. They describe how activation of the renin-angiotensin system may promote free radical production in vascular diseases which may contribute to the development of heart failure. They then consider how angiotensin receptor blockers may attenuate vascular free radical production and oxidative stress and how these actions may contribute to the therapeutic effects of these drugs in CHF.

Chapter 11 explores the interplay of the microvasculature with oxidative stress, coronary flow, reperfusion injury, the vulnerable plaque, and the acute coronary syndrome. In chapter 12, Drs. Zheng, Krum, and Katz critically review the role of reactive oxygen species in the pathogenesis of endothelial dysfunction by citing relevant experimental and clinical studies, cellular effects of reactive oxygen species which may impact on endothelial function—considering an effect via cell signaling, altered nitric oxide synthase (eNOS) expression or eNOS availability, and the potential effects of specific antioxidant therapeutic interventions on vascular function in heart failure.

The antioxidant vitamins A, C, and E have long been linked with reducing oxidative stress in biological systems. In the final chapter, Drs. Qin and Liang provide an excellent review of the clinical and laboratory evidence of antioxidant vitamins and their experimental and clinical roles in reducing the incidence of apoptosis and progression of heart failure.

The division of this book into these three sections and their component chapters was chosen to provide the most comprehensive review of the subject with contributions from the recognized experts in the field. Inevitably, and perhaps beneficially, there is some overlap among chapters. For instance, the subject of apoptosis and heart failure overlaps the experimental and therapeutic discussions. Similarly, given the important role of endothelial function in heart failure and oxidative stress, different chapters address this topic in both therapeutic and experimental areas. Rather than being a problem, I view this as a strength of the book by showing the complementary nature of the chapter distinctions that were made in order to provide an orderly sequencing to this book. I have attempted by chapter assignment and editing to minimize overlap and instead mold the chapters into a comprehensive whole. Any failure to achieve that is my sole responsibility and not that of any chapter authors.

It is our hope that this book will not only review the topic of oxidative stress and heart failure for investigators and clinicians, but also spur further research and clinical applications in this field.

Marrick Kukin
Valentin Fuster
New York, NY

Contributors

William T. Abraham, MD, FACP, FACC Professor of Medicine, Chief, Division of Cardiology, The Ohio State University Heart Center, Columbus, OH

Jill J.F. Belch, MD, FRCP Professor of Vascular Medicine, Department of Medicine, Ninewells Hospital and Medical School, Dundee, Scotland, UK

Colin Berry, MBChB, PhD, MRCP Registrar in Cardiology and Medicine, Medical Research Council Training Fellow, Clinical Research Initiative in Heart Failure, University of Glasgow, Glasgow, Scotland, UK

Michael R. Bristow, MD, PhD Professor of Medicine, Head, Division of Cardiology, University of Colorado Health Sciences Center, Denver, CO

Wilson S. Colucci, MD Thomas J. Ryan Professor of Medicine and Chief, Cardiovascular Medicine, Boston University Medical Center, Boston, MA

Gary S. Francis, MD Director, Coronary Intensive Care Unit, Department of Cardiovascular Medicine, Cleveland Clinic Foundation, Cleveland, OH

Valentin Fuster, MD, PhD Richard Gorlin, MD/Heart Research Foundation Professor of Cardiology, Mount Sinai School of Medicine; Director, The Zena and Michael A. Wiener Cardiovascular Institute, Mount Sinai Medical Center, New York, NY

Mardi Gomberg-Maitland, MD, MSc Faculty, Department of Cardiology, Zena and Michael A. Wiener Cardiovascular Institute, Mount Sinai Medical Center, New York, NY

Stuart D. Katz, MD Associate Professor of Internal Medicine, Yale University School of Medicine, New Haven, CT

Neelam Khaper, PhD CIHR Fellow in Cardiovascular Research, Heart and Stroke/Richard Lewar Centre of Excellence, University of Toronto; Division of Cardiology, Toronto General Hospital, University Health Network, Toronto, Canada

Henry Krum, MBBS, PhD, FRACP Associate Professor of Medicine, Head of Clinical Pharmacology, Monash University, Melbourne, Australia

Marrick L. Kukin, MD, FACC Associate Professor of Medicine, Mount Sinai School of Medicine; Director, Heart Failure Program, The Zena and Michael A. Wiener Cardiovascular Institute, Mount Sinai Medical Center, New York, NY

Chang-seng Liang, MD, PhD, FACC Professor of Medicine, University of Rochester School of Medicine and Dentistry; Attending Physician, University of Rochester Medical Center/Strong Memorial Hospital, Rochester, NY

Peter Liu, MD Heart and Stroke/Polo Chair Professor of Medicine, Heart and Stroke/Richard Lewar Centre of Excellence, University of Toronto; Division of Cardiology, Toronto General Hospital, University Health Network, Toronto, Canada

John McMurray, BSc(Hons), MBChB, MD, FRCP, FESC, FACC Professor of Medical Cardiology, Clinical Research Initiative in Heart Failure, University of Glasgow, Glasgow, Scotland, UK

David R. Pimentel, MD Instructor of Medicine, Cardiovascular Section, Department of Medicine, Boston University School of Medicine, Boston, MA

Fuzhong Qin, MD, PhD Research Assistant Professor, University of Rochester School of Medicine and Dentistry, Rochester, NY

Hani N. Sabbah, PhD Professor of Medicine, Director, Cardiovascular Research, Henry Ford Hospital, Detroit, MI

Douglas B. Sawyer, MD, PhD Assistant Professor of Medicine, Cardiovascular Section, Department of Medicine, Boston University School of Medicine, Boston, MA

Mona Shawky, MD CIHR Fellow in Cardiovascular Research, Heart and Stroke/Richard Lewar Centre of Excellence, University of Toronto; Division of Cardiology, Toronto General Hospital, University Health Network, Toronto, Canada

Balkrishna Singh, MD, FACC Assistant Professor of Medicine, Division of Cardiology, University of Arkansas for Medical Sciences, Little Rock, AR

Krisha Singh, PhD Associate Professor, Department of Physiology, East Tennessee State University, Johnson City, TN

Deborah A. Siwik, PhD Instructor of Medicine, Cardiovascular Section, Department of Medicine, Boston University School of Medicine, Boston, MA

Allan D. Struthers, MD, FRCP   Professor of Cardiovascular Medicine and Therapeutics, Department of Clinical Pharmacology, Ninewells Hospital and Medical School, Dundee, Scotland, UK

W.H. Wilson Tang, MD   Fellow in Cardiology, Department of Cardiovascular Medicine, Cleveland Clinic Foundation, Cleveland, OH

Elaine J. Tanhehco, PhD   Department of Medicine, Division of Cardiovascular Medicine, Henry Ford Heart and Vascular Institute, Detroit, MI

Tatiana Tsvetkova, MD   Fellow, Cardiology, University of Colorado Health Sciences Center, Denver, CO

Frederick A. Villamena, PhD   Postdoctoral Fellow, Davis Heart and Lung Institute, Department of Medicine, The Ohio State University College of Medicine, Columbus, OH

Kenneth Y.K. Wong, MA (Oxon), BM BCh (Oxon), MRCP (UK)   British Heart Foundation Clinical Research Fellow and Honorary SpR, Department of Clinical Pharmacology, Ninewells Hospital and Medical School, Dundee, Scotland, UK

Lei Xiao, PhD   Instructor of Medicine, Cardiovascular Section, Department of Medicine, Boston University School of Medicine, Boston, MA

Haoyi Zheng, MD   Postdoctoral Research Associate, Yale University School of Medicine, New Haven, CT; Attending Physician of Cardiology, Peking Union Medical College, Beijing, P.R. China

Jay L. Zweier, MD   Director, Davis Heart and Lung Research Institute, Professor of Internal Medicine, John H. and Mildred C. Lumley Chair in Medicine, The Ohio State University College of Medicine, Columbus, OH

Abbreviations Used in This Book

AAPH = 2,2-azobis [2-amidino propane] dihydrochloride
ACE = angiotensin-converting enzyme
ADP = adenosine diphosphate
ALVD = asymptomatic left ventricular dysfunction
ANP = atrial natriuretic peptide
ARB = angiotensin II receptor blocker
ASK1 = apoptosis signal-regulating kinase
ATP = adenosine triphosphate
BNP = brain natriuretic peptide
BzPO = benzoyl peroxide
Cdk = cyclin-dependent kinase
CHF = congestive heart failure
COX = cyclooxygenase
DCM = dilated cardiomyopathy
DDC = diethyldithiocarbamic acid
DMPO = dimethyl pyrrolidine oxide
DPI = diphenylene iodonium
EDRF = endothelium-derived relaxing factor
EHNA = erythro-9-(2-hydroxy-3-nonyl) adenine
eNOS = endothelial nitric oxide synthase
EPR = electron paramagnetic resonance
ERK = extracellular signal-regulated kinase
Fe-MGD = Fe^{2+}-N-methyl-D-glucamine dithiocarbamate
GPx = glutathione peroxidase
GSH = glutathione
HIF-1 = hypoxia-inducible factor 1
HUVEC = human umbilical vein endothelial cell
ICAM-1 = intercellular adhesion molecule-1
ICE = interleukin-converting enzyme
iNOS = inducible nitric oxide synthase
JNK = Jun kinase
L-NMMA = N-monomethyl-L-arginine
LPO = lipoxygenase
LVEF = left ventricular ejection fraction
LVH = left ventricular hypertrophy
MAPK = mitogen-activated protein kinase
MAPKK = mitogen-activated protein kinase kinase

MDA = malondialdehyde
MI = myocardial infarction
MMP = matrix metalloproteinase
MPO = myeloperoxidase
NADH = nicotinamide adenine dinucleotide
NAD(P)H = nicotinamide adenine dinucleotide phosphate
NO = nitric oxide
NOS = nitric oxide synthase
   eNOS, NOS3 = endothelial nitric oxide synthase
   iNOS, NOS2 = inducible nitric oxide synthase
   nNOS, NOS1 = neuronal nitric oxide synthase
NT = nucleotide transport
OFR = oxygen free radical
PAT = phenylazotriphenylmethane
PGHS = prostaglandin synthase
PHE = percentage of hemolysed erythrocytes
PKC = protein kinase C
RAAS = renin-angiotensin-aldosterone system
ROS = reactive oxygen species
SAPK = stress-activated protein kinase
sCR1 = soluble complement receptor type 1
SHR = spontaneously hypertensive rat
SOD = superoxide dismutase
   CuZnSOD = copper- and zinc-containing superoxide dismutase
   FeSOD = iron-containing superoxide dismutase
   MnSOD = manganese-containing superoxide dismutase
SAPK = stress-activated protein kinase
TAS = total antioxidant status
TBARS = thiobarbituric acid reactive substance
VEGF = vascular endothelial growth factor
VSMC = vascular smooth muscle cell
XO = xanthine oxidase
XXO xanthine plus xanthine oxidase

Contents

I. Current Concepts in Heart Failure

II. Pathophysiology, Clinical, and Laboratory Evidence of Oxidative Stress in Heart Failure

III. Therapeutic Pathways and Modulation of Oxidative Stress

I

Current Concepts in Heart Failure

• 1 •

Natural History of Heart Failure

W.H. Wilson Tang, MD, and Gary S. Francis, MD

Introduction: The Burden of
Heart Failure Syndrome

Heart failure has been recognized as a major health problem in the world, affecting up to 2.5% of the adult population.[1,2] From the latest figures in the United States, the syndrome of heart failure affects approximately 4.8 million Americans, producing 550,000 new cases each year.[3] These numbers are predicted to increase by 50–70% in the next few decades, even though there have been recent trends of improvement in survival and hospitalization rates.[4,5] Once symptomatic heart failure develops, the outlook for the patient is often particularly poor, with an average 5-year mortality reaching as high as 75% in men and 62% in women— a prognosis that is even worse than most cancers.[6,7]

During this period of disease progression, recurring symptoms and comorbid conditions have a significant adverse impact on the patients' quality of life, which is often characterized by extensive adverse drug effects, invasive procedures, as well as frequent clinic visits and hospitalizations. The result is escalating health care expenditure for the diagnosis and management of heart failure, with the latest conservative estimate in excess of $23.2 billion per year in the United States (or 11% of total expenditure for heart diseases).[3,8] Perhaps the most poignant or telling updated estimates of disease burden of heart failure come from trends in heart failure hospitalization, which made up two-thirds of the expenditure.[3] The latest National Hospital Discharge Survey estimated an increase in hospitalizations from 377,000 in 1979 to more than 962,000 in 1999 for a principal diagnosis of heart failure, an astounding

From: Kukin ML, Fuster V (eds). *Oxidative Stress and Cardiac Failure*. Armonk, NY: Futura Publishing Co., Inc. ©2003.

160% increase over the past two decades.[3] This is accompanied by a 145% increase in heart failure deaths, with the 1999 overall death rate being 18.8%.[3] After a previous hospital discharge for heart failure, readmission rates of 30–50% within 3–6 months have also been reported, regardless of the presence or absence of left ventricular dysfunction.[9–12] Furthermore, the estimated annual number of hospitalizations for any diagnosis of heart failure increased from 1.7 million in 1985 to over 2.6 million in 1995 in the United States.[13] This burden is definitely going to increase further as patients with heart failure survive longer, more drugs and devices become available, and those with minimally symptomatic left ventricular dysfunction are recognized and treated earlier in their natural history.[7]

In recent years, therapeutic advances and better control of cardiac risk factors have led to improved survival of postinfarction patients and perhaps an increase in the size of the elderly population with heart failure.[8] There has also been an expanding interest in developing new medical and surgical strategies to manage this devastating and costly condition. Effective management strategies and knowledge of the underlying pathophysiology require a thorough understanding of the natural history. Therapeutic options that provide the best outcomes at various stages of the disease can then be determined. This chapter reviews our current understanding of the natural history of heart failure based on a wide variety of data sources, and highlights the substantial diversity in etiology, presentation, and clinical course of the heart failure syndrome.

Defining the Natural History of Heart Failure

The lack of a consensus definition of heart failure reflects the complexity of the syndrome.[14] Heart failure is a heterogeneous clinical syndrome that represents a constellation of signs and symptoms usually associated with congestion and circulatory failure. It has many etiologies, and therefore there is substantial variation in the natural history. As the syndrome progresses into the final stages, the natural history tends to unfold in a "final common pathway" with features that are common to most patients. The pace of heart failure progression, however, can vary markedly depending on the etiology. For example, a young woman with primary pulmonary hypertension may have a relatively rapid course culminating in severe right heart failure within 2 to 3 years, while a patient with chronic aortic regurgitation may have subtle or no symptoms for decades and ultimately develop mild to moderate heart failure that is readily controlled by medical or surgical therapy. Therefore, the early natural history of heart failure is characterized by marked heterogeneity and is largely driven by etiological considerations. In contrast, the later stages of heart failure share common features and tend to unfold in a more uniform, predictable manner.

Clinical Presentation

A clinically useful definition of heart failure is necessary if an attempt is to be made to describe the frequency and characteristics of heart failure within a population. Historically when clinical diagnoses were largely made at the bedside, the definition of heart failure was limited to a constellation of clinical signs and symptoms of "congestion," which develop as a consequence of venous congestion and salt and water retention.[15] However, some clinical features of heart failure (such as dyspnea and cardiomegaly) are relatively sensitive but not specific, whereas others (such as edema, ventricular gallop sound, and neck vein distension) are highly specific but relatively insensitive.[16,17] The quality and quantity of symptoms often vary among patients, and most signs and symptoms of heart failure are not independent predictors of outcomes.[18] Overall, there is poor correlation between the clinical signs and symptoms of heart failure and the objective measures of circulatory, ventilatory, neurohormonal, or metabolic dysfunction.[19]

Several scoring systems have been used in population-based studies to establish the diagnosis of heart failure and to determine its severity, but their validity is in question because there is no true "gold standard" (Table 1). In a series of patients suspected of heart failure by general practitioners, only 34% were later confirmed to have heart failure by cardiologists, and about half of prescriptions for "heart failure" are believed to be inappropriate.[20] It is likely that a substantial degree of misdiagnosis of heart failure is common, with symptoms confounded by obesity, advanced lung diseases, or unrecognized ischemic heart diseases.[21] At the other end of the spectrum, up to 50% of patients with "atypical" or even typical signs and symptoms of heart failure on admission may be missed and these patients are unlikely to receive appropriate therapy for heart failure.[22]

Ventricular Dysfunction

Ventricular dysfunction (dilatation and contractile abnormalities) as the primary structural basis for the development of the heart failure syndrome has been described for over 40 years.[23] The primary "lesion" of chronic heart failure is left ventricular remodeling, a process characterized by progressive chamber enlargement and impaired systolic dysfunction.[24] In population studies, up to 90% of patients with left ventricular dysfunction (left ventricular ejection fraction, or LVEF $\leq$35%) have underlying cardiovascular disease, hypertension, or diabetes.[25] However,

Table 1
Diagnosis of Heart Failure by Clinical Scoring Systems

	Framingham[46]	NHANES[51]
Clinical History		
Paroxysmal nocturnal dyspnea	Major	
Orthopnea	Major	
Weight loss (≥4.5 kg in 5 days after Rx)	Major/minor	
Ankle edema	Minor	2
Night cough	Minor	
Dyspnea on exertion/shortness of breath	Minor	1 #–2 ##
Tachycardia (≥120 bpm)	Minor	1 (≤110 bpm)–2 (>110 bpm)
Physical Examination		
Neck vein distention	Major	1
Rales	Major	1 (basal)–2 (> basal)
S3 gallop	Major	
Increased JVP (>16 mm H$_2$0)	Major	
Circulation time (>25 sec)	Major	
Hepatojugular reflex	Major	
Hepatomegaly	Minor	2 (+ neck distention)
Diagnostic tests		
Cardiomegaly (CXR)	Major	
Acute pulmonary edema (CXR)	Major	
Pleural effusion (CXR)	Minor	3 (+ alveolar fluid/edema)
Interstitial edema (CXR)		2
Pulmonary vein cephalization (CXR)		1
Vital capacity (>33% reduced from max)	Minor	

Heart failure definition:
Framingham – 2 major criteria
    or 1 major plus 2 minor criteria;
NHANES – score ≥3.

#Shortness of breath when hurrying on level/slight uphill or walking on level at ordinary pace.
##Stop for breathing on own pace or after 100 yards on level.
CXR = chest x-ray; bpm = beats per minute; Rx = therapy; max = maximum.

the onset of symptoms of heart failure may occur at all levels of ventricular dysfunction. Furthermore, the time course of the natural progression is highly variable. Some patients with deteriorating ventricular dysfunction may even die before developing any symptoms of overt heart failure.[26] Relying on self-reporting is therefore inadequate. This point is highlighted in the findings from the SOLVD (Studies Of Left Ventricular Dysfunction) Registry where patients with ventricular dysfunction (LVEF <45%) were recruited to participate in clinical trials to determine the efficacy of enalapril in heart failure. In 6273 consecutive patients largely screened from echocardiography laboratories, approximately 80% had mild or no symptoms (New York Heart Association functional class, or NYHA I or II).[27] In the SOLVD Registry, only 32% of patients had pulmonary rales, 26% had edema, and 20% had elevated jugular venous distension on clinical examination at the time of enrollment. Therefore, the mechanism whereby patients with heart failure are screened for a large trial, in this case using busy echocardiography laboratories, may have a major influence on both the registry and the type of patients entering the trial.

The availability of modern imaging modalities has revealed widespread discrepancies between the clinical diagnosis of heart failure and underlying ventricular dysfunction. In a recent British series of patients that were being treated for presumed heart failure based on their presenting symptoms, only 36% of men and 18% of women had definitive evidence of impaired ventricular function by echocardiography.[28] Those presenting with typical heart failure symptoms and preserved systolic function are often labeled as having diastolic heart failure (otherwise known as isolated "diastolic dysfunction"). Our understanding of diastolic heart failure has been limited by the difficulty in establishing a precise definition, the requirement for echocardiographic data, and the lack of clinical trials that demonstrate effective therapeutic strategies.[29–31] Nevertheless, diastolic heart failure has pathophysiological derangements similar to patients with systolic dysfunction, such as neuroendocrine activation (raised serum brain natriuretic peptide and norepinephrine levels), and severely reduced exercise capacity and quality of life.[32] Diastolic heart failure can be isolated, but usually coexists with systolic dysfunction. The natural history of diastolic heart failure is somewhat more benign than that of systolic heart failure, but recurrent pulmonary edema is a particularly poor prognostic sign.[33]

Recent studies using echocardiography and biochemical screening assays such as serum brain natriuretic peptide (BNP) have led to the realization that there is a patient population with no clinical heart failure but obvious ventricular dysfunction.[34–36] This condition, otherwise known as asymptomatic left ventricular dysfunction (ALVD), is believed to be at least as prevalent as overt heart failure.[37] When characteristics of ALVD patients are explored, patients are found to be more "under-recognized" than "asymptomatic," as many patients have subtle symptoms following detailed assessment. When comparing patients with ALVD to healthy, age-matched control subjects, ALVD is associated with shorter exercise times on treadmill testing, and lower questionnaire scores for assessing physical functioning.[38] Such patients are at risk for developing heart failure.[39–41] It is likely that patients with ALVD may pass through a "latent" phase with impaired systolic function before developing overt symptoms of heart failure. The concept of continuum from asymptomatic ventricular dysfunction to heart failure is supported by the finding of a surprisingly high incidence of "silent" or undetected myocardial infarction in the community, where up to 30% of such cases have been unrecognized due to the lack of presenting symptoms.[42] Such patients are at risk for developing heart failure. Indeed, recent population-based studies of ALVD have demonstrated that ischemic heart disease may accompany ventricular dysfunction by echocardiography in up to 78% of these cases.[25,43] A lower prevalence of "asymptomatic" ventricular dysfunction seen in the Rotterdam study may also be explained by a lower percentage of patients with ischemic diseases.[34] The term "ventricular dysfunction" should not be used interchangeably with "heart failure"—heart failure implies signs and symptoms of congestion with salt and water retention that are present at rest or with exercise.

Defining Epidemiology and Risk Profiles in Heart Failure

Methodology Considerations

Varying methods of case ascertainment in epidemiological and clinical studies have limited our ability to interpret the true natural history of heart failure.[2,8] There are three main data sources: (1) population-based studies, (2) referral-based studies, and (3) clinical trial databases. They each have their strengths and weaknesses and may complement each other in providing insights into the natural history of heart failure. However, examination of these three types of databases can lead to different but often complementary conclusions.

Population-Based Studies

Most estimates of heart failure epidemiology are limited to population-based studies with well-defined regional communities (such as Framingham, Massachusetts, or Olmsted County, Minnesota). Population-based studies, extracted from the "real world," are regarded as one of the most reliable ways to study the natural history of disease in a population and have greatly shaped our overall understanding of the frequency and risk factors for developing heart failure. Population-based studies are designed to survey a cross-section of the total general population and to dissect out various factors that are associated with the onset and development of heart failure. In particular, population-attributable risks (which take into account both the hazard ratio and the prevalence of the predisposing condition in the general population) can be derived from these studies to assess the potential of developing symptomatic heart failure (Table 2).

Table 2
Population-Attributable Risks (PAR) in Developing Heart Failure
from Major Population-Based Studies

Risk Factors	Framingham Heart Study[46]			Cardiovascular Health Study[201]			NHANES I Epidemiology Study[202]		
	HR	Prev	PAR	RR	Prev	PAR	RR	Prev	PAR
Hypertension	M 2.1 F 3.4	M 60% F 62%	M 39% F 59%	1.4	41%	13%	M 1.3 F 1.5	M 47% F 41%	M 9% F 12%
Coronary artery disease	M 6.3 F 6.0	M 10% F 3%	M 34% F 13%	1.9	17%	13%	M 8.1 F 8.2	M 85% F 84%	M 68% F 56%
Angina	M 1.4 F 1.7	M 11% F 9%	M 5% F 5%	—	—	—	—	—	—
Diabetes mellitus	M 1.8 F 3.7	M 8% F 5%	M 6% F 12%	1.8	12%	8%	M 1.8 F 1.8	M 66% F 62%	M 3% F 3%
Left ventricular hypertrophy (ECG)	M 2.2 F 2.9	M 4% F 3%	M 4% F 5%	2.3	5%	6%	—	—	—
Valvular heart disease	M 2.5 F 2.1	M 5% F 8%	M 7% F 8%	—	—	—	M 1.7 F 1.4	M 62% F 45%	M 3% F 2%
Renal insufficiency	—	—	—	1.8	8%	6%	—	—	—
Low FEV$_1$	—	—	—	1.4	19%	6%	—	—	—
Cerebrovascular disease	—	—	—	1.5	5%	3%	—	—	—
Peripheral vascular disease	—	—	—	1.8	13%	9%	—	—	—

continues

Table 2
Population-Attributable Risks (PAR) in Developing Heart Failure
from Major Population-Based Studies (*Continued*)

Risk Factors	Framingham Heart Study[46]			Cardiovascular Health Study[201]			NHANES I Epidemiology Study[202]		
	HR	Prev	PAR	RR	Prev	PAR	RR	Prev	PAR
Atrial fibrillation (ECG)	—	—	—	2.1	2%	2%	—	—	—
Cigarette smoking	—	—	—	—	—	—	M 1.5 F 1.9	M 45% F 39%	M 16% F 22%
Low physical activity	—	—	—	—	—	—	M 1.1 F 1.3	M 45% F 37%	M 9% F 13%
Male sex	—	—	—	—	—	—	1.2	41%	9%
Overweight	—	—	—	—	—	—	M 1.2 F 1.3	M 45% F 39%	M 6% F 10%
< High school education	—	—	—	—	—	—	M 1.2 F 1.3	M 41% F 36%	M 9% F 10%

Prev = prevalence; HR = hazard ratio (Framingham only); RR = relative risk (CHS & NHANES); M = male; F = female; FEV$_1$ = forced expiratory volume in 1 second.
Blank spaces represent data not reported.

Of course, recognition of these risk factors has important implications for prevention.

Regional populations have the advantage of controlling for overall practice patterns or environmental influences concerning the diagnosis and management of heart failure in a relatively constrained population. Although these studies allow a rare glimpse into the natural progression of heart failure that is relatively free of selection biases, most population-based studies use nonspecific and variable definitions of heart failure. In addition, only relatively small numbers of "incident" and "prevalent" cases are usually identified.

Careful population-based studies that explore the nature of heart failure onset and progression in the community require substantial follow-up (more than 40 years in the Framingham Study), consistent and reliable data collecting processes, and sophisticated analytical techniques. Due to the extended duration of these longitudinal studies, the impact of evolving trends regarding recent therapeutic advances in the management of heart failure can be difficult problems to correct for, but statistical models are helpful. In addition, population-based studies that utilize a unified medical record system and hospital registries may have further potential selection bias by retrospectively identifying patients who sought medical attention or were hospitalized—a patient population that is likely to be more symptomatic. As useful as the population-based studies are, they are not perfect.

Referral-Based Studies

Referral-based studies (such as the Duke databank) are usually performed in a shorter time period, thereby having the advantage of evaluating the impact of contemporary therapeutic strategies on the natural history of heart failure in the community setting. Referral-based studies usually have more selection bias based on the relatively more symptomatic patients who seek medical attention in the community. These studies are also biased toward entry of patients with "index events," such as acute myocardial infarction or valvular dysfunction, and thereby tend to underestimate the epidemiology of patients with minimal symptoms. On the other hand, referral-based studies have the advantage of following a relatively large, community-based heart failure population to examine specific disease characteristics. Confounding factors and outcome measures are often more difficult to assess and control in this setting.

Clinical Trial Databases

Clinical trials are rich repositories of data that allow one to examine specific aspects of heart failure and the differential responses to therapy.

The primary objective of clinical trials is to address the treatment effects of new therapeutics. However, there can be a wide range of inclusion criteria. Sometimes entry criteria are applicable only to a small group of patients, usually younger, more compliant, more educated, and accessible. Large numbers of patients are often screened and excluded from clinical trials, raising doubt that patients in the trials are truly representative of the "real world." The majority of clinical trials in heart failure select patients based on the presence of ventricular dysfunction (often using LVEF criteria from imaging studies). In addition, subjective biases are often present when patients are "cherry-picked" to be enrolled in clinical trials, where investigators may have preconceived notions about the study drug and high hopes of demonstrating clinical benefits for their patients. For example, the relatively large proportion of nonischemic cardiomyopathy patients enrolled in recent beta-blocker heart failure trials may be a reflection of the belief that these drugs might provide selective benefit for this patient population (selection bias). This can also occur in transplantation referral centers where highly selected patients are recruited (population bias).[44,45] There is a widespread belief, whether true or not, that clinical trials do not represent the "real world" of medicine, but are made up of a highly selected and nonrepresentative group of patients. Nevertheless, the availability of a large heart failure study population within a short duration allows a contemporary perspective of heart failure epidemiology to be established.

Epidemiology of Heart Failure

Several excellent population-based studies have described the epidemiology of symptomatic heart failure in regional populations. The Framingham Heart Study is the "gold-standard" prospective cohort study that follows 5209 healthy Framingham residents and their 4196 offspring.[1,46,47] After four decades of systematic follow-up, a total of 498 men and 487 women have developed symptomatic heart failure, with the prevalence rate estimated to be 8 per 1000 persons at ages 50–59 years, increasing to 66–79 per 1000 at ages 80–89 years.[1] During this period, the incidence of heart failure has nearly doubled with each increasing decade of age (from 2 per 1000 persons per year at ages 35–64 years, up to 12 per 1000 persons per year at ages 65–94 years).[46] More contemporary data come from two London studies, quoting an age-adjusted incidence rate of 1.3 new symptomatic heart failure cases per 1000 persons per year (ranging from 0.02 cases per 1000 persons per year in those aged 25–34 years to 11.6 in those aged 85 years and over).[36,48] These findings are consistent among several nationwide surveys and population-based studies (Tables 3 and 4).[34,49–55]

Echocardiographic observational studies have confirmed that up to

Table 3
Prevalence of Heart Failure: Large-Scale Population-Based Studies

Study (start year)	Design	Age Group*	Prevalence per 1000 Total	Male	Female	PLVSF
Framingham MA, USA (1948)[1,46]	10,344 Framingham residents, 47% men, 44 yr longitudinal follow-up with periodic exam, 985 prevalent cases by 1998 identified.	50–59	8	8	8	
		60–69	23	–	–	
		70–79	49	–	–	
		80–89	91	66	79	
		≥45	–	24	25	
		Total (30+)	–	*7.4*	*7.7*	*51%*
Goteborg, Sweden (1963)[53]	973 men born in 1913, prospective periodic exam, 84 HF cases identified.	50–54	–	21	–	NR
		55–60	–	32	–	
		61–67	–	130	–	
NHANES-I, USA (1971)[51]	14,407 subjects, age 25–74 yr, HF diagnosed by self-report, and 6913 persons by clinical exam score.	*Self report:* 25–54	4	4	3	
		55–64	21	22	20	
		65–74	34	37	32	
		Total (25–74)	*11*	*11*	*10*	*NR*
		Clinical: 25–54	11	8	13	
		55–64	37	45	30	
		65–74	45	48	43	
		Total (25–74)	*20*	*19*	*20*	*NR*
NHANES-II, USA (1976)[52]	10,450 subjects age 25–75 yr, HF diagnosed by self-report and clinical score.	*Self-report:*	10.4	–	–	NR
		Clinical: 55–64	–	24.8	26.5	
		65–75	–	50.8	52.8	
		Total (25–74)	*17.8*	–	–	*NR*
Rochester MN, USA (1981)[50]	Rochester residents age ≤74 yr, retrospective chart review, 113 prevalent cases identified.	45–54	–	0.8	1.5	
		55–64	–	9.7	5.2	
		65–74	–	26.8	19.4	
		Total (≤74)	*2.7*	*3.3*	*2.1*	*NR*
Rochester MN, USA (1986)[49]	2122 Rochester residents age ≥35 yr from stratified random sampling, 48% men, questionnaire & chart review, 41 HF cases identified.	35–54	1	1	1	
		55–64	5	5	1	
		65–74	12	23	0	
		75+	76	69	80	
		Total (35+)	*19.3*	*17.6*	*20.9*	*43%*

continues

Table 3
Prevalence of Heart Failure: Large-Scale
Population-Based Studies (*Continued*)

Study (start year)	Design	Age Group*	Prevalence per 1000 Total	Male	Female	PLVSF
London, UK (1988)[55]	30,204 subjects in 3 GP practices, retrospective chart review of diuretics-treated patients, identified 117 HF cases.	<65 ≥65 *Total (all)*	0.6 28 *3.9*	– – –	– – –	*NR*
NHANES-III, USA (1988)[3,203]	16,679 subjects, age ≥20 yr, HF diagnosed by self-report and clinical score (preliminary data, not formally presented).	35–44 45–54 55–64 65–74 ≥75 *Total (NHW)* *Total (NHB)*	– – – – – *–* *–*	7 18 62 68 98 *23* *35*	5 13 34 66 97 *15* *31*	*NR* *NR*
Cardio-vascular Health Study, USA (1989)[54]	5201 subjects, age ≥65 yr, HF by self-report and drug use or clinical records.	65–69 70–74 75–79 80–84 85+ *Total (65+)*	– – – – – *20*	22 19 32 32 29 *24.4*	12 15 24 25 22 *16.6*	*55%*
Rotterdam, the Netherlands (1990)[34]	5540 subjects age 55–95 yr with echo screening for LV dysfunction and HF (71% PLVSF).	55–64 65–74 75–84 85–94 *Total (55+)*	7 27 130 117 *39*	7 37 144 59 *31*	6 16 121 140 *30*	*71%*
Strong Heart Study, USA (1993)[204]	3184 subjects, age 47–81 yr (mean 60 yr), screened by echo & exam for HF and LV dysfunction.	*Total (47–81)*	*30*	*42*	*17*	*53%*
Copen-hagen, Denmark (1993)[205]	2158 subjects, age ≥50 yr, screened by questionnaire.	40–49 50–59 60–69 70–79 ≥80 *Total (50+)*	5 15 48 93 117 *64*	– – – – – *–*	– – – – – *–*	*71%*

continues

Table 3
Prevalence of Heart Failure: Large-Scale
Population-Based Studies (*Continued*)

Study (start year)	Design	Age Group*	Prevalence per 1000 Total	Male	Female	PLVSF
Notting-hamshire, UK (1994)[206]	Prevalence esti-mate based on diuretics prescrip-tion data from Nottinghamshire.	30–39 50–59 70–79 *Total* *(30+)*	0.1 5.5 42 *13*	– – – –	– – – –	*NR*
Västerås, Sweden (1997)[207]	433 subjects, age 75 yr, screened by echo & exam for HF and LV dysfunction.	*Total* *(75)*	*67*	*95*	*40*	*46%*

NHANES = National Heath and Nutritional Examination Survey; HF = heart failure; PLVSF = preserved LV systolic function; NR = not reported; NHW = non-Hispanic whites; NHB = non-Hispanic blacks.
Blank spaces denote data not reported in the literature.
*Values in brackets represent age group, NHANES III data include ages 20 and above.

Table 4
Incidence of Heart Failure: Large-Scale Population-Based Studies

Study	Year (f/u)	Design	Age Group	Incidence per 1000 per annum Total	Male	Female
Framingham MA, USA[1,46]	1948 (40+ yr)	10,344 Framingham residents, 47% men, longitudinal follow-up with periodic exam, 652 prevalent cases identified.	50–59 80–89 ≥45 *Total* *(all)*	– – – –	3 27 7.2 *2.3*	2 22 4.7 *1.4*
Goteborg, Sweden[53]	1963 (17 yr)	973 men born in 1913, 84 HF cases identi-fied by exam.	50–54 61–67	– –	1.5 10.2	– –
East Fin-land[208]	1986 (?)	Retrospective chart/drug review of 37,600 subjects, 75 HF cases identified using Framingham criteria.	45–54 55–64 65–74 *Total* *(45–75)*	– – – –	2.2 3.3 7.7 *4.1*	0.2 2.2 2.9 *1.6*

continues

Table 4
Incidence of Heart Failure: Large-Scale
Population-Based Studies (*Continued*)

Study	Year (f/u)	Design	Age Group	Incidence per 1000 per annum Total	Male	Female
Rochester, MN, USA[50]	1981–2 (7 yr)	Rochester residents age >74 yr, retrospective chart review, 113 prevalent cases identified.	45–49	–	1	0
			50–54	–	1	0
			55–59	–	3	1
			60–64	–	6	2
			65–69	–	16	5
			70–74	–	9	10
			Total (0–74)	*1.1*	*1.6*	*0.7*
Cardiovascular Health Study, USA[201]	1989 (6 yr)	5626 independently living elderly, 597 HF by self-report, drug use or clinical records, and 95% with baseline normal left ventricular function.	65–69	10.6	–	–
			70–74	17.2	–	–
			75–80	26.3	–	–
			80+	42.5	–	–
			Total (65+)	*19.3*	*26.2*	*14.6*
Lorraine-EPICAL, France[196]	1994 (1–2 yr)	1.59 million Lorraine residents age 20–80y, prospective hospitalization records, 499 HF cases (358 incident) identified with advanced HF (NYHA III-IV).	20–30	0.01	0.02	0.01
			30–40	0.02	0.02	0.02
			40–50	0.09	0.16	0.02
			50–60	0.27	0.47	0.07
			60–70	0.60	0.98	0.28
			70–80	0.94	1.48	0.58
			Total (20–80)	*0.23*	–	–
Hillingdon, London, UK[36]	1995 (2 yr)	151,000 patients in Hillingdon, admitted or seen at rapid access clinic for HF, 220 new HF cases identified over 20 months.	25–34	0.02	0	0.04
			35–44	0.2	0.2	0.2
			45–54	0.2	0.3	0.1
			55–64	1.2	1.7	0.7
			65–74	3.0	3.9	2.3
			75–84	7.4	9.8	5.9
			85+	11.6	16.8	9.6
			Total (25+)	*1.3*	*1.4*	*1.2*
Bromley, London, UK[48]	1995 (1.5 yr)	292,000 patients in Bromley, admitted or seen at rapid access clinic for HF, 332 new HF cases identified over 15 months.	25–34	–	0	0
			35–44	–	0.04	0
			45–54	–	0.38	0.08
			55–64	–	1.71	0.64
			65–74	–	3.30	1.74
			75–84	–	8.10	5.45
			85+	–	10.44	5.99
			Total (25+)	*1.2*	–	–

continues

Table 4
Incidence of Heart Failure: Large-Scale
Population-Based Studies (*Continued*)

Study	Year (f/u)	Design	Age Group	Incidence per 1000 per annum Total	Male	Female
General	1996	3 million British resi-	40–44	–	0.24	0.16
Practice	(2 yr)	dents from 2000	45–49	–	0.72	0.11
Research		general practices,	50–54	–	0.70	0.32
Database,		identify patients age	55–59	–	2.13	0.85
UK[209]		40–84 yr newly	60–64	–	4.47	2.43
		diagnosed with HF.	65–69	–	6.38	4.59
			70–74	–	11.28	7.86
			75–79	–	19.24	15.48
			80–84	–	31.17	22.09
			Total (40+)	*4.2*	*4.4*	*3.9*

f/u = follow-up; yr = years; HF = heart failure; NYHA = New York Heart Association class.
Blank spaces denote data not reported in the literature.

half of all patients who present with symptomatic heart failure have left ventricular systolic dysfunction.[33,56] This observation has also been validated by a 30–50% prevalence rate of heart failure with left ventricular systolic dysfunction seen in recent referral-based studies in the primary care setting.[57] On the other hand, heart failure with preserved systolic function is especially prevalent in the elderly population. In the Cardiovascular Health Study where 8.8% of the 4842 elderly participants had signs and symptoms of heart failure, definite left ventricular systolic dysfunction was found only in 31% and 10% cases of symptomatic heart failure in men and women, respectively.[58] A recent French survey in heart failure hospitalizations also found a high proportion of heart failure patients (>50%) admitted with relatively preserved left ventricular systolic function (ejection fraction >40%), especially in women and in the elderly.[59] So-called "diastolic heart failure" is more prevalent in the elderly, in women, and in African American inner-city urban residents.[58,60,61]

Epidemiology of Ventricular Dysfunction

Ventricular dysfunction is rather prevalent in the general population, with estimates ranging from 2% to 7% in the adult population.[34,43,62,63] Again, these figures vary depending on the definitions used, the population being studied, and the types of measurements being made (Table 5).[25] Up to 40–60% are minimally symptomatic and can be easily

Table 5
Prevalence of Left Ventricular Dysfunction:
Large-Scale Population-Based Studies

Study (start year)	Design	Definition	Age Group	Prevalence			
				Total	Male	Female	ALVD
Cardio-vascular Health Study, USA (1989)[67]	5201 subjects, age 65–100, screened by echo & exam.	Subjective assessment ("abnormal")	65–69	23	–	–	
			70–74	36	–	–	
			75–79	52	–	–	
			≥80	55	–	–	
			Total (65+)	*37*	*6.3*	*1.8*	*NR*
Rotterdam, The Netherlands (1990)[34]	1698 subjects, age 55–95 yr (mean 65 yr), screened by echo & HF.	FS ≤ 25%	55–64	23	37	12	
			65–74	53	76	31	
			75–84	48	69	33	
			85–94	103	100	105	
			Total (55+)	*37*	*55*	*22*	*60%*
Augsburg, Germany (1992)[62]	1866 subjects age 25–75 yr (mean 50y), screened by echo & exam (MONICA).	EF <48%	*Total (25–75)*	*28*	*32*	*23*	*42%*
Glasgow Clinical Research Initiative, UK (1992)[25]	1640 subjects age 25–74 yr (mean 50 yr), screened by echo.	EF ≤30%	25–34	–	0	0	
			35–44	–	7	0	
			45–54	–	58	24	
			55–64	–	57	20	
			65–74	56	64	49	
			Total (25+)	*29*	–	–	*48%*
		EF ≤35%	*Total (25+)*	*77*	–	–	*77%*
Strong Heart Study, USA (1993)[210]	3184 subjects, age 45–74 yr (mean 60 yr), screened by echo & exam.	EF 40–54%	*Total (45–74)*	*111*	*177*	*72*	*95%*
		EF <40%	*Total (45–74)*	*29*	*47*	*18*	*72%*
Copen-hagen, Denmark (1993)[205]	2158 subjects, age ≥50 yr, screened by echo/ques-tionnaire.	LWMI ≤1.5 or FS <0.26	*Total (50+)*	*29*	–	–	*34%*

continues

Table 5
Prevalence of Left Ventricular Dysfunction:
Large-Scale Population-Based Studies (*Continued*)

Study (start year)	Design	Definition	Age Group	Prevalence Total	Male	Female	ALVD
ECHOES, Birmingham, UK (1995)[145]	3960 subjects age ≥45 yr, screened by echo.	EF <40%	45–54	3	–	–	
			75–84	37	–	–	
			Total (45+)	*18*	–	–	*47%*
		EF 40–50%	*Total (45+)*	*35*	–	–	*61%*
North Glasgow, UK (1995)[43]	1009 subjects, age 55–74 yr, 750 with echo EF.	EF ≤35%	55–59	46	54	39	
			60–64	54	76	31	
			65–69	54	71	40	
			70–74	120	180	52	
			Total (55–74)	*67*	*94*	*40*	*54%*
Bromley, London, UK (1995)[48]	292,000 subjects in Bromley, 332 new HF cases identified over 15 months, 311 with echo.	FS ≥25, LVIDd <5.6	<75	14	–	–	
			75+	19	–	–	
			Total (all)	*17*	–	–	*NR*
		FS ≥20, LVIDd<6	*Total (all)*	*27*	–	–	*NR*
Olmsted County MN, USA (1997)[63]	2042 Olmsted County residents, age >45 yr, screened by echo & chart review.	Any LVSD*	BSEF	51	79	28	
			LVEF	62	96	31	
			Total (both)	*48*	*87*	*18*	*62%*
		Significant LVSD*	BSEF	17	28	8	
			LVEF	35	57	15	
			Total (both)	*22*	*36*	*11*	*61%*
Västerås, Sweden (1997)[207]	433 subjects, age 75 yr, screened by echo & exam for HF.	LVEF<43%	*Total (75)*	*89*	–	–	*NR*
		LVWMI <1.7%	*Total (75)*	*68*	*102*	*34*	*46%*

ALVD = asymptomatic left ventricular dysfunction; LVEF = left ventricular ejection fraction (visual estimates); BSEF = biplane Simpson's ejection fraction; EF = ejection fraction; FS = fractional shortening; LVIDd = left ventricular internal dimensions (diastole); LVSD = left ventricular systolic dysfunction; LVWMI = left ventricular wall motion index; ECHOES = Echocardiographic Heart Of England Screening study.
Blank spaces denote data not reported in the literature.
* Any LVSD if <2 standard deviations (LVEF <52% or BSEF<49%); significant LVSD if ≤3 standard deviations (LVEF<40% or BSEF<40%).

overlooked in the general practice setting.[64] By considering only strict echocardiographic criteria, some degree of diastolic dysfunction was noted in up to 25% of patients with heart failure and preserved systolic function and in up to 80% in those with reduced systolic function.[63] On the other hand, only an estimated 15% of patients with heart failure under 65 years of age were likely to suffer from isolated diastolic heart failure.[36] By extrapolation, isolated diastolic heart failure may be rare (<0.1% in general population) in patients under 65 years old, but is much more common in patients over 65 years old (up to 1–3% in the population).[65]

There are currently no data regarding the incidence of emerging ventricular dysfunction in the general population, although among patients who develop left ventricular systolic dysfunction, up to 50–75% have underlying ischemic heart disease.[25,43] In addition, up to a 5-fold increase in the risk of developing ventricular dysfunction has been observed in patients with previous peripheral vascular or cerebrovascular diseases.[66] It is well recognized that there are individuals who are at increased risk of developing ventricular dysfunction. They often have risk factors that directly or indirectly cause intrinsic myocardial damage, such as long-standing underlying coronary artery disease, poorly controlled hypertension especially with left ventricular hypertrophy (LVH), diabetes mellitus, valvular abnormalities, and alcohol or drug misuse. These "risk factors" often predate the development of overt heart failure and may create regional or global myocardial damage that can accumulate over time to cause substantial ventricular dysfunction. In addition, some of these "risk factors" may develop into "comorbidities" as heart failure progresses, such as worsening mitral regurgitation from ventricular dilation or arrhythmia from worsening heart failure. These at-risk patients should therefore be identified promptly and screened for ventricular dysfunction while aggressively treated with angiotensin-converting enzyme (ACE) inhibitors and beta-blockers to control or reverse their cardiac risks.

Demographic Risk Factors

Age

Increasing age is consistently associated with increased risk of developing heart failure and ventricular dysfunction and carries an increase in morbidity and mortality.[25,39,67] In the Olmsted County database, 88% of the 216-incident heart failure cases identified in 1991–1992 were over 65 years of age.[50] Although the overall incidence of heart failure has been steady over the past several decades, a significant increase in the incidence of heart failure has been found among the elderly population (≥75 years).[68] Due to age-related changes in the cardiovascular system, elderly patients are more likely to have advanced heart failure at the time of initial presentation, and may be less likely to receive effective drugs.[69,70] In addition, more than half of them suffer from two or more comorbid conditions,[71] and may have a poorer prognosis.[72,73] Hospital admissions and readmissions rates are also higher in the elderly.[5,74,75] In the latest National Hospital Discharge Survey, almost 78% of men and 85% of women hospitalized with heart failure are aged ≥65 years, making heart failure the most common reason for hospitalization for this age group.[13]

Most early clinical trials of heart failure excluded elderly patients, especially those with multiple comorbidities. The rationale was that many would die of noncardiac causes (such as cancer), which might then obscure the true impact of the drugs tested in the trials. This strategy has made it difficult to translate clinical trial results into everyday practice, where a large majority of heart failure patients are elderly. Investigators now recognize that elderly patients should participate in clinical trials, and age exclusions are not as commonly mandated by today's standards. In fact, some contemporary trials such as the ELITE (Evaluation of Losartan In The Elderly) study specifically enrolled elderly patients.[76] Recent cohort and subgroup analyses have also validated the comparable benefits of various drugs in the elderly heart failure population.[77]

Gender and Ethnicity

Gender and ethnic differences in heart failure prevalence have been highlighted in the latest NHANES-III survey (1988–1994), which identified 3.5% of non-Hispanic black men suffering from heart failure ages 20 and older, as compared to 3.1% of non-Hispanic black women, 2.3% of non-Hispanic white men, or 1.5% of non-Hispanic white women.[78,79] In the Framingham database, the age-adjusted incidence rate of symptomatic heart failure in women was almost one-third less than that in men, as women were often assumed to be less vulnerable to developing coronary artery disease than men.[1] However, women who sustained myocardial infarction were found to be more likely to develop heart failure.[80] Hypertension, valvular diseases, obesity, and diabetes mellitus have also been identified as stronger risk factors for heart failure in women than in men.[81,82] Women often present with more signs and symptoms of heart failure,[83] and have long been thought to have a better prognosis (as women are thought to have less ischemic heart failure and better adaptations to their illness),[84–86] even though recent studies have questioned this notion.[27,87,88]

Several epidemiological databases have concurred with the findings that heart failure occurs at an earlier age in African Americans than in Caucasians, with relatively lower documented ischemic etiologies and more prevalent uncontrolled hypertension, left ventricular hypertrophy, and diabetes mellitus.[89–91] In contrast, adjusted survival rates have been found to be similar among African Americans, Hispanics, and Caucasians in hospital series.[92–94] Unfortunately, African American or Hispanic patients with heart failure have been under-represented in population-based studies or clinical trials, making any conclusive insights difficult.

There is recent interest in determining discrepancies in response to therapy based on differences in gender and ethnicity. Lower effectiveness of ACE inhibitors with more drug discontinuations and underprescriptions in women has been suggested. Recent reports of better therapeutic responses to hydralazine/nitrates than to ACE inhibitors,[95] similar responses to carvedilol,[96] and lower efficacy of enalapril[97] and bucindolol in the African American subgroup may require validation in prospective clinical trials.[98,99] BiDil® (NitroMed Inc, Bedford MA), which combines two vasodilators with a nitric oxide source (isosorbide dinitrate and hydralazine), will be tested with other drugs in over 600 African American patients in a multicenter study.[100]

Family History

It has recently become apparent that up to 30% of patients with dilated cardiomyopathy may have family members similarly involved, a process known as familial dilated cardiomyopathy.[101,102] It is likely that there are complex genetic predispositions.[103,104] Although no standardized criteria have been established to determine the diagnosis of familial dilated cardiomyopathy,[105] echocardiographic and metabolic screenings have demonstrated a high prevalence of ALVD in first-degree relatives of some patients with heart failure, with more aggressive disease progression at a younger age.[101,106] Often, they present with left ventricular dilitation, and up to 30% subsequently develop heart failure.[107] A familial cause has been shown in 50% of patients with hypertrophic cardiomyopathy, in 35% with dilated cardiomyopathy, and in 30% with arrhythmogenic left ventricular dysplasia; they often have a high risk for major arrhythmic events.[104] A family history of heart failure is therefore an important risk factor in addition to other cardiovascular risk factors, such as coronary artery disease, diabetes mellitus, and hypertension.

Determining Comorbidities in Heart Failure

Traditionally, the description of the natural history of heart failure requires an understanding of the underlying etiology, with the idea that different causes of heart failure (such as "ischemic" versus "nonischemic") may result in variations in natural history. The etiology is sometimes determined by casual association between comorbid conditions and the presence of heart failure symptoms, and may even become misleading as the disease progresses. For example, patients with dilated cardiomyopathy who drink alcohol are often labeled as "alcoholic cardiomyopathy," or those with idiopathic dilated cardiomyopathy are often told they have "a virus" that damaged their heart.

Risk factor identification and correction at an early stage is clearly a more effective public health policy than waiting for overt heart failure to appear and then instituting treatment. Population-based studies such as the Framingham and the Olmsted County studies have provided the greatest insights into longitudinal risk factors of developing symptomatic heart failure in the general population.[1,108,109] However, some of these findings have changed throughout the decades. In particular, uncontrolled hypertension and valvular diseases have declined steadily since the 1950s, concomitant with an increase in the incidence of coronary artery disease and diabetes mellitus. From 1950 to 1998 in the Framingham Heart Study, the odds of developing heart failure with a prior history of myocardial infarction increased by 26% in men per decade and 48% per decade in women; and the odds of developing heart failure with diabetes increased by 42% in men per decade.[110] Also, many of these studies were conducted before the widespread use of neurohormonal antagonists, and therefore much of our understanding of the impact of comorbid conditions still relies on insights from referral-based series and clinical trial data (Table 6).

Myocardial Ischemia

Myocardial ischemia has long been considered to be an increasingly common cause of heart failure and ventricular dysfunction. It is also a major precipitating factor for the exacerbation of heart failure. "Ischemic heart failure" is often limited to a clinical (with ischemic chest pain symptoms) or an angiographic (associated with significant stenosis in epicardial coronary arteries) definition, and "ischemic cardiomyopathy" is often loosely defined.[111] Clinically, symptoms are often indistinguishable from patients with nonischemic heart failure, although the prognosis may be worse.[112] Some patients with a large acute myocardial infarction develop immediate pump failure resulting from irreversible loss of myocardium. Others survive to develop transient or persistent ventricular dysfunction. Subsequent progression of ventricular dysfunction from the index event may account for a substantial group of patients with ischemic heart disease.

From the Framingham data, a clinical history of angina by itself posed a 2- to 3-fold risk increase in developing heart failure, while in the case of myocardial infarction, heart failure developed in 23% of men and in 35% of women over time (a 4- to 8-fold risk increase in risk of developing heart failure).[46,109,113] Clinical evidence of coronary artery disease was

Table 6
Etiology and Risk Factors of Symptomatic Heart Failure

Study	Size	Male	Age	NYHA	ICM	HTN	DM	AF	AM*
Population-based studies									
Framingham MA, USA[1]	985	51%	70	I-IV	54%	74%	19%	—	43%
Olmsted County MN, USA[56]	216	58%	77	I-IV	40%	52%	—	24%	23%
CHS, USA[58]	425	48%	79	I-IV	43%	50%	28%	14%	—
EPICAL, France[196]	499	76%	65	III-IV	46%	20%	26%	26%	35%
Hillingdon, UK[36,188]	220	54%	76	I-IV	36%	14%	16%	31%	38%
Scottish NHS database[194]	66,547	47%	75	II-IV	26%	—	3%	3%	45%
Bromley, UK[48]	332	54%	?	I-IV	29% # 52% †	9% # 4% †	—	—	—
GPRD, UK[209]	938	52%	73	I-IV	37%	22%	14%	—	—
Large-scale mortality trials									
CONSENSUS[211]	253	71%	71	IV	73%	22%	23%	50%	36%
VHeFT-II[212]	804	100%	61	II-III	53%	48%	20%	14%	13%
SOLVD-T[122]	2569	80%	61	II-III	71%	18%	26%	10%	10%
SOLVD-P[41]	4228	89%	59	I-II	83%	9%	15%	4%	5%
SOLVD Registry[27]	6063	74%	62	I-IV	69%	7%	23%	14%	—
DIG[213]	6800	78%	64	II-III	71%	45%	28%	0%¶	13%
US Carvedilol[45]	1094	77%	58	II-III	48%	—	28%	12%	11%
PROMISE[214]	1088	78%	64	III-IV	54%	—	—	—	48%
ATLAS[215]	3164	80%	64	II-III	65%	20%	20%	18%	12%
MERIT-HF[216]	3991	77%	64	II-III	65%	44%	25%	17%	11%
CIBIS-II[44]	2647	81%	61	II-IV	50%	16%	12%	21%	13%
RALES[217]	1663	73%	65	III-IV	55%	—	25%	—	25%
ELITE-II[218]	3152	70%	71	II-III	59%	49%	24%	30%	11%
BEST[219]	2523	78%	60	II-IV	58%	59%	36%	11%	17%
DIAMOND-CHF[220]	1518	69%	70	II-IV	67%	15%	12%	26%	11%
COPERNICUS[221]	2289	80%	63	III-IV	67%	—	26%	—	19%

continues

Table 6
Etiology and Risk Factors of Symptomatic
Heart Failure (*Continued*)

Study	Size	Male	Age	NYHA	ICM	HTN	DM	AF	AM *
Val-HeFT[222]	5010	80%	63	II-III	57%	7%	24%	12%	10%
CAPRI-CORN[223]	1959	73%	63	I-III	100%	54%	22%	—	12%

Age expressed as mean or median age.
* Annualized mortality (AM) extrapolated from studies based on (mortality rate) ÷ (study duration); in clinical trials AM based on study group treated with vasodilators/ACE inhibitors only (treatment group in early trials, control group in later).
# Etiology based on clinical history.
†Etiology based on angiographic and myocardial perfusion data.
¶Atrial fibrillation is one of the exclusion criteria for trial entry in the DIG trial; incidence of developing supraventricular tachycardia during the study period (mean duration of 37 months) was 11.1%.
Blank spaces denote data not reported in the literature.
CHS = Cardiovascular Health Study; NHS = National Health Service (administrative database); EPICAL = Epidemiologie de l'Insuffisance Cardiaque Avancee en Lorraine; GPRD = General Practice Research Database; CONSENSUS = Cooperative North Scandinavian Enalapril Survival Study; SOLVD = Studies Of Left Ventricular Dysfunction (T = treatment arm; P = prevention arm); V-HeFT = Vasodilator Heart Failure Trial; DIG = Digitalis Investigation Group study; PROMISE = Prospective Randomized Milrinone Survival Evaluation trial; ATLAS = Assessment of Treatment with Lisinopril And Survival trial; MERIT-HF = Metoprolol Controlled-Release Randomized Intervention Trial in Heart Failure; CIBIS = Cardiac Insufficiency Bisoprolol Study; RALES = Randomized Aldactone Evaluation Study; ELITE = Evaluation of Losartan In The Elderly study; DIAMOND = Dofetilide in patients with congestive heart failure and left ventricular dysfunction: safety aspects and effects on atrial fibrillation; BEST = Beta-blocker Evaluation Survival Trial; COPERNICUS = Carvedilol Prospective Randomized Cumulative Survival trial; Val-HeFT = Valsartan in Heart Failure Trial; CAPRICORN = Carvedilol Post-infarct Survival Control in LV Dysfunction; NYHA = New York Heart Association functional class; ICM = ischemic cardiomyopathy; HTN = hypertension; IDCM = idiopathic dilated cardiomyopathy; DM = diabetes mellitus; AF = atrial fibrillation/flutter.

found in 46% of men and in 27% of women preceding the development of heart failure. However, due to the lack of myocardial viability and perfusion assessments in this population study, it is impossible to determine whether ischemia was a manifestation of reduced oxygen supply resulting from progressive coronary artery disease or due to increased oxygen demand as might result from LVH. As more coronary artery disease is diagnosed by objective measurements (such as exercise stress testing and angiography), the true proportion of ischemic causes of heart failure is substantial. Recent data from the Alberta database of 566 consecutively referred heart failure patients highlighted this point by finding 67% of patients with an ischemic etiology (with 78% having systolic dysfunction)[114]—a trend similar to that seen in major clinical trial registries.[27]

The notion that ischemic heart disease may play a larger role in heart failure than anticipated from population-based studies comes from trials that directly evaluated ventricular dysfunction. In one population-based study, a high prevalence of ischemic heart disease was demonstrated in patients with symptomatic (95%) as well as in patients with asymptomatic (71%) ventricular dysfunction.[37] Multivariate analysis from a recent population-based study in North Glasgow also revealed the importance of both angina and prior myocardial infarction in increased risk of developing ventricular dysfunction.[43] In prospective autopsy series, 31% of patients with clinically determined nonischemic heart failure had autopsy-documented significant ischemic heart disease, and the cause of death may be directly linked to ischemic events.[115] Among those patients with myocardial infarction as the cause of death, 79% had no prior diagnosis of ischemic heart disease, and many experienced sudden death with no immediate antecedent history of chest pain.

Recent studies have also pointed out that underdiagnosis or misdiagnosis of ischemic heart disease in the heart failure population is common if angiographic evaluation was not undertaken as part of the heart failure work-up. In a retrospective series of patients with presumed idiopathic dilated cardiomyopathy, up to 34% were proven by angiography to have ischemic heart failure.[116] In the SOLVD trials, over 10% of patients who had nonischemic heart failure subsequently experienced myocardial infarction within the 40-month follow-up period.[117]

Hypertension and Left Ventricular Hypertrophy

One of the most consistent findings in the Framingham database is the importance of hypertension as the underlying cause of heart failure, even though symptomatic heart failure developed in only approximately 12% of men and 8% of women who manifested hypertension in the general population. Nevertheless, up to 76% of men and 79% of women with symptomatic heart failure had preexisting hypertension in Framingham.[1,46] A previous history of hypertension was as prevalent (if not more) in clinical studies as well as in observational series, even though most patients presented with normal or even low blood pressure at the onset of heart failure. Due to the high prevalence of hypertension, especially in the African American and elderly populations, and the associated risk for developing ischemic heart diseases and diastolic dysfunction, hypertension is considered to be the most significant risk factor for developing symptomatic heart failure. The impact of better blood pressure control in reducing the prevalence of heart failure progression is also clear.[118]

Left ventricular hypertrophy, often a major complication of uncontrolled hypertension, may progress into frank heart failure with or without preexisting hypertension. About 20% of symptomatic cases of heart failure have antecedent electrocardiographic evidence of LVH (a 15-fold increase in heart failure risk), and 60–70% have echocardiographic evidence of LVH. Echocardiographic determinants of left ventricular dilatation from the Framingham database have also been shown to correlate with an increase in risk of developing heart failure.[40] These observations stress the importance of echocardiography in the detection of patients with LVH who are at risk of developing heart failure, and the potential for reversal of the disease process.

Although hypertension and ischemic heart disease can independently lead to heart failure progression, their interrelationship in the pathophysiology of heart failure makes it difficult to understand their quantitative contribution to the syndrome. Many patients with ischemic heart failure often have preexisting hypertension (34–52% of hypertensive patients from the Framingham data have interim myocardial infarction[1]), and having ischemic heart failure does not render a patient immune from a separate cardiomyopathic process caused by uncontrolled hypertension. In fact, it is conceivable that patients with preexisting hypertension are 5- to 6-fold more likely to develop heart failure following an ischemic event, supporting a "multi-hit" hypothesis. Retrospective data from the GUSTO (Global Utilization of Streptokinase and Tissue plasminogen activator in Occluded coronary arteries) study also shows that when patients develop heart failure after acute coronary syndrome (estimated incidence of 4.4%), they were more likely to be older or female, or to have a history of hypertension, myocardial infarction, and/or diabetes mellitus.[119]

Diabetes Mellitus and Glucose Intolerance

Patients with insulin resistance or type 2 diabetes have a particularly high risk for heart failure and a poor prognosis once they develop heart failure.[120] Data from the Framingham study indicate that heart failure develops in approximately 16% of men and 18% of women less than age 65 years who have diabetes mellitus, while impaired glucose tolerance increases the incidence of heart failure by 4- and 8-fold in men and women, respectively.[1] Older persons with diabetes mellitus had a 1.3 times higher chance of developing heart failure than those without diabetes mellitus after controlling for the confounding effects of other prognostic variables.[121] Diabetic patients accounted for approximately 25% of the total population of the major heart failure trials, and both ACE inhibitors and beta-blockers have been shown to be equally effective in this population.[122–125] However, in both the SOLVD and the RESOLVD (Randomized Evaluation of Strategies for Left Ventricular Dysfunction) studies, diabetic status was found to be an independent risk factor for death in patients with heart failure.[122, 126]

Diabetes mellitus is an independent risk factor for coronary artery disease, even in its asymptomatic form. In the GUSTO trials, heart failure was twice as common in diabetic as in the nondiabetic population following acute myocardial infarction[127,128] or following acute coronary syndromes.[129] Diabetic patients often carry a particularly poor prognosis following acute myocardial infarction.[130] Interestingly, this increased mortality risk seemed to be associated with increased risk in developing heart failure, but was independent of worsening ventricular dysfunction.[131,132] There is recent clinical evidence to suggest that alterations in the myocardium precede overt heart failure in diabetic patients. Multivariate analyses from population-based studies suggest that diabetes remains an independent contributor to increased left ventricular mass and wall thickness by echocardiography (especially in women).[133–135] These changes are not totally accounted for by age, gender, body habitus, race, or blood pressure differences.[134,136] The patients also have greater arterial stiffness and reduced systolic function at rest or during stress (suggesting reduced cardiac reserve).[137,138] Although direct, concrete evidence is still lacking, most experts now believe that a distinctive entity of diabetic cardiomyopathy does exist as a "vulnerable" alteration to the myocardium in the setting of impaired glycemic control and insulin resistance. However, the gross anatomic, histological, and echocardiographic morphological features of early diabetic cardiomyopathy are often indistinguishable from that of idiopathic dilated cardiomyopathy. Both idiopathic dilated cardiomyopathy and diabetes may share many similar pathophysiological processes (such as endothelial dysfunction or oxidative stress) that can contribute to their combined disease progression and clinical deterioration. The presence of coexisting risk factors (such as hypertension and dyslipidemia) coupled with the occurrence of major index events (such as myocardial infarction) can lead to the development of overt heart failure that is often difficult to treat.

Poor glycemic control may be associated with an increased risk of developing heart failure.[139] In the clinical setting, every 1% increase in the baseline glycosylated hemoglobulin level translates into a 15% increase in the risk of developing heart failure.[140] On the other hand, the presence of heart failure itself has also been found to pose a higher risk for developing diabetes mellitus after controlling for confounding effects of age, gender, and hypertension.[121] Insulin resistance relates to the severity and etiology of heart failure.[141] There is evidence from an elderly Italian heart failure population that the incidence of new-onset diabetes is 29% compared with 18% in matched controls during a 3-year follow-up.[142] These observations can be explained in two ways. First, undiagnosed glucose abnormalities are common in heart failure patients. In the recent RESOLVD substudy that systematically evaluated fasting plasma glucose and insulin levels, up to 43% of patients had documented glucose abnormalities, with 8% having previously undiagnosed diabetes mellitus and 9% having impaired glucose tolerance.[143] Second, heart failure and overt diabetes share a common continuum of cardiovascular risks (such as endothelial dysfunction or insulin resistance). Indeed, increased adrenergic drive in heart failure itself has been shown to raise free fatty acid oxidation and insulin resistance, and has been suggested as a cause of impaired peripheral vasodilation and vascular activity resulting from diminished nitric oxide production, increased left ventricular afterload, and increased atherogenicity.[142,144]

Valvular Diseases

Valvular diseases are common not only as a cause of heart failure but also as an important comorbid condition. In a British series of 7000 patients screened by echocardiography, secondary valvular abnormalities were found in 32% of patients with a previous diagnosis of heart failure (among whom only 30% had systolic dysfunction).[145] Functional mitral regurgitation is an especially common consequence of end-stage heart failure, and may affect almost all heart failure patients as a preterminal or terminal event.[146] Mitral regurgitation can develop from incomplete leaflet coaptation due to mitral annular dilation and cordal tethering, or papillary muscle dysfunction in ischemic cardiomyopathy. With advances in surgical techniques, mitral valve repair and reconstruction with annuloplasty rings have shown promise in improving clinical outcomes in patients with severe mitral regurgitation and advanced heart failure. Significant tricuspid regurgitation is also a common complication, especially with right heart failure and severe secondary pulmonary hypertension. It is nearly always present in end-stage heart failure. The indications and timing of valvular surgery in heart failure patients remain largely subjective.

Rhythm Disturbances

Abnormal rhythm control is often under-recognized as an important contributor to the development of heart failure. This occurs by precipitating acute decompensation of otherwise quiescent heart failure (up to 24% in one series[147]), or it actually causes myocardial impairment (so-called "tachycardia-induced cardiomyopathy"[148]). As heart failure progresses, myocardial tissue also becomes more vulnerable to arrhythmias. The prevalence of arrhythmia increases as a result of heightened neurohormonal activation and progressive chamber "remodeling" with alterations in refractory periods.[149]

Atrial fibrillation is a common problem in heart failure, usually as a result of enlargement and remodeling of the atria. It is well recognized as a major cause of heart failure exacerbation due to the development of various deleterious hemodynamic consequences, including a rapid ventricular heart rate. It has been reported that atrial fibrillation is present in 10% of patients with mild heart failure (New York Heart Association functional class, NYHA class I-II) compared to 40% in patients with advanced heart failure (NYHA class III-IV).[150] It is especially common in the elderly population in the presence of ventricular dysfunction.[59,151] The incidence of new-onset supraventricular tachycardia in patients with heart failure who manifest baseline sinus rhythm in the Digitalis Investigation Group (DIG) was 11% in the 3-year period of follow-up. It occurs more commonly in men, in the elderly, and in patients with longer heart failure duration and larger ventricular dimensions.[152]

The presence of heart failure and ventricular dysfunction (as measured by reduced left ventricular fractional shortening) was suggested to be a significant risk factor for developing atrial fibrillation, with a 5-fold increased risk in Framingham.[153,154] However, it is unclear whether atrial fibrillation is an independent risk factor for cardiac mortality in the setting of heart failure. Multivariate analyses from clinical trial databases[155] and from hospital series[150] have not supported this notion. On the other hand, total mortality and risk of sudden death were lowered by conversion to sinus rhythm in patients with heart failure. In the DIG trial, atrial fibrillation was associated with an increased risk of mortality, stroke, and heart failure hospitalizations.[152]

Ambulatory electrocardiograms revealed that >60% of patients with heart failure have >30 premature ventricular contractions per hour, and 50% have nonsustained ventricular tachycardia.[156] Up to 30–40% of the mortality in heart failure is attributable to arrhythmic sudden cardiac death, with a higher proportion of sudden cardiac death in patients with milder forms of heart failure (NYHA class I-II).[157] Despite the high incidence of ventricular tachyarrhythmias causing sudden cardiac deaths, bradyarrhythmias and electromechanical dissociation may account for up to 30% of sudden cardiac deaths during advanced heart failure.[158]

Among patients with sick sinus syndrome, the prevalence of heart failure is high, ranging from 10% to 20%. Improvement in heart failure symptoms has been reported following pacemaker implantation in patients with sick sinus syndrome and sinus bradycardia.[159–161] Still unresolved is the problem of asynchrony associated with bundle branch block due to ventricular dilatation causing delayed conduction and pump inefficiency (up to 25–30% of the heart failure population). New strategies using biventricular pacing techniques are promising, and are currently undergoing widespread clinical investigation.[162]

Other Comorbid Conditions

Recent attention has been given to other major comorbid conditions that are prevalent in patients with heart failure. Poor renal function not only independently affects the prognosis of patients with heart failure, but limits the prescription of medications that are known to be beneficial (such as ACE inhibitors) or prevents adequate diuresis for symptomatic relief.[163–165] Acute worsening of renal function following admission for decompensated heart failure is common and may be associated with poorer prognosis.[166] On the other hand, anemia has also been reported in small studies to be a relatively common finding in chronic heart failure. Anemia often becomes worse as the severity of heart failure increases, and is associated with a poorer prognosis.[165,167,168] Other common comorbid conditions in patients with heart failure that are potentially treatable include thyroid disorders,[169,170] sleep disorders (such as sleep apnea[171,172]), nutritional disorders (such as thiamine deficiency in long-standing diuretic use[173,174]) or other noncardiac vascular diseases (such as cerebrovascular or peripheral vascular disease[175]).

Defining Disease Progression and Prognosis

Heart Failure Exacerbations and Relapses

Once pronounced symptoms develop, the natural course of heart failure is believed to follow a highly variable course involving progressive ventricular dysfunction, symptomatic deterioration, and the development of the aforementioned comorbid conditions. Rather than having persistent symptoms, it is characteristic for patients with heart failure to have "exacerbations" from time to time during the course of their illness. Most exacerbations occur in the form of acute cardiogenic pulmonary edema, a clinical entity signifying the abnormal accumulation of extravascular lung fluid caused by leakage of fluid from the pulmonary capillaries and venules into the pulmonary interstitium and alveoli.[176] Patients often present with dramatic acute onset of dyspnea secondary to altered gas exchange and poor pulmonary compliance. The underlying mechanisms and etiology of such "relapses" are poorly understood, but a number of precipitating factors are known (Table 7). These factors include excess fluid or salt intake, noncompliance with prescribed medical regimens, or direct burden on the already dysfunctional heart (such as myocardial ischemia, rhythm disturbances, and volume or pressure overload from valvular abnormalities or uncontrolled hypertension).[177] Concomitant medications and adverse drug interactions are frequent culprits.[178,179] In studies in the elderly and African American heart failure populations, up to 50% may have one or more preventable causes, including medication (15%) or diet (18%) noncompliance, inadequate discharge planning (15%) or follow-up (20%), failed social support systems (21%), or failure to seek medical attention promptly when symptoms recurred (20%).[10,180] A recent retrospective analysis also

Table 7
Common Precipitating Factors of Heart Failure

Myocardial ischemia or infarction
Dietary sodium excess or excess fluid intake
Medication noncompliance
Iatrogenic volume overload
Arrhythmia (atrial fibrillation/flutter, ventricular tachyarrhythmias, bradyarrhythmias)
Comorbidities (fever, infections/sepsis, thyroid dysfunction, anemia, renal insuf-
    ficiency, thiamine deficiency, pulmonary embolism, hypoxemia, uncontrolled
    hypertension)
Adverse drug effects (alcohol, negative inotropic agents such as beta-blockers,
    clonidine, and calcium channel blockers, antiarrhythmic drugs, nonsteroidal anti-
    inflammatory drugs and corticosteroids, thiazolidinediones)

highlighted a history of chronic obstructive pulmonary disease as an important predictor of rehospitalization, which may reflect a lower ventilatory reserve.[181] Similar findings are seen in the diastolic heart failure population, with precipitating factors being labile hypertension, infection (26%), ischemia (17%), anemia (4%), renal insufficiency (5%), arrhythmia (30%), and other comorbidities (10%).[182] However, no clear cause of decompensation can be identified in up to 40–50% of the patients.[59]

Reversibility of Ventricular Dysfunction

It has long been observed that disease progression varies considerably among heart failure patients, even with similar degrees of ventricular dysfunction or clinical presentations. Some patients will have a transient course of ventricular dysfunction that will reverse (a process known as "reverse remodeling"). In recent case series, up to 20–25% of patients have marked improvement following beta-blocker therapy.[183,184] Early reports have suggested that a history of hypertension, less severe left ventricular dysfunction by echocardiographic parameters, and certain etiologies such as alcoholic cardiomyopathy, severe insulin resistance, or myocarditis may predict a higher likelihood of reverse remodeling with or without medical therapy.[183–185] More importantly, normalization in ventricular function following therapy has been correlated with improvement in survival.[186,187]

Prognosis

The prognosis of heart failure remains dismal, despite a long list of successful clinical trials (see Table 6). On average, new effective therapies prolong life by only 6–18 months. In the Framingham study, only 25% of men and 38% of women were alive 5 years after their diagnoses of heart failure, with a median survival of only 1.66 years in men and 3.17 years in woman.[6] These figures are substantially worse than the data of most clinical trials. Closer analysis may reveal that heart failure definitions in population-based studies are vastly different and nonspecific, and may also reflect the presence of sampling bias. Especially in ischemic heart failure, mortality rates are often significant within the first 3–6 months following the onset of heart failure (in the Hillingdon study, survival rates were 81% at 1 month, 75% at 3 months, and 70% at 6 months[188]). Patients with impaired left ventricular function and documented coronary artery disease have significantly higher mortality rates than those with no coronary disease in the large Duke cardiac catherization database.[189] Indeed, adjusted median survival rates from the Framingham database improved to 3.2 years in men and 5.4 years in women, respectively, when patients who die within 90 days following heart failure onset were excluded—figures that were comparable with clinical trial results.[6] Recent efforts using administrative data have also found a significant increase in prevalent cases of heart failure of 1/1000 for women and 0.9/1000 for men from 1989 to 1999.[190]

The notion as to whether substantial advances in technology and therapeutics have improved the prognosis of heart failure in the general population has recently been questioned.[4,65] Longitudinal follow-up studies from nationwide surveys including NHANES-I (1971–1986)[51] and NHANES-II (1976–1992),[52] as well as population-based studies from Framingham (1948–1988),[6] Olmsted (1981–1991),[191] and Wooster (1975–1995)[192] have demonstrated remarkably similar long-term mortality rates over the past four decades after adjusting for age, gender, and NYHA classes (Table 6). From the Hillingdon study (in the "modern era" of heart failure management), the 16-month follow-up of the 220 new heart failure cases found similar 12- and 18-month survival rates when compared to those of the historical population-based studies (62% and 57%, respectively).[188] Recently, however, data from the Framingham study have highlighted a decrease in cardiovascular mortality based on risk factor modifications, rather than due to a reduction in the incidence of heart failure.[118] A landmark hospital-based retrospective series of 737 consecutive patients with advanced heart failure found a reduction in mortality risk from 33% in 1986–1988 to 16% in 1991–1993.[193] Retrospective analyses performed in the Scottish system of hospital discharge records further demonstrated a 15–26% reduction of case fatality rates between 1986 and 1995,[194] and a 5–23% relative risk reduction in 3-year mortality risk from 1984 to 1992.[4,195] Of note, the mortality rates observed in the Scottish studies still remained higher than those seen in most clinical trials (adjusted 1-year mortality rate of 44.5% versus 11–25%, respectively), which may reflect an older heart failure population with underutilization of "proven" therapies and higher comorbidity rates. Recent data from the

EPICAL (Epidemiologie de l'Insuffisance Cardiaque Avancee en Lorraine, 1994–1995) study are encouraging, although the 1-year mortality rate remains high at 35% in a patient population with advanced heart failure (NYHA class III-IV, LVEF <30%).[196] Various predictors of mortality have been identified from a number of sources, but the validity of these models has only rarely been verified.[197] When dealing with individual patients, predicting prognosis is notoriously difficult. Specific projections regarding prognosis are therefore best avoided.

Long-term follow-up of patients with isolated diastolic heart failure in the Framingham population reveals that this subgroup experiences a 4-fold higher mortality risk compared to that of normal controls (annual unadjusted mortality rate of 8.7%).[198] Various studies have shown that despite similar hospitalization rates, diastolic heart failure may have a similar[56,114] or lower mortality risk[198,199] when compared with that of systolic dysfunction, depending on age and disease severity. Patients with diastolic heart failure seem to be at risk for the development of sudden pulmonary edema. There are no randomized controlled trials to guide therapy, and the treatment is largely predicated on the etiology.

Conclusions

This chapter summarizes the changing picture of heart failure as abstracted from population studies, registries, and clinical trials. Extensive data from epidemiological studies and large-scale clinical trials have repeatedly pointed out that heart failure is a heterogeneous condition with a wide range of predisposing factors, clinical manifestations, and natural history of disease progression. Like anemia, it is a syndrome with a highly variable natural history. We are beginning to recognize the magnitude of this highly prevalent problem, which clusters in a population with advancing age. In subsets of patients, such as those with valvular and ischemic heart disease, prognosis has improved over the past 50 years with advances in surgical techniques and perioperative management. We should recognize that we are just entering the age of enlightenment in terms of the natural history of heart failure. Despite much progress in our understanding of the underlying pathophysiology, there is a need to focus on more "upstream" modifiable risk factors, so that preventive measures can be implemented to make a larger impact on reducing morbidity and mortality of heart failure.[200] Prevention is a far more powerful force in dealing with this epidemic than employing our currently available drug therapies for established heart failure.[179] Further public health effects are required to identify and treat patients in the earliest stages of the natural history of heart failure if we are to successfully manage this epidemic.

References

1. Ho KK, Pinsky JL, Kannel WB, et al. The epidemiology of heart failure. The Framingham Study. J Am Coll Cardiol 1993;22:6A–13A.
2. Cowie MR, Mosterd A, Wood DA, et al. The epidemiology of heart failure. Eur Heart J 1997;18:208–225.
3. American Heart Association. 2002 heart and stroke statistics update. Dallas, Texas: American Heart Association, 2001.
4. Khand A, Gemmel I, Clark AL, et al. Is the prognosis of heart failure improving? J Am Coll Cardiol 2000;36:2284–2286.
5. Stewart S, MacIntyre K, MacLeod MM, et al. Trends in hospitalization for heart failure in Scotland, 1990–1996. An epidemic that has reached its peak? Eur Heart J 2001;22:209–217.
6. Ho KK, Anderson KM, Kannel WB, et al. Survival after the onset of congestive heart failure in Framingham Heart Study subjects. Circulation 1993; 88: 107–115.
7. McMurray JJ, Petrie MC, Murdoch DR, et al. Clinical epidemiology of heart failure: public and private health burden. Eur Heart J 1998;19(Suppl)9–16.
8. Massie BM, Shah NB. Evolving trends in the epidemiologic factors of heart failure: rationale for preventive strategies and comprehensive disease management. Am Heart J 1997;133:703–712.
9. Gooding J, Jette AM. Hospital readmissions among the elderly. J Am Geriatr Soc 1985;33:595–601.
10. Vinson JM, Rich MW, Sperry JC, et al. Early readmission of elderly patients with congestive heart failure. J Am Geriatr Soc 1990;38:1290–1295.
11. Chin MH, Goldman L. Correlates of early hospital readmission or death in patients with congestive heart failure. Am J Cardiol 1997;79:1640–1644.
12. Stamos TD, Thomas S, Thomas JT, et al. The rate of re-admission is similar for congestive heart failure patients with normal and abnormal systolic function [abstract]. J Am Coll Cardiol 2001;37:198A.
13. Haldeman GA, Croft JB, Giles WH, et al. Hospitalization of patients with heart failure: National Hospital Discharge Survey, 1985 to 1995. Am Heart J 1999;137:352–360.
14. Purcell IF, Poole-Wilson PA. Heart failure: why and how to define it? Eur J Heart Fail 1999;1:7–10.
15. Struthers AD. The diagnosis of heart failure. Heart 2000;84:334–338.
16. Butman SM, Ewy GA, Standen JR, et al. Bedside cardiovascular examination in patients with severe chronic heart failure: importance of rest or inducible jugular venous distension. J Am Coll Cardiol 1993;22:968–974.
17. Harlan WR, Obermann A, Grimm R, et al. Chronic congestive heart failure in coronary artery disease: clinical criteria. Ann Intern Med 1977;86:133–138.
18. Brophy JM, Dagenais GR, McSherry F, et al. A prediction model for mortality and hospitalizations based on a cohort of 7,274 patients with congestive heart failure [abstract]. J Am Coll Cardiol 2001;37:157A.
19. Wilson JR, Rayos G, Yeoh TK, et al. Dissociation between exertional symptoms and circulatory function in patients with heart failure. Circulation 1995; 92:47–53.
20. Remes J, Miettinen H, Reunanen A, et al. Validity of clinical diagnosis of heart failure in primary health care. Eur Heart J 1991;12:315–321.
21. Caruana L, Petrie MC, Davie AP, et al. Do patients with suspected heart failure and preserved left ventricular systolic function suffer from "diastolic

heart failure" or from misdiagnosis? A prospective descriptive study. Br Med J 2000;321:215–219.

22. Akosah KO, Moncher K, Schaper A, et al. Congestive heart failure in the community: missed diagnosis and missed opportunities [abstract]. J Am Coll Cardiol 2001;37:511A.

23. Linzbach AJ. Heart failure from the point of view of quantitative anatomy. Am J Cardiol 1960;5:370–382.

24. Francis GS. Neurohumoral activation and progression of heart failure: hypothetical and clinical considerations. J Cardiovasc Pharmacol 1998;32:S16–S21.

25. McDonagh TA, Morrison CE, Lawrence A, et al. Symptomatic and asymptomatic left-ventricular systolic dysfunction in an urban population. Lancet 1997;350:829–833.

26. Cleland JG. From left ventricular dysfunction to heart failure. Arch Mal Coeur Vaiss 1996;89:1397–1402.

27. Bourassa MG, Gurne O, Bangdiwala SI, et al. Natural history and patterns of current practice in heart failure. J Am Coll Cardiol 1993;22:14A–19A.

28. Francis CM, Caruana L, Kearney P, et al. Open access echocardiography in management of heart failure in the community. Br Med J 1995;310:634–636.

29. Hart CY, Redfield MM. Diastolic heart failure in the community. Curr Cardiol Rep 2000;2:461–469.

30. Petrie MC, Caruana L, Berry C, et al. "Diastolic heart failure" or heart failure caused by subtle left ventricular systolic dysfunction? Heart 2002;87:29–31.

31. Chen HH, Lainchbury JG, Senni M, et al. Two-dimensional and doppler echocardiographic features in new-onset diastolic heart failure: a community-based study [abstract]. J Am Coll Cardiol 2001;37:210A.

32. Kitzman DW, Brubaker P, Anderson RT, et al. Isolated diastolic heart failure: Does it exist? Characterization of an important syndrome among the elderly [abstract]. J Am Coll Cardiol 2000;35:193.

33. Vasan RS, Benjamin EJ, Levy D. Prevalence, clinical features and prognosis of diastolic heart failure: an epidemiologic perspective. J Am Coll Cardiol 1995;26:1565–1574.

34. Mosterd A, Hoes AW, de Bruyne MC, et al. Prevalence of heart failure and left ventricular dysfunction in the general population. The Rotterdam Study. Eur Heart J 1999;20:447–455.

35. McDonagh TA, Robb SD, Murdoch DR, et al. Biochemical detection of left-ventricular systolic dysfunction. Lancet 1998;351:9–13.

36. Cowie MR, Wood DA, Coats AJ, et al. Incidence and aetiology of heart failure: a population-based study. Eur Heart J 1999;20:421–428.

37. McDonagh T. Asymptomatic left ventricular dysfunction in the community. Curr Cardiol Rep 2000;2:470–474.

38. Robb SD, McDonagh TA, Morrison CE, et al. The effects of symptomatic and asymptomatic left ventricular systolic dysfunction on effort capacity and quality of life in 55- to 74-year-olds from an urban population [abstract P1624]. Eur Heart J 2000;21:291.

39. Lauer MS, Evans JC, Levy D. Prognostic implications of subclinical left ventricular dilatation and systolic dysfunction in men free of overt cardiovascular disease (the Framingham Heart Study). Am J Cardiol 1992;70:1180–1184.

40. Vasan RS, Larson MG, Benjamin EJ, et al. Left ventricular dilatation and the risk of congestive heart failure in people without myocardial infarction. N Engl J Med 1997;336:1350–1355.

41. The SOLVD Investigators. Effect of enalapril on mortality and the develop-

ment of heart failure in asymptomatic patients with reduced left ventricular ejection fractions. N Engl J Med 1992;327:685–691.

42. Sigurdsson E, Thorgeirsson G, Sigvaldason H, et al. Unrecognized myocardial infarction: epidemiology, clinical characteristics, and the prognostic role of angina pectoris. The Reykjavik Study. Ann Intern Med 1995;122:96–102.
43. Robb SD, McDonagh TA, Morrison CE, et al. Prevalence and aetiological associates of left ventricular systolic dysfunction in the population of North Glasgow aged 55 to 74 years [abstract P2870]. Eur Heart J 2000;21:531.
44. The Cardiac Insufficiency Bisoprolol Study II (CIBIS-II). A randomised trial. Lancet 1999;353:9–13.
45. Packer M, Bristow MR, Cohn JN, et al. The effect of carvedilol on morbidity and mortality in patients with chronic heart failure. U.S. Carvedilol Heart Failure Study Group. N Engl J Med 1996;334:1349–1355.
46. McKee PA, Castelli WP, McNamara PM, et al. The natural history of congestive heart failure. The Framingham Study. N Engl J Med 1971;285:1441–1446.
47. Kannel WB: Vital epidemiologic clues in heart failure. J Clin Epidemiol 2000;53:229–235.
48. Fox KF, Cowie MR, Wood DA, et al. Coronary artery disease as the cause of incident heart failure in the population. Eur Heart J 2001;22:228–236.
49. Phillips SJ, Whisnant JP, O'Fallon WM, et al. Prevalence of cardiovascular disease and diabetes mellitus in residents of Rochester, Minnesota. Mayo Clin Proc 1990;65:344–359.
50. Rodeheffer RJ, Jacobsen SJ, Gersh BJ, et al. The incidence and prevalence of congestive heart failure in Rochester, Minnesota. Mayo Clin Proc 1993;68:1143–1150.
51. Schocken DD, Arrieta MI, Leaverton PE, et al. Prevalence and mortality rate of congestive heart failure in the United States. J Am Coll Cardiol 1992;20:301–306.
52. Schocken DD, Sharma K, Schwartz S, et al. Population-based prevalence and mortality of heart failure in the United States: data from NHANES II with 12–16 years follow-up [abstract #2080]. Circulation 1999;100:I-396.
53. Eriksson H, Svardsudd K, Larsson B, et al. Risk factors for heart failure in the general population: the study of men born in 1913. Eur Heart J 1989; 10: 647–656.
54. Mittelmark MB, Psaty BM, Rautaharju PM, et al. Prevalence of cardiovascular diseases among older adults. The Cardiovascular Health Study. Am J Epidemiol 1993;137:311–317.
55. Parameshwar J, Shackell MM, Richardson A, et al. Prevalence of heart failure in three general practices in northwest London. Br J Gen Pract 1992;42: 287–289.
56. Senni M, Tribouilloy CM, Rodeheffer RJ, et al. Congestive heart failure in the community: a study of all incident cases in Olmsted County, Minnesota, in 1991. Circulation 1998;98:2282–2289.
57. Diller PM, Smucker DR, David B, et al. Congestive heart failure due to diastolic or systolic dysfunction: frequency and patient characteristics in an ambulatory setting. Arch Fam Med 1999;8:414–420.
58. Kitzman DW, Gardin JM, Gottdiener JS, et al. Importance of heart failure with preserved systolic function in patients ≥65 years of age. Am J Cardiol 2001;87:413–419.
59. Cohen-Solal A, Desnos M, Delahaye F, et al. A national survey of heart failure in French hospitals. Eur Heart J 2001;21:763–769.

60. Ofili EO, Mayberry R, Alema-Mensah E, et al. Gender differences and practice implications of risk factors for frequent hospitalization for heart failure in an urban center serving predominantly African American patients. Am J Cardiol 1999;83:1350–1355.
61. Alexander M, Grumbach K, Remy L, et al. Congestive heart failure hospitalizations and survival in California: patterns according to race/ethnicity. Am Heart J 1999;137:919–927.
62. Schunkert H, Broeckel U, Hense HW, et al. Left-ventricular dysfunction. Lancet 1998;351:372.
63. Redfield MM, Burnett JC, Jacobsen SJ, et al. Prevalence of left ventricular systolic and diastolic dysfunction in Olmsted County, MN, a population-based, cross-sectional Doppler-echocardiographic survey [abstract]. J Am Coll Cardiol 2001;37:145A.
64. Morgan S, Smith H, Simpson I, et al. Prevalence and clinical characteristics of left ventricular dysfunction among elderly patients in general practice setting: cross-sectional survey. Br Med J 1999;318:368–372.
65. Cleland JGF, Clark AL. Has the survival of the heart failure population changed? Lessons from trials. Am J Cardiol 1999;83:112D–119D.
66. Kelly R, McWalter R, Stonebridge P, et al. Should we screen for asymptomatic left ventricular systolic dysfunction in patients with their first stroke, transient ischaemic attack, or overt peripheral vascular disease? [abstract]. Eur Heart J 2000;21:292.
67. Gardin JM, Siscovick D, Anton-Culver H, et al. Sex, age, and disease affect echocardiographic left ventricular mass and systolic function in the free-living elderly. The Cardiovascular Health Study. Circulation 1995;91:1739–1748.
68. Barker WH, Getchell W, Mullooly J, et al. Changing congestive heart failure incidence in an older population, 1970–74 and 1990–94 [abstract P45]. Circulation 2001;103:1359.
69. Pulignano G, Del Sindaco D, Maggioni AP, et al. Heart failure in the elderly in hospital cardiology units: data from the Italian network on congestive heart failure [abstract]. Eur Heart J 1999;20:661.
70. Rich MW. Epidemiology, pathophysiology, and etiology of congestive heart failure in older adults. J Am Geriatr Soc 1997;45:968–974.
71. McGann PE. Comorbidity in heart failure in the elderly. Clin Geriatr Med 2000;16:631–648.
72. Cicoira M, Varney S, Florea V, et al. Chronic heart failure in the very elderly: survival and prognostic factors in 186 patients over 70 years of age [abstract]. Eur Heart J 1999;20:91.
73. Croft JB, Giles WH, Pollard RA, et al. Heart failure survival among older adults in the United States: a poor prognosis for an emerging epidemic in the Medicare population. Arch Intern Med 1999;159:505–510.
74. McMurray J, McDonagh T, Morrison CE, et al. Trends in hospitalization for heart failure in Scotland 1980–1990. Eur Heart J 1993;14:1158–1162.
75. Graves E, Gillum B. 1994 Summary: National Hospital Discharge Survey: advance data. National Center for Health Statistics 1996;278:1–12.
76. Pitt B, Segal R, Martinez F, et al. Randomized trial of losartan versus captopril in patients over 65 with heart failure (Evaluation of Losartan In The Elderly study, ELITE). Lancet 1997;349:747–752.
77. Gambassi G, Lapane KL, Sgadari A, et al. Effects of angiotensin-converting enzyme inhibitors and digoxin on health outcomes of very old patients with heart failure. Arch Intern Med 2000;160:53–60.

78. Phase I, National Health and Nutrition Examination Survey (NHANES-III), 1988–91. Bethesda, MD: National Center for Health Statistics and the American Heart Association, 1995.
79. Richardson AD, Piepho RW. Effect of race on hypertension and antihypertensive therapy. Int J Clin Pharmacol Ther 2000;38:75–79.
80. Tofler GH, Stone PH, Mueller JE, et al. Effects of gender and race on prognosis after myocardial infarction: adverse prognosis for women, particularly black women. J Am Coll Cardiol 1987;9:473–482.
81. Fox KF, Cowie MR, Wood DA, et al. Aetiology of heart failure in women aged <75 years in the population [abstract]. Eur Heart J 1999;20:655.
82. Petrie MC, Dawson NF, Murdoch DR, et al. Failure of women's hearts. Circulation 1999;99:2334–2341.
83. Johnstone D, Limacher M, Rousseau M, et al. Clinical characteristics of patients in the Studies of Left Ventricular Dysfunction. Am J Cardiol 1992;70:894–900.
84. Adams KF Jr, Dunlap SH, Sueta CA, et al. Relation between gender, etiology and survival in patients with symptomatic heart failure. J Am Coll Cardiol 1996;28:1781–1788.
85. Simon T, Mary-Krause M, Funck-Brentano C, et al. Sex difference in the prognosis of congestive heart failure: results from the Cardiac Insufficiency Bisoprolol Study (CIBIS II). Circulation 2001;103:375–380.
86. Evangelista LS, Kagawa-Singer M, Dracup K: Gender differences in health perceptions and meaning in persons living with heart failure. Heart Lung 2001;30:167–176.
87. Tacchi D, Mayans CV, Cimbaro Canela JP, et al. Heart failure in women: clinical, epidemiological and prognostic differences in relation with men: substudy of national survey of heart failure in Argentina (CONAREC VI Study) [abstract]. Eur Heart J 1999;20:659.
88. Opasich C, Tavazzi L, Lucci D, et al. Comparison of one-year outcome in women versus men with chronic congestive heart failure. Am J Cardiol 2000;86:353–357.
89. Mathew J, Davidson S, Narra L, et al. Etiology and characteristics of congestive heart failure in blacks. Am J Cardiol 1996;78:1447–1450.
90. Dries DL, Exner DV, Gersh BJ, et al. Racial differences in the outcome of left ventricular dysfunction. N Engl J Med 1999;340:609–616.
91. Afzal A, Ananthasubramaniam K, Sharma N, et al. Racial differences in patients with heart failure. Clin Cardiol 1999;22:791–794.
92. Dunlap SH, Sueta CA, Schwartz TA, et al. Survival rates are similar between African Americans and other races with heart failure [abstract]. J Am Coll Cardiol 2000;35:177.
93. Aronow WS, Ahn C, Kronzon I: Comparison of incidences of congestive heart failure in older African Americans, Hispanics, and whites. Am J Cardiol 1999;84:611–612.
94. Demirovic J, Prineas R, Rudolph M. Epidemiology of congestive heart failure in three ethnic groups. Congest Heart Fail 2001;7:93–96.
95. Carson P, Ziesche S, Johnson G, et al. Racial differences in response to therapy for heart failure: analysis of the vasodilator-heart failure trials. Vasodilator-Heart Failure Trial Study Group. J Card Fail 1999;5:178–187.
96. Yancy CW, Fowler MB, Colucci WS, et al. Race and the response to adrenergic blockade with carvedilol in patients with chronic heart failure. N Engl J Med 2001;344:1358–1365.
97. Exner DV, Dries DL, Domanski MJ, et al. Lesser response to angiotensin-

converting-enzyme inhibitor therapy in black as compared with white patients with left ventricular dysfunction. N Engl J Med 2001;344:1351–1357.

98. Wood AJ. Racial differences in the response to drugs: pointers to genetic differences. N Engl J Med 2001;344:1394–1396.

99. Yancy CW. Heart failure in African Americans: a cardiovascular enigma. J Card Fail 2000;6:183–186.

100. Franciosa JA, Taylor AL, Cohn JN, et al. African-American Heart Failure Trial (A-HeFT): rationale, design and methodology. J Card Fail. In press.

101. Baig MK, Goldman JH, Caforio AL, et al. Familial dilated cardiomyopathy: cardiac abnormalities are common in asymptomatic relatives and may represent early disease. J Am Coll Cardiol 1998;31:195–201.

102. Grunig E, Tasman JA, Kucherer H, et al. Frequency and phenotypes of familial dilated cardiomyopathy. J Am Coll Cardiol 1998;31:186–194.

103. Sinagra G, Di Lenarda A, Brodsky GL, et al. Current perspective new insights into the molecular basis of familial dilated cardiomyopathy. Ital Heart J 2001;2:280–286.

104. Franz WM, Muller OJ, Katus HA. Cardiomyopathies: from genetics to the prospect of treatment. Lancet 2001;358:1627–1637.

105. Hershberger RE, Ni H, Crispell KA. Familial dilated cardiomyopathy: echocardiographic diagnostic criteria for classification of family members as affected. J Card Fail 1999;5:203–212.

106. Valantine HA, Hunt SA, Fowler MB, et al. Frequency of familial nature of dilated cardiomyopathy and usefulness of cardiac transplantation in this subset. Am J Cardiol 1989;63:959–963.

107. Michels VV, Moll PP, Miller FA, et al. The frequency of familial dilated cardiomyopathy in a series of patients with idiopathic dilated cardiomyopathy. N Engl J Med 1992;326:77–82.

108. Kannel WB, Ho KK, Thom T. Changing epidemiological features of cardiac failure. Br Heart J 1994;72:S3–S9.

109. Kannel WB. Current status of the epidemiology of heart failure. Curr Cardiol Rep 1999;1:11–19.

110. Levy D, Vasan RS, Benjamin EJ, et al. Temporal trends in heart failure risk factors from 1950–1998 [abstract #2005]. Circulation 2000;102:II-412.

111. Felker GM, Shaw LK, O'Connor CM. A standardized definition of ischemic cardiomyopathy for use in clinical research. J Am Coll Cardiol 2002;39:210–218.

112. Hare JM, Walford GD, Hruban RH, et al. Ischemic cardiomyopathy: endomyocardial biopsy and ventriculographic evaluation of patients with congestive heart failure, dilated cardiomyopathy and coronary artery disease. J Am Coll Cardiol 1992;20:1318–1325.

113. Kannel WB. Epidemiological aspects of heart failure. Cardiol Clin 1989;7:1–9.

114. McAlister FA, Teo KK, Taher M, et al. Insights into the contemporary epidemiology and outpatient management of congestive heart failure. Am Heart J 1999;138:87–94.

115. Uretsky BF, Thygesen K, Armstrong PW, et al. Acute coronary findings at autopsy in heart failure patients with sudden death: results from the Assessment of Treatment with Lisinopril And Survival (ATLAS) trial. Circulation 2000;102:611–666.

116. Brookes CI, Hart P, Keogh BE, et al. Angiography and the etiology of heart failure. Postgrad Med J 1995;71:480–482.

117. Yusuf S, Pepine CJ, Garces C, et al. Effect of enalapril on myocardial infarction and unstable angina in patients with low ejection fractions. Lancet 1992;340:1173–1178.
118. Sytkowski PA, Kannel WB, D'Agostino RB. Changes in risk factors and the decline in mortality from cardiovascular disease. The Framingham Heart Study. N Engl J Med 1990;322:1635–1641.
119. Shah MR, Bahit MC, Granger CB, et al. Clinical features of patients with heart failure after an acute coronary syndrome: findings from GUSTO-IIb [abstract]. J Am Coll Cardiol 2000;35:212.
120. Tang WH, Young JB. Cardiomyopathy and heart failure in diabetes. Endocrinol Metab Clin North Am 2001;30:1031–1046.
121. Aronow WS, Ahn C. Incidence of heart failure in 2,737 older persons with and without diabetes mellitus. Chest 1999;115:867–868.
122. The SOLVD Investigators. Effect of enalapril on survival in patients with reduced left ventricular ejection fractions and congestive heart failure. N Engl J Med 1992;325:293–302.
123. Heart Outcomes Prevention Evaluation (HOPE) Study Investigators. Effect of ramipril on cardiovascular and microvascular outcomes in people with diabetes mellitus: results of the HOPE study and MICRO-HOPE substudy. Lancet 2000;355:253–259.
124. Bristow M, Gilbert E, Abraham W, et al. Effect of carvedilol on LV function and mortality in diabetic versus nondiabetic patients with ischemia or non-ischemic dilated cardiomyopathy [abstract]. Circulation 1996;94:I-664.
125. Deedwania PC, Giles TD, Ghali JK, et al. Safety and efficacy of treatment with metoprolol CR/XL in diabetic patients with heart failure [abstract]. Circulation 2000;102:II-779.
126. McKelvie R, Yusuf S, Pericak D, et al. Comparison of candesartan, enalapril, and their combination in congestive heart failure. Randomized Evaluation of Strategies for Left Ventricular Dysfunction (RESOLVD) Pilot Study. Circulation 1999;100:1056–1064.
127. Timmis AD. Diabetic heart disease: clinical considerations. Heart 2001;85: 463–469.
128. Mak K, Moliterno D, Granger C, et al. Influence of diabetes mellitus on clinical outcome in the thrombolytic era of acute myocardial infarction. GUSTO-I Investigators. Global Utilization of Streptokinase and Tissue Plasminogen Activator for Occluded Coronary Arteries. J Am Coll Cardiol 1997;30:171–179.
129. McGuire DK, Emanuelsson H, Granger CB, et al. Influence of diabetes mellitus on clinical outcomes across the spectrum of acute coronary syndromes: findings from the GUSTO-IIb Study. Eur Heart J 2000;21:1750–1758.
130. Malmberg K. Prospective randomised study of intensive insulin treatment on long-term survival after acute myocardial infarction in patients with diabetes mellitus. DIGAMI (Diabetes Mellitus, Insulin Glucose Infusion in Acute Myocardial Infarction) Study Group. Br Med J 1997;314:1512–1515.
131. Solomon SD, St. John Sutton MG, Rouleau J-L, et al. Left ventricular remodeling does not explain the increased incidence of congestive heart failure in diabetics. The SAVE experience [abstract #116]. Circulation 1999; 102:II-28.
132. Stone PH, Muller JE, Hartwell T, et al. The effect of diabetes mellitus on prognosis and serial left ventricular function after acute myocardial infarction: contribution of both coronary disease and diastolic left ventricu-

lar dysfunction to the adverse prognosis. J Am Coll Cardiol 1989;14:49–57.

133. Galderisi M, Anderson KM, Wilson PWF, et al. Echocardiographic evidence for the existence of a distinct diabetic cardiomyopathy (The Framingham Heart Study). Am J Cardiol 1991;68:85–89.

134. Devereux RB, Roman MJ, Paranicas M, et al. Impact of diabetes on cardiac structure and function. The Strong Heart Study. Circulation 2000;101:2271–2276.

135. Lee M, Gardin JM, Lynch JC, et al. Diabetes mellitus and echocardiographic left ventricular function in free-living elderly men and women. The Cardiovascular Health Study. Am Heart J 1997;133:36–43.

136. Palmieri V, Bella JN, Arnett DK, et al. Does diabetes affect LV structure and systolic function independent of blood pressure, age and gender? A population sample-based study from the Hypertension Genetic Epidemiology Network (HyperGEN) Study. Circulation 2001;103:102–107.

137. Mustonen JN, Uusitupa MI, Laakso M, et al. Left ventricular systolic dysfunction in middle-aged patients with diabetes mellitus. Am J Cardiol 1994; 73:1202–1208.

138. Mildenberger RR, Bar-Shlomo B, Druck MN, et al. Clinically unrecognized dysfunction in young diabetic patients. J Am Coll Cardiol 1984;1984:234–238.

139. Iribarren C, Karter AJ, Go AS, et al. Glycemic control and heart failure among adult patients with diabetes. Circulation 2001;103:2668–2673.

140. Chae C, Glynn R, Manson J, et al. Diabetes predicts congestive heart failure risk in the elderly [abstract]. Circulation 1998;98:721.

141. Swan J, Anker S, Walton C, et al. Insulin resistance in chronic heart failure: relation to severity and etiology of heart failure. J Am Coll Cardiol 1997; 30: 527–532.

142. Amato L, Paolisso G, Cacciatore F, et al. Congestive heart failure predicts the development of non-insulin-dependent diabetes mellitus in the elderly. The Osservatorio Geriatrico Regione Campania Group. Diabetes Metab 1997;23:213–218.

143. Suskin N, McKelvie RS, Burns RJ, et al. Glucose and insulin abnormalities relate to functional capacity in patients with congestive heart failure. Eur Heart J 2000;21:1368–1375.

144. Scherrer U, Sartori C. Insulin as a vascular and sympathoexcitatory hormone: implications for blood pressure regulation, insulin sensitivity and cardiovascular morbidity. Circulation 1997;96:4104–4113.

145. Davies M, Hobbs F, Davis R, et al. Prevalence of left-ventricular systolic dysfunction and heart failure in the Echocardiographic Heart of England Screening study: a population-based study. Lancet 2001;358:439–444.

146. Smolens IA, Pagani FD, Bolling SF. Mitral valve repair in heart failure. Eur J Heart Fail 2000;2:365–371.

147. Opasich C, Febo O, Riccardi PG, et al. Concomitant factors of decompensation in chronic heart failure. Am J Cardiol 1996;78:354–357.

148. Redfield MM, Kay GN, Jenkins LS, et al. Tachycardia-related cardiomyopathy: a common cause of ventricular dysfunction in patients with atrial fibrillation referred for atrioventricular ablation. Mayo Clin Proc 2000;75: 790–795.

149. De Ferrari GM, Tavazzi L. The role of arrhythmia in the progression of heart failure. Eur J Heart Fail 1999;1:35–40.

150. Middlekauff HR, Stevenson WG, Stevenson LW. Prognostic significance of

atrial fibrillation in advanced heart failure: a study of 390 patients. Circulation 1991;84:40–48.

151. Cohen-Solal A, Delahave F, Emeriau JP, et al. Who are the patients hospitalized for heart failure in France today? [abstract]. Eur Heart J 1998;19: 248A.

152. Mathew J, Hunsberger S, Fleg J, et al. Incidence, predictive factors, and prognostic significance of supraventricular tachyarrhythmias in congestive heart failure. Chest 2000;118:914–922.

153. Benjamin EJ, Wolf PA, D'Agostino RB, et al. Impact of atrial fibrillation on the risk of death. The Framingham Heart Study. Circulation 1998;98:946–952.

154. Vaziri SM, Larson MG, Benjamin EJ, et al. Echocardiographic predictors of nonrheumatic atrial fibrillation. The Framingham Heart Study. Circulation 1994;89:724–730.

155. Carson PE, Johnson MR, Dunkman WB, et al. The influence of atrial fibrillation on prognosis in mild to moderate heart failure. The V-HeFT Studies. Circulation 1993;87:102–110.

156. Singh SN: Congestive heart failure and arrhythmias: therapeutic modalities. J Cardiovasc Electrophysiol 1997;8:88–97.

157. Leier CV, Alvarez RJ, Binkley PF. The problem of ventricular dysrhythmias and sudden death mortality in heart failure: the impact of current therapy. Cardiology 2000;93:56–69.

158. Luu M, Stevenson WG, Stevenson LW, et al. Diverse mechanisms of unexpected cardiac arrest in advanced heart failure. Circulation 1989;80:1675–1680.

159. Nielsen JC, Andersen HR, Mortensen PT. Heart failure and echocardiographic changes during long-term follow-up of patients with sick sinus syndrome randomized to single-chamber atrial or ventricular pacing. Circulation 1988;97:978–995.

160. Alboni P, Brignole M, Menozzi C, et al. Is sinus bradycardia a factor facilitating overt heart failure? Eur Heart J 1999;20:252–255.

161. Alboni P, Menozzi C, Brignole M. Effects of permanent pacemaker and oral theophylline in sick sinus syndrome. The THEOPACE study: a randomized controlled trial. Circulation 1997;96:260–266.

162. Pavia SV, Wilkoff BL. Biventricular pacing for heart failure. Cardiol Clin 2001;19:637–651.

163. Knight EL, Glynn RJ, McIntyre KM, et al. Predictors of decreased renal function in patients with heart failure during angiotensin-converting enzyme inhibitor therapy: results from the Studies Of Left Ventricular Dysfunction (SOLVD). Am Heart J 1999;138:849–855.

164. Dries DL, Exner DV, Domanski MJ, et al. The prognostic implications of renal insufficiency in asymptomatic and symptomatic patients with left ventricular systolic dysfunction. J Am Coll Cardiol 2000;35:681–689.

165. Al-Ahmad A, Rand WM, Manjunath G, et al. Reduced kidney function and anemia as risk factors for mortality in patients with left ventricular dysfunction. J Am Coll Cardiol 2001;38:955–962.

166. Krumholz HM, Chen YT, Vaccarino V, et al. Correlates and impact on outcomes of worsening renal function in patients ≥65 years of age with heart failure. Am J Cardiol 2000;85:1110–1113.

167. Volpe M, Tritto C, Testa U, et al. Blood levels of erythropoietin in congestive heart failure and correlation with clinical, hemodynamic, and hormonal profiles. Am J Cardiol 1994;74:468–473.

168. Silverberg DS, Wexler D, Sheps D, et al. The effect of correction of mild ane-

mia in severe, resistant congestive heart failure using subcutaneous erythropoietin and intravenous iron: a randomized controlled study. J Am Coll Cardiol 2001;37:1775–1780.

169. Hamilton MA, Stevenson LW. Thyroid hormone abnormalities in heart failure: possibilities for therapy. Thyroid 1996;6:527–529.

170. Opasich C, Pacini F, Ambrosino N, et al. Sick euthyroid syndrome in patients with moderate-to-severe chronic heart failure. Eur Heart J 1996;17:1860–1866.

171. Yan AT, Bradley TD, Liu PP. The role of continuous positive airway pressure in the treatment of congestive heart failure. Chest 2001;120:1675–1685.

172. Obenza Nishime E, Liu LC, Coulter TD, et al. Heart failure and sleep-related breathing disorders. Cardiol Rev 2000;8:191–201.

173. Suter PM, Haller J, Hany A, et al. Diuretic use: a risk for subclinical thiamine deficiency in elderly patients. J Nutr Health Aging 2000;4:69–71.

174. Bohmer T. How prevalent is thiamine deficiency in heart failure patients? Nutr Rev 2001;59:342–344.

175. Kelly R, Staines A, MacWalter R, et al. The prevalence of treatable left ventricular systolic dysfunction in patients who present with noncardiac vascular episodes: a case-control study. J Am Coll Cardiol 2002;39:219–224.

176. Johnson MR. Acute pulmonary edema. Curr Treat Options Cardiovasc Med 1999;1:269–276.

177. Feenstra J, Grobbee DE, Jonkman FA, et al. Prevention of relapse in patients with congestive heart failure: the role of precipitating factors. Heart 1998;80:432–436.

178. Feenstra J, Heerdink ER, Grobbee DE, et al. Association of non-steroidal anti-inflammatory drugs with first occurrence of heart failure and with relapsing heart failure. The Rotterdam Study. Arch Intern Med 2002;162:265–270.

179. Tang WH, Francis GS. Polypharmacy of heart failure: creating a rational pharmacotherapeutic protocol. Cardiol Clin 2001;19:583–596.

180. Ghali JK, Kadakia S, Cooper R, et al. Precipitating factors leading to decompensation of heart failure: traits among urban blacks. Arch Intern Med 1988;148:2013–2016.

181. Harjai KJ, Thompson HW, Turgut T, et al. Simple clinical variables are markers of the propensity for readmission in patients hospitalized with heart failure. Am J Cardiol 2001;87:234–237.

182. Chen HH, Lainchbury JG, Senni M, et al. Diastolic heart failure in the community: underlying cardiovascular diseases and precipitating factors [abstract #3769]. Circulation 2000;102:II-780.

183. Metra M, Nodari S, Boldi E, et al. Marked improvement in left ventricular function after long-term beta-blockade in patients with heart failure: clinical characteristics and prognostic significance [abstract #3046]. Circulation 2000;102:II-628.

184. Tang WHW, Prikazsky LM, Fowler MB. Insulin resistance is associated with the reversal of left ventricular remodeling following carvedilol [abstract]. Circulation 2000;102:II-719.

185. Francis GS, Johnson TH, Ziesche S, et al. Marked spontaneous improvement in ejection fraction in patients with congestive heart failure. Am J Med 1990;89:303–307.

186. Tang WHW, Larson MS, Vagelos RH, et al. Reverse remodeling following

long-term carvedilol therapy is associated with improvement in survival. The Stanford Carvedilol Echocardiographic Registry [abstract #1062MP-121]. J Am Coll Cardiol 2002;39:141A.

187. Kawai K, Takaoka H, Hata K, et al. Prevalence, predictors, and prognosis of reversal of maladaptive remodeling with intensive medical therapy in idiopathic dilated cardiomyopathy. Am J Cardiol 1999;84:671–676.

188. Cowie MR, Wood DA, Coats AJ, et al. Survival of patients with a new diagnosis of heart failure: a population-based study. Heart 2000;83:505–510.

189. Bart BA, Shaw LK, McCants CB, et al. Clinical determinants of mortality in patients with angiographically diagnosed ischemic or nonischemic cardiomyopathy. J Am Coll Cardiol 1997;30:1002–1008.

190. McCullough PA, Philbin EF, Spertus JA, et al. Confirmation of a heart failure epidemic: findings from the Resource Utilization Among Congestive Heart Failure (REACH) study. J Am Coll Cardiol 2002;39:60–69.

191. Senni M, Tribouilloy CM, Rodeheffer RJ, et al. Congestive heart failure in the community: trends in incidence and survival in a 10-year period. Arch Intern Med 1999;159:29–34.

192. Spencer FA, Meyer TE, Goldberg RJ, et al. Twenty-year trends (1975–1995) in the incidence, in-hospital and long-term death rates associated with heart failure complicating acute myocardial infarction: a community-wide perspective. J Am Coll Cardiol 1999;35:1378–1387.

193. Stevenson WG, Stevenson LW, Middlekauff HR, et al. Improving survival for patients with advanced heart failure: a study of 737 consecutive patients. J Am Coll Cardiol 1995;26:1417–1423.

194. MacIntyre K, Capewell S, Stewart S, et al. Evidence of improving prognosis in heart failure: trends in case fatality in 66,547 patients hospitalized between 1986 and 1995. Circulation 2000;102:1126–1131.

195. Cleland JGF, Gemmell I, Aleem K, et al. Is the prognosis of heart failure improving? Eur J Heart Fail 1999;1:229–241.

196. Zannad F, Braincon S, Juilliere Y, et al. Incidence, clinical and etiologic features, and outcomes of advanced chronic heart failure. The EPICAL Study. Epidemiologie de l'Insuffisance Cardiaque Avancee en Lorraine. J Am Coll Cardiol 1999;33:734–742.

197. Cowburn PJ, Cleland JG, Coats AJ, et al. Risk stratification in chronic heart failure. Eur Heart J 1998;19:696–710.

198. Vasan RS, Larson MG, Benjamin EJ, et al. Congestive heart failure in subjects with normal versus reduced left ventricular ejection fraction: prevalence and mortality in a population-based cohort. J Am Coll Cardiol 1999;33:1948–1955.

199. Philbin EF, Erb T, Jenkins P. The natural history of heart failure with preserved left ventricular systolic function [abstract #977–156]. J Am Coll Cardiol 1997;29:245A.

200. Braunwald E, Bristow MR. Congestive heart failure: fifty years of progress. Circulation 2000;102:IV4–IV23.

201. Gottdiener JS, Arnold AM, Aurigemma GP, et al. Predictors of congestive heart failure in the elderly. The Cardiovascular Health Study. J Am Coll Cardiol 2000;35:1628–1637.

202. He J, Ogden LG, Bazzano LA, et al. Risk factors for congestive heart failure in US men and women. NHANES I epidemiologic follow-up study. Arch Intern Med 2001;161:996–1002.

203. Vargas CM, Burt VL, Gillum RF. Cardiovascular disease in the NHANES III. Ann Epidemiol 1997;7:523–525.
204. Devereux RB, Roman MJ, Liu JE, et al. Congestive heart failure despite normal left ventricular systolic function in a population-based sample. The Strong Heart Study. Am J Cardiol 2000;86:1090–1096.
205. Nielsen OW, Hilden J, Larsen CT, et al. Cross-sectional study estimating prevalence of heart failure and left ventricular systolic dysfunction in community patients at risk. Heart 2001;86:172–178.
206. Clarke KW, Gray D, Hamptom JR. How common is heart failure? Evidence from PACT (Prescribing Analysis and Cost) data in Nottingham. J Public Health Med 1995;17:459–464.
207. Hedberg P, Lonnberg I, Jonason T, et al. Left ventricular systolic dysfunction in 75-year-old men and women: a population-based study. Eur Heart J 2001;22:676–683.
208. Remes J, Reunanen A, Aromaa A, et al. Incidence of heart failure in eastern Finland: a population-based surveillance study. Eur Heart J 1992;13:588–593.
209. Johansson S, Wallander M, Ruigomez A, et al. Incidence of newly diagnosed heart failure in UK general practice. Eur J Heart Fail 2001;3:225–231.
210. Devereux RB, Roman MJ, Paranicas M, et al. A population-based assessment of left ventricular systolic dysfunction in middle-aged and older adults. The Strong Heart Study. Am Heart J 2001;141:439–446.
211. The CONSENSUS Trial Study Group. Effects of enalapril on mortality in severe congestive heart failure: results of the Cooperative North Scandinavian Enalapril Survival Study (CONSENSUS). N Engl J Med 1987;316:1429–1435.
212. Cohn JN, Johnson G, Ziesche S, et al. A comparison of enalapril with hydralazine-isosorbide dinitrate in the treatment of chronic congestive heart failure. N Engl J Med 1991;325:303–310.
213. The Digitalis Investigation Group. The effect of digoxin on mortality and morbidity in patients with heart failure. N Engl J Med 1997;336:525–533.
214. Packer M, Carver JR, Rodeheffer RJ, et al. Effect of oral milrinone on mortality in severe chronic heart failure. The PROMISE Study Research Group. N Engl J Med 1991;325:1468–1475.
215. Packer M, Poole-Wilson P, Armstrong P, et al. Comparative effects of low and high doses of the angiotensin-converting enzyme inhibitor, lisinopril, on morbidity and mortality in chronic heart failure. Circulation 1999;100:2312–2318.
216. MERIT-HF Study Group: Effect of metoprolol CR/XL in chronic heart failure. Metoprolol CR/XL Randomized Intervention Trial in Congestive Heart Failure (MERIT-HF). Lancet 1999;353:2001–2007.
217. Pitt B, Zannad F, Remme WJ, et al. The effect of spironolactone on morbidity and mortality in patients with severe heart failure. Randomized Aldactone Evaluation Study Investigators. N Engl J Med 1999;341:709–717.
218. Pitt B, Poole-Wilson PA, Segal R, et al. Effect of losartan compared with captopril on mortality in patients with symptomatic heart failure. Randomized trial—the Losartan Heart Failure Survival Study ELITE II. Lancet 2000;355:1582–1587.
219. A trial of the beta-blocker bucindolol in patients with advanced chronic heart failure. N Engl J Med 2001;344:1659–1667.
220. Torp-Pedersen C, Moller M, Bloch-Thomsen PE, et al. Dofetilide in patients with congestive heart failure and left ventricular dysfunction. Danish In-

vestigations of Arrhythmia and Mortality on Dofetilide Study Group. N Engl J Med 1999;341:857–865.
221. Packer M, Coats AJ, Fowler MB, et al. Effect of carvedilol on survival in severe chronic heart failure. N Engl J Med 2001;344:1651–1658.
222. Cohn JN, Tognoni G. A randomized trial of the angiotensin-receptor blocker valsartan in chronic heart failure. N Engl J Med 2001;345:1667–1675.
223. Dargie HJ: Effect of carvedilol on outcome after myocardial infarction in patients with left-ventricular dysfunction. The CAPRICORN randomised trial. Lancet 2001;357:1385–1390.

• 2 •

Pathophysiology of Chronic Heart Failure

Tatiana Tsvetkova, MD,
and Michael R. Bristow, MD, PhD

The Chronic Heart Failure Syndrome

Chronic heart failure is a clinical syndrome resulting from cardiac pump dysfunction. As befits the critical nature of adequate circulatory support to most bodily functions, the chronic heart failure syndrome itself can manifest in any number of ways, including symptoms or signs of low cardiac output (fatigue, weakness, light-headedness, cool extremities), high filling pressures (breathlessness, abdominal discomfort, edema, rales, jugular venous distention), arrhythmias, embolic phenomena, or hypertrophy. Pump dysfunction can result from abnormalities in any component of the heart, including valves, coronary vessels, pericardium, electrophysiological tissue, and myocardium. However, the vast majority of cases of chronic heart failure result from myocardial dysfunction that results from a cardiomyopathic process, which is the topic of this chapter.

The Dilated Cardiomyopathy Phenotype

The most common cause of myocardial dysfunction is a primary or secondary dilated cardiomyopathy, as defined by the 1995 W.H.O. Classification.[1] The other components of the W.H.O. Classification[1] (hypertrophic, restrictive, arrhythmogenic right ventricular, and unclassified)

From: Kukin ML, Fuster V (eds). *Oxidative Stress and Cardiac Failure.* Armonk, NY: Futura Publishing Co., Inc. ©2003.

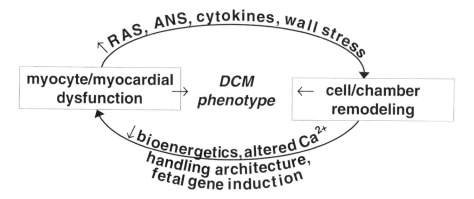

Figure 1. Relationship between the primary pathophysiological processes that are responsible for the DCM phenotype: contractile dysfunction and remodeling.

make up a small minority of cardiomyopathy cases. Therefore, the focus of this chapter is on the dilated cardiomyopathy (DCM) phenotype. As depicted in Figure 1, two interrelated general processes—chamber remodeling and myocardial contractile dysfunction—play critical and interrelated roles in the development and progression of primary and secondary DCMs.[2,3] Although both are the products of changes that occur at the cardiac myocyte level, changes in the interstitium also contribute.[4]

General Pathophysiology of DCMs: Interaction of Remodeling and Contractile Dysfunction as the Major Components of the DCM Phenotype

Remodeling/Pathologic Hypertrophy

In the remodeling process, cardiac myocytes become longer with less of a proportional increase in transverse diameter, which explains the increase in chamber diameter without an increase in wall thickness that characterizes the DCM phenotype.[5,6] Although this adjustment does increase the number of contractile elements as new sarcomeres are laid down in series, the law of LaPlace dictates that wall stress will be markedly increased. This will decrease contractile function, as may the altered cytoarchitecture of the remodeled myocyte that causes Ca^{2+} handling mechanisms to become dysfunctional.[7] In addition, as was detailed 20 years ago in rat models,[8] in the failing human heart the process of pathologic hypertrophy is accompanied by a qualitative change in the expression of genes regulating cell growth and contractile function.[9-13] This constellation of changes in myocardial gene expression resembles the pre-

Table 1
Changes in Myocardial Gene Expression

Gene Expressed	Normal/Nonfailing	Fetal	FHH
ANP/BNP	↓⤬	↑↑	↑↑
SERCA-2	↑	↓	↓,↔
α-MyHC	↑	↓	↓
β-MyHC	↑	↑↑	↑↑

natal pattern of expression, and hence the term "induction of fetal gene expression" is used to describe these changes. Some of the specific changes are shown in Table 1. Based on work done in rodent models,[8,14,15] it is likely that this mechanism of fetal gene induction contributes to the development of myocardial failure in the context of pathologic hypertrophy, as depicted in Figure 1. Thus, remodeling of cardiac myocytes results in the desired increase in contractile elements, but the process of pathologic hypertrophy also results in contractile dysfunction.

Contractile Dysfunction

The DCM phenotype may also be initiated by the development of contractile dysfunction. In this phenotype, systolic contractile dysfunction predominates, but diastolic dysfunction is also invariably found. In transgenic mice with intrinsic contractile dysfunction due to overexpression of the SR function inhibitory protein phospholamban, the ultimate result is the development of pathologic hypertrophy and remodeling.[16] In this genetic model, adrenergic activation occurs to compensate for the depressed contractile dysfunction, but ultimately the adverse effects of this mechanism produce a cardiomyopathy.[16] In the human heart, pure contractile or global pump dysfunction without remodeling can be identified in subjects presenting with acute, new-onset heart failure. Examples are the presentations of adriamycin cardiomyopathy, postpartum cardiomyopathy, myocarditis, or after a first, large myocardial infarction where ventricular size is initially normal. All of these presentations are accompanied by high heart rates since an increase in stroke volume is not available for increasing cardiac output. If the patient survives, ultimately remodeling and pathologic hypertrophy will occur in all of these cases where contractile dysfunction persists. As shown in Figure 1, in addition to adrenergic activation, other signal transduction pathways are activated to produce pathologic hypertrophy and remodeling. Some of these are the renin-angiotensin system, increased endothelin-1 production, and wall stress–stretch-activated pathways.

Table 2
Categories of Contractile Function

INTRINSIC (*Function in the absence of neural, hormonal or cytokine influence*)	**MODULATABLE** (*Function which may be stimulated or inhibited by extrinsic factors including neuro-transmitters, cytokines or hormones*)
• Contractile proteins • E-C coupling mechanisms • Bioenergetics • R-G-adenylyl cyclase pathways • Cytoskeleton • Sarcomere and cell remodeling	• R-G-adenylyl cyclase pathways • R-G-phospholipase C pathways

It is useful to subdivide contractile function and dysfunction into two different categories: intrinsic and modulatable (Table 2).[17] *Intrinsic function* is defined as the systolic or diastolic contractile function in isolated heart or cell preparations where neural and hormonal influences have been eliminated, and *modulatable function* is contractile function re-cruitable by rapid-response neural and hormonal mechanisms activated to increase cardiac performance in times of increased demand. The heart is unique among critical organs in that it has the ability to rapidly and markedly (by 2- to 5-fold) increase its performance above a basal level of function, utilizing modulatable function mechanisms. In the human heart, beta-adrenergic mechanisms are the main source of modulatable function.[17,18] Modulatable function mechanisms support the periodic increases in daily activities confronting both normal and chronic heart failure patients, and they are also the same compensatory mechanisms activated to support reduction in intrinsic function in chronic heart failure. The validity of subdividing myocardial function into these two categories is supported by the observations that both types of function independently predict prognosis.[19]

Effect of Components of the DCM Phenotype on the Natural History of Chronic Heart Failure

The processes of contractile dysfunction and remodeling are progressive in most patients with established chronic heart failure,[19] and the pace[20] and degree[21] of progression are directly related to prognosis. In clinical practice, instrinsic systolic function is estimated by the ejection fraction, and modulatable function is estimated by peak VO_2. However, the left ventricular ejection fraction (LVEF), which is measured by radionuclide, angiographic, or echocardiographic techniques, measures both remodeling function and systolic function. The LVEF measures remodeling because end-diastolic volume is the denominator of the calculation, and it measures basal systolic function because end-systolic volume appears in the numerator of the ejection fraction equation (stroke volume/end-diastolic volume). Since the LVEF is ordinarily measured at rest, the function measurement includes intrinsic systolic function + the degree of modulatable function present under basal conditions. In most circumstances, intrinsic function would be the major component of function measured at rest.

Since LVEF and peak VO_2 independently predict prognosis in chronic heart failure, it can be concluded that the processes of remodeling, intrinsic function, and modulatable function all exert an effect on outcome. A corollary of this observation is that heart failure therapies should be directed at one or all of these abnormalities, without exacerbating effects on the others.

Compensatory Mechanisms Activated to Support the Failing Heart

How is contractile dysfunction converted into pathologic hypertrophy, and vice versa (Figure 1)? The answers are found within the mechanisms that are activated to support the failing heart. When the heart begins to fail, either because of an initial process that decreases global pump function or as the result of secondary contractile dysfunction arising in the setting of pathologic hypertrophy, the possibilities for stabilizing myocardial performance are limited (Figure 2). These are: (1) an increase

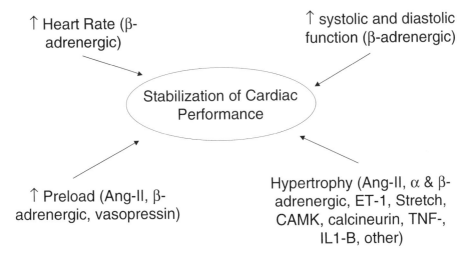

Figure 2. Compensatory mechanisms activated to support the failing heart.

in heart rate, (2) an increase in contractile function, (3) volume expansion via vasopressin and aldosterone production and release, to increase preload which results in a higher position on the Frank-Starling curve, and (4) increasing the number of contractile elements and chamber volume through cell and chamber hypertrophy. As described below, the majority of these physiological and structural adjustments are mediated by activation of so-called neurohormonal mechanisms, which in reality include increased production/release of neurotransmitters, hormones, and cytokines.

Neurohumoral Adaptations in Chronic Heart Failure

The principal neurohormonal systems activated in the response to chronic heart failure are the adrenergic nervous system, the renin-angiotensin-aldosterone system, and antidiuretic hormone (arginine vasopressin).[22,23] Other biological substances are also profoundly altered in this setting, including the vasoconstrictor autocrine/paracrine peptide endothelin-1 and the vasodilators atrial natriuretic peptide and nitric oxide. These neurohormonal changes are seen with both systolic and diastolic dysfunction, but have been extensively investigated only in the former.

Adrenergic Nervous System

One of the first responses to a decrease in cardiac output (sensed as a fall in blood pressure, an increase in filling pressures, and by other means) is activation of the adrenergic nervous system, resulting in both increased release and decreased uptake of norepinephrine at adrenergic nerve endings. Downregulation of peripheral alpha-2 receptor function, which normally inhibits norepinephrine release, may contribute to adrenergic activation in heart failure.[24]

Adrenergic activation plays a major role in the compensatory mechanisms listed in Figure 2. The increase in heart rate and contractile function is predominantly beta-adrenergic, beta-receptor stimulation is a major source of nonosmotic release of vasopressin, and beta-adrenergic and possibly alpha-adrenergic mechanisms contribute to pathologic hypertrophy. Based on these realities, it is no surprise that modulation of the adrenergic nervous system can have a major favorable[25] or adverse[26] effect on the natural history of chronic heart failure.

Increased adrenergic activity also leads to systemic vasoconstriction and enhanced venous tone, both of which initially contribute to the maintenance of blood pressure. Renal vasoconstriction (mediated by both norepinephrine and angiotensin II) occurs primarily at the efferent arteriole, producing an increase in filtration fraction that allows glomerular filtration to be relatively well maintained despite a fall in renal blood flow. Both norepinephrine and angiotensin II also stimulate proximal tubular sodium reabsorption, which contributes to the sodium retention characteristic of heart failure.

In addition to systemic adrenergic activation, there is also a selective increase in cardiac activity. This effect has been demonstrated by increased cardiac norepinephrine spillover (i.e., elevated norepinephrine levels in cardiac veins).[27] The chronic increase in cardiac adrenergic activity can also lead to downregulation of cardiac beta-adrenergic receptor signal transduction and direct adverse effects on cardiac myocytes, including cellular Ca^{2+} accumulation[28] and the induction of apoptosis.[29] The adverse effect on beta-adrenergic signal transduction contributes to a reduction in peak VO_2,[18] intracellular Ca^{2+} accumulation predisposes to arrhythmias and activation of Ca^{2+}-dependent genes involved in pathologic hypertrophy, and apoptosis directly contributes to loss of contractile function and the development of replacement fibrosis. It appears that beta-1-adrenergic stimulation is the primary influence on apoptosis[30,31] and activation of pathologic hypertrophy.[10] These concepts are summarized in Figure 3.

Renin-Angiotensin-Aldosterone System

Most factors that stimulate renin release—decreased stretch of the glomerular afferent arteriole, reduced delivery of chloride to the macula densa, and increased beta-1-adrenergic activity—are activated in chronic heart failure. There is also evidence that angiotensin II can be synthesized locally at a variety of tissue sites including the kidney, vascular endothelium, adrenal gland, and brain.

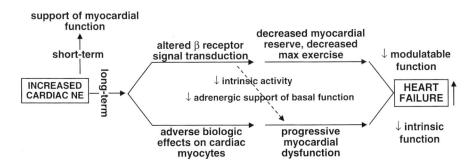

Figure 3. Role of adrenergic mechanisms in the natural history of chronic heart failure.

In addition to activation of the systemic renin-angiotensin system in heart failure, there is evidence of local cardiac angiotensin II, angiotensin-converting enzyme (ACE), and aldosterone production with adverse effects on cardiac function and the promotion of pathologic hypertrophy; their production is in proportion to the severity of heart failure.[32] Within this construct, renin is not produced locally, but increased amounts originally generated in the kidneys are taken up from the circulation.

Angiotensin II has actions similar to norepinephrine in chronic heart failure, increasing sodium reabsorption (an effect mediated in part by enhanced release of aldosterone) and inducing systemic and renal vasoconstriction.[33-35] Stretch of cardiac myocytes results in the autocrine release of angiotensin II.[33] This response is associated with upregulation of fetal proteins and is inhibited by ACE inhibitors and angiotensin II receptor blockers (ARBs). Stretch-induced angiotensin II release also leads to a 5- to 8-fold increase in apoptosis of myocytes, which occurs 4–24 hours after the induction of stretch.[34]

Arginine Vasopressin

Activation of the carotid sinus baroreceptors by the low cardiac output in heart failure leads to enhanced release of vasopressin and stimulation of thirst. Elevated levels of vasopressin may contribute to the increase in systemic vascular resistance in chronic heart failure and also promote water retention by enhancing water reabsorption in the collecting tubules. The combination of decreased water excretion and increased water intake via thirst often leads to a fall in the plasma sodium concentration. The severity of these defects tends to parallel the severity of the heart failure. As a result, the degree of hyponatremia is an important predictor of survival in these patients.

Atrial and Brain Natriuretic Peptides

Atrial natriuretic peptide (ANP) is released primarily from the atria but also from the ventricles in response to volume expansion that appears to be sensed as an increase in stretch. ANP release is increased in heart failure. Plasma ANP levels rise early in the course of the disease and have been used as a marker for the diagnosis of asymptomatic left ventricular dysfunction.[35,36] With chronic and more advanced heart failure, ventricular cell release of ANP becomes more prominent. In addition, brain natriuretic peptide (BNP), an analogous peptide, is selectively produced in the ventricle in response to high ventricular filling pressures[38] and in established pathologic hypertrophy. ANP is antiproliferative and induces apoptosis in isolated cardiac myocytes, which may be mediated through reduced expression of Mcl-1, a homolog of the antiapoptotic protein Bcl-2.[38]

Tumor Necrosis Factor-Alpha

Plasma levels of tumor necrosis factor-alpha (TNF-α) are elevated in patients with heart failure.[39] TNF-α is produced in failing human cardiac myocytes[40] and has been shown to contribute to the development of remodeling.[41,42] TNF-α induces apoptosis in isolated rat cardiomyocytes,[43] but may also protect against apoptosis in certain situations.[44]

Endothelin-1

Endothelin-1 is a 21-amino acid peptide ordinarily produced by the vascular endothelium, which is the most potent naturally occurring vasoconstrictor that has been identified.[45] Experimental evidence indicates that endothelin-1 contributes to the regulation of myocardial function, vascular tone, and peripheral resistance in chronic heart failure.[46-48] Endothelin (ET) can bind to two receptors, ET_A and ET_B, found in multiple tissues and cells including vascular smooth muscle, cardiac myocytes, and fibroblasts. In vascular smooth muscle, the ET_A receptor mediates vasoconstriction, while the ET_B receptor, found predominantly in endothelial cells, mediates vasodilatation through the production of NO and prostacyclin.[46] Both ET_A and ET_B receptors exist within the human myocardium, with only ET_A receptors predominating in failing ventricles.[49,50] In addition to its vasoconstrictor effects, endothelin-1 decreases renal blood flow, glomerular filtration, and salt and water excretion and aldosterone secretion via ET_A receptor mechanisms,[51] but increases renal blood flow, glomerular filtration, and natriuresis via ET_B receptor pathways.[52] Experimental studies suggest that ET is released in part from cardiac myocytes and coronary vascular endothelium.[53,54] Given these considerations, it is not surprising that endothelin-1 levels are directly related to adverse outcomes in chronic heart failure.[55]

The deleterious vascular effects of ET in chronic heart failure may be partially counteracted by its ET_A-receptor-mediated positive inotropic activity.[55] This effect may be mediated, in part, by increased sensitivity of the myofilaments to calcium.[56] Inhibition of the ET_B receptor may have adverse effects on cardiac and renal hemodynamics as a result of vasoconstriction, although it may prevent volume retention through inhibition of aldosterone secretion.[57-59]

Therapeutic Approach to the Pathophysiology of DCM

Given the above considerations, it is obvious that the positive feedback loop described in Figure 1 needs to be interrupted to improve the natural history of the most common cause of chronic heart failure. In its most general sense, this means using an agent or treatment that either improves contractile function or reverses pathologic hypertrophy and remodeling.

Improving Natural History by Improving Contractile Function

There is ample evidence that improvement in contractile function can produce a beneficial effect on the natural history of chronic heart failure, in both model systems and humans. Certain transgenic manipulations resulting in improved contractile function improve survival in mice,[60,61] "biological" improvement in contractile function by beta-blocking agents is associated with dramatic improvements in natural history,[3] and devices that improve pump function are associated with improvement in surrogates of clinical outcome.[62] On the other hand, with the exception of digoxin,[63] positive inotropic agents have not improved chronic heart failure natural history, and have usually worsened it in large-scale trials.[64,65] The basis for this is that the pharmacological mechanism of the inotropic agents being used has produced adverse effects, particularly proarrhythmic, which have overridden any beneficial effect of the compounds. It remains to be seen whether newer approaches, including lower doses of phosphodiesterase inhibitors combined with beta-blocking agents[66] or novel mechanisms can produce the favorable effects on chronic heart failure natural history that would be predicted from DCM pathophysiology.

Improving Natural History by Preventing or Reversing Pathologic Hypertrophy and Remodeling

There is also ample evidence that preventing or reversing pathologic hypertrophy has a favorable effect on the natural history of chronic heart failure resulting from a DCM phenotype uncomplicated by a situation that requires increased hypertrophy to normalize wall stress, such as aortic stenosis. The data include ACE inhibitor heart chronic heart failure[67-69] and post-MI trials,[70-72] and beta-blocker chronic heart failure[25,73] and post-MI[74] trials. The data with ACE inhibitors are more compelling in support of the hypothesis that preventing remodeling is beneficial, since contractile function is not affected.[75] With beta-blocking agents, which have been administered on a background of ACE inhibition in clinical trials, contractile function appears to be favorably affected before remodeling/hypertrophy is reversed.[3] This makes it difficult to assign the primary mechanism to remodeling reversal. However, with beta-blockade, a molecular marker of pathologic hypertrophy, beta-myosin heavy chain, decreases as markers of contractile function increase in subjects who improve their ejection fractions.[10] Therefore, the effect of beta-blockade is likely to be on both improvements in contractile function and reversal of pathologic hypertrophy.

With ACE inhibition and beta-blockade, the prevention or reversal in remodeling has been effected by blocking single, albeit powerful, neurohormonal pathways. These and other growth-promoting pathways such as endothelin-1 converge intracellularly on distal, "final common pathway" regulators of the hypertrophic response. Some of these are calcineurin[74] and the MEF2-HDAC[75] system. This emerging reality has led to the idea that preventing or reversing hypertrophy would be much more effective if rate-limiting steps in these distal activators could be inhibited, and this approach is now being taken by several groups of investigators.

References

1. Richardson P, McKenna W, Bristow MR, et al. Report of the 1995 World Health Organization/International Society and Federation of Cardiology Task Force on the Definition and Classification of Cardiomyopathies. Circulation 1996;93:841–842.
2. Bristow MR. Why does the myocardium fail? New insights from basic science. Lancet 1998;352:(Suppl I):8–14.
3. Eichhorn EJ, Bristow MR. Medical therapy can improve the biologic properties of the chronically failing heart: a new era in the treatment of heart failure. Circulation 1996;94:2285–2296.
4. Weber KT. Extracellular matrix remodeling in heart failure: a role for de novo angiotensin II generation. Circulation 1997;96:4065–4082.
5. Gerdes AM, Kellerman SE, Moore JA, et al. Structural remodeling of cardiac myocytes from patients with chronic ischemic heart disease. Circulation 1992;86:426–430.
6. Gerdes AM, Kellerman SE, Schocken DD. Implications of cardiomyocyte remodeling in heart dysfunction. In: Dhalla NS, Beamish RE, Takeda N, et al., eds. The Failing Heart. Raven Press, NY, 1995; 197–205.
7. Gomez AM, Valdivia HH, Cheng H, et al. Defective excitation-contraction coupling in experimental cardiac hypertrophy and heart failure. Science 1997;276:800–806.
8. Swynghedauw B. Developmental and functional adaptation of contractile proteins in cardiac and skeletal muscles. Physiol Rev 1986;66:710–771.
9. Lowes BD, Minobe WA, Abraham WT, et al. Changes in gene expression in the intact human heart: downregulation of a-myosin heavy chain in hypertrophied, failing ventricular myocardium. J Clin Invest 1997;100:2315–2324.
10. Lowes BD, Gilbert EM, Abraham WT, et al. Molecular remodeling accompanies phenotypic improvement in dilated cardiomyopathy treated with beta-adrenergic blocking agents. N Engl J Med, in press.
11. Nakao K, Minobe WA, Roden RL, et al. Myosin heavy chain gene expression in human heart failure. J Clin Invest 1997;100:2362–2370.
12. Mercadier JJ, Lompre AM, Duc P, et al. Altered sarcoplasmic reticulum Ca-ATPase gene expression in the human ventricle during end-stage heart failure. J Clin Invest 1990;85:305–309.

13. Miyata S, Minobe WA, Bristow MR, et al. Myosin heavy chain isoform expression in the failing and non-failing human heart. Circ Res 2000;86:386–390.
14. Nadal-Ginard B, Mahdavi V. Molecular basis of cardiac performance: plasticity of the myocardium generated through protein isoform switches. J Clin Invest 1989;84:1693–1700.
15. Chang KC, Figueredo VM, Schreur JHM, et al. Thyroid hormone improves function and Ca^{2+} handling in pressure overload hypertrophy. J Clin Invest 1997;100:1742–1749.
16. Dash R, Kadambi V, Schmidt AG, et al. Interactions between phospholamban and beta-adrenergic drive may lead to cardiomyopathy and early mortality. Circulation 2001;103:889–896.
17. Bristow MR, Gilbert EM. Improvement in cardiac myocyte function by biologic effects of medical therapy: a new concept in the treatment of heart failure. Eur Heart J 1995;16:20–31.
18. White M, Yanowitz F, Gilbert EM, et al. Role of beta-adrenergic receptor downregulation in the peak exercise response in patients with heart failure due to idiopathic dilated cardiomyopathy. Am J Cardiol 1995;76:1271–1276.
19. Cohn JN, Johnson GR, Shabetai R, et al., for the V-HeFT VA Cooperative Studies Group. Ejection fraction, peak exercise oxygen consumption, cardiothoracic ratio, ventricular arrhythmias, and plasma norepinephrine as determinants of prognosis in heart failure. Circulation 1993;87(Suppl VI):VI-5–VI-16.
20. Cohn JN. Structural basis for heart failure: ventricular remodeling and its pharmacological inhibition. Circulation 1995;91:2504–2507.
21. Cintron C, Johnson G, Francis G, et al. Prognostic significance of serial changes in left ventricular ejection fraction in patients with congestive heart failure. Circulation 1993;87(Suppl VI):17–23.
22. Francis GS, Goldsmith SR, Levine TB, et al. The neurohumoral axis in congestive heart failure. Ann Intern Med 1984;101:370.
23. Dzau VJ. Renal and circulatory mechanisms in congestive heart failure. Kidney Int 1987;31:1402.
24. Aggarwal A, Esler MD, Socratous F, et al. Evidence for functional presynaptic alpha-2 adrenoceptors and their downregulation in human heart failure. J Am Coll Cardiol 2001;37:1246.
25. Bristow MR. Beta-adrenergic receptor blockade in chronic heart failure. Circulation 2000;101:558–569.
26. Coats AJ. Heart failure 99: the MOXCON story. Int J Cardiol 1999;71:109–111.
27. Kaye DM, Lambert GW, Lefkovits J, et al. Neurochemical evidence of cardiac sympathetic activation and increased central nervous system norepinephrine turnover in severe congestive heart failure. J Am Coll Cardiol 1994;23:570.
28. Mann D, Kent R, Parsons B, et al. Adrenergic effects on the biology of the adult mammalian cardiocyte. Circulation 1992;85:790–804.
29. Communal C, Singh K, Pimentel DR, et al. Norepinephrine stimulates apoptosis in adult rat ventricular myocytes by activation of the β-adrenergic pathway. Circulation 1998;98:1329.
30. Communal C, Singh K, Sawyer DB, et al. Opposing effects of β_1- and β_2-adrenergic receptors on cardiac myocyte apoptosis: role of a pertussis-toxin sensitive G protein. Circulation 1999;100:2210–2212.
31. Bisognano JD, Weinberger HD, Bohlmeyer TJ, et al. Myocardial-directed

overexpression of the human β_1-adrenergic receptor in transgenic mice. J Mol Cell Cardiol 2000;32:817–830.
32. Mizuno Y, Yoshimura M, Yasue H, et al. Aldosterone production is activated in failing ventricle in humans. Circulation (Online) 2001;103:72.
33. Lerman A, Gibbons RJ, Rodeheffer RJ, et al. Circulating N terminal atrial natriuretic peptide as an indicator marker for symptomless left ventricular dysfunction. Lancet 1993;341:1105.
34. Motwani JG, McAlpine H, Kennedy N, et al. Plasma brain natriuretic peptide as an indicator for angiotensin-converting enzyme inhibition after myocardial infarction. Lancet 1993;341:1109.
35. Schunkert H, Ingelfinger JR, Hirsch AT, et al. Evidence for tissue specific activation of renal angiotensinogen mRNA expression in chronic stable experimental heart failure. J Clin Invest 1992;90:1523.
36. Nagata, S. Apoptosis by death factor. Cell 1997;88:355.
37. Lee MA, Bohm M, Paul M. Tissue renin-angiotensin systems: their role in cardiovascular disease. Circulation 1993;87:IV7.
38. Wu CF, Bishopric NH, Pratt RE. Atrial natriuretic peptide induces apoptosis in neonatal rat cardiac myocytes. J Biol Chem 1997;272:14860.
39. Levine B, Kalman J, Mayer L, et al. Elevated circulating levels of tumor necrosis factor in severe chronic heart failure. N Engl J Med 1990;323(4):236–241.
40. Torre-Amione G, Kapadia S, Lee J, et al. Tumor necrosis factor alpha and tumor necrosis factor receptors in the failing human heart. Circulation 1996;93(4):704–711.
41. Bozkurt B, Kribbs SB, Clubb FJ, et al. Pathophysiologically relevant concentrations of tumor necrosis factor-alpha promote progressive left ventricular dysfunction and remodeling in rats. Circulation 1998;97(14):1382–1391.
42. Kubota T, McTieman CF, Frye CS, et al. Dilated cardiomyopathy in transgenic mice with cardiac-specific overexpression of tumor necrosis factor alpha. Circ Res 1997;81(4):627–635.
43. Krown KA, Paige MT, Nguyen C, et al. Tumor necrosis factor alpha-induced apoptosis in cardiac myocytes: involvement of the sphingolipid signaling cascade in cardiac cell death. J Clin Invest 1996;29(6):1214–1220.
44. Kurrelmeyer KM, Michael LH, Baumgarten G, et al. Endogenous tumor necrosis factor protects the adult cardiac myocyte against ischemic-induced apoptosis in a murine model of acute myocardial infarction. Proc Natl Acad Sci USA 2000;97(10):5456–5461.
45. Yanagisawa M, Kurihara H, Kimura S, et al. A novel potent vasoconstrictor peptide produced by vascular endothelial cells. Nature 1988;332:411.
46. Kirchengast M, Munter K. Endothelin-1 and endothelin receptor antagonists in cardiovascular remodeling (review). Proc Soc Exp Biol Med 1999;312:325.
47. Wada A, Tsutamoto T, Fukai D, et al. Comparison of the effects of selective endothelin ET_A and ET_B receptor antagonists in congestive heart failure. J Am Coll Cardiol 1997;30:1385.
48. Kiowski W, Sutsch G, Hunziker P, et al. Evidence for endothelin-1-mediated vasoconstriction in severe chronic heart failure. Lancet 1995;346:732.
49. Ponicke K, Vogelsang M, Heinroth M, et al. Endothelin receptors in the failing and nonfailing human heart. Circulation 1998;97:744.
50. Asano K, Zisman LS, Bohlmeyer TJ, et al. Upregulated endothelin ET, and downregulated ET, receptors in the failing human heart. Circulation 1998;98(Suppl I):420.

51. Schmetterer L, Dallinger S, Bobr B, et al. Systemic and renal effects on an ET(A) receptor subtype-specific antagonist in healthy subjects. Br J Pharmacol 1998;124(5):930–934.
52. Renal tubular effects of endothelin-B receptor signaling: its role in cardiovascular homeostasis and extracellular volume regulation (review). Curr Opin Nephrol Hyperten 2000;9(4):435–439.
53. Sakai S, Miyauchi T, Sakurai T, et al. Endogenous endothelin-1 participates in the maintenance of cardiac function in rats with congestive heart failure: marked increase in endothelin-1 production in the failing heart. Circulation 1996; 93:1214.
54. Cannan CR, Burnett JC, Lerman A. Enhanced coronary vasoconstriction to endothelin-B-receptor activation in experimental congestive heart failure. Circulation 1996;93:646.
55. Pousset F, Isnard R, Lechatt P, et al. Prognostic value of plasma endothelin-1 in patients with chronic heart failure. Eur Heart J 1997;18:254.
56. Kramer BK, Smith TW, Kelly RA. Endothelin and increased contractility in adult rat ventricular myocytes. Circ Res 1991;68:269.
57. Mulder P, Richard V, Derumeaux G, et al. Role of endogenous endothelin in chronic heart failure: effect of long-term treatment with an endothelin antagonist on survival, hemodynamics, and cardiac remodeling. Circulation 1997;96:1976.
58. Fraccarollo D, Hu K, Galuppo P, et al. Chronic endothelin receptor blockade attenuates progressive ventricular dilatation and improves cardiac function in rats with myocardial infarction: possible involvement of myocardial endothelin system in ventricular remodeling. Circulation 1997;96:3963.
59. Spinale FG, Walker JD, Mukherjee R, et al. Concomitant endothelin receptor subtype-A blockade during the progession of pacing-induced congestive heart failure in rabbits: beneficial effects on left ventricular and myocyte function. Circulation 1997;95:1918.
60. Arber S, Hunter JJ, Ross J Jr, et al. MLP-deficient mice exhibit a disruption of cardiac cytoarchitectural organization, dilated cardiomyopathy, and heart failure. Cell 1997;88(3):393–403.
61. Freeman K, Lerman I, Kranias EG, et al. Alterations in cardiac adrenergic signaling and calcium cycling differentially affect the progression of cardiomyopathy. J Clin Invest 2001;107:967–974.
62. Abraham W. Rationale and design of a randomized clinical trial to assess the safety and efficacy of cardiac resynchronization therapy in patients with advanced heart failure: the Multicenter InSync Randomized Clinical Evaluation (MIRACLE). J Card Fail 2000;6(4):369–380.
63. Garg R, Gorlin R, Smith T, et al. The effect of digoxin on mortality and morbidity in patients with heart failure. The Digitalis Investigation Group. N Engl J Med 1997;336(8):525–533.
64. Teerlink JR, Jalauddin M, Anderson S, et al. Ambulatory ventricular arrhythmias in patients with heart failure do not specifically predict an increased risk of sudden death. PROMISE (Prospective Randomized Milrinone Survival Evaluation) investigators. Circulation 2000;101(1):40–46.
65. Cohn J, Goldstein S, Greenber B, et al. A dose-dependent increase in mortality with vesnarinone among patients with severe heart failure. Vesnarinone Trial Investigators. N Engl J Med 1998;339(25):1810–1816.
66. Shakar SF, Abraham WT, Gilbert EM, et al. Combined oral positive inotropic and beta-blocker therapy for the treatment of refractory Class IV heart failure. J Am Coll Cardiol 1998;31:1336–1340.

67. The CONSENSUS Trial Study Group. Effects of enalapril on mortality in severe congestive heart failure: results of the Cooperative North Scandinavian Enalapril Survival Study (CONSENSUS). N Engl J Med 1987;316:429–435.
68. The SOLVD Investigators. Effect of enalapril on survival in patients with reduced left ventricular ejection fractions and congestive heart failure. N Engl J Med 1991;325:293–302.
69. The SOLVD Investigators. Effect of enalapril on mortality and the development of heart failure in asymptomatic patients with reduced left ventricular ejection fractions. N Engl J Med 1992;327:685–691.
70. Pfeffer MA, Braunwald E, Moye LA, et al. Effect of captopril on mortality and morbidity in patients with left ventricular dysfunction after myocardial infarction: results of the survival and ventricular enlargement trial. The SAVE Investigators. N Engl J Med 1992;327:669–677.
71. The Acute Infarction Ramipril Efficacy (AIRE) Study Investigators. Effect of ramipril on mortality and morbidity of survivors of acute myocardial infarction with clinical evidence of heart failure. Lancet 1993;342:821–828.
72. Kober L, Torp-Pedersen C, Carlsen JE, et al. A clinical trial of the angiotensin-converting-enzyme inhibitor trandolapril in patients with left ventricular dysfunction after myocardial infarction. Trandolapril Cardiac Evaluation (TRACE) Study Group. N Engl J Med 1995;333:1670–1676.
73. Packer M, Coats AJ, Fowler MB, et al. Effect of carvedilol on survival in severe chronic heart failure. N Engl J Med 2001;344:1651–1658.
74. Dargie, HJ. Effect of carvediolol on outcome after myocardial infarction in patients with left ventricular dysfunction. The CAPRICORN randomised trial. Lancet 2001;357(9266):1385–1390.
75. Greenberg B, Quinones MA, Koilpillai C, et al. Effects of long-term therapy on cardiac structure and function in patients with left ventricular dysfunction: results of the SOLVD echocardiography substudy. Circulation 1995;91:2573–2581.

II

Pathophysiology, Clinical, and Laboratory Evidence of Oxidative Stress in Heart Failure

• 3 •

Chemistry of Free Radicals in Biological Systems

Jay L. Zweier, MD, and
Frederick A. Villamena, PhD

Introduction

Over the last two decades, it has become clear that free radicals are critical mediators of cardiovascular function and disease. A large body of literature has accumulated, demonstrating that oxygen free radicals (OFRs) and reactive oxygen species (ROS) are key mediators of heart damage in acute myocardial infarction and are of particular importance in ischemia-reperfusion injury. It has also been reported that these oxidants are important mediators of cardiomyopathy and heart failure. For all major etiologies of heart failure including postischemic, hypertensive, alcohol-induced, postviral, autoimmune, and adriamycin-induced, OFRs have been invoked as critical mediators. OFRs are also of importance in the etiology of arteriosclerosis as well as in the process of acute plaque rupture. In recent years, there has also been increasing evidence that free radicals have a critical role in the pathogenesis of hypertension and vascular dysfunction.

In biological tissues, OFRs and ROS are formed by a variety of specific molecular and cellular mechanisms. These pathways are activated under a variety of disease conditions. Figure 1 shows a general view, depicting the common pathways of OFR generation, and how these radicals are transformed from one species to another or detoxified by antioxidant enzymes. As shown, failure to eliminate these active species leads to cellular injury.

From: Kukin ML, Fuster V (eds). *Oxidative Stress and Cardiac Failure.* Armonk, NY: Futura Publishing Co., Inc. ©2003.

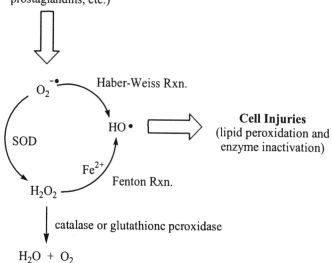

Radical Sources
(xanthine oxidase, mitochondrial respiration,
nuetrophils and macrophages, catecholamine oxidation,
prostaglandins, etc.)

Figure 1. Summary of the pathways of superoxide and hydroxyl radical production and their enzymatic degradation.

Chemistry of Free Radicals

Free radicals or simply radicals are species that contain one or more unpaired electrons that could be in the form of neutral molecules (e.g., $NO\cdot$, $HO\cdot$), ions ($O_2^-\cdot$, $GSSG^-\cdot$), or atoms ($Cl\cdot$, $H\cdot$). Free radicals were studied as important intermediates in gas phase reactions in the 1920s, or as intermediates in some organic reactions in the 1930s.[1] By the 1940s, the development of electron paramagnetic resonance (EPR) spectroscopy paved the way for the direct measurement and characterization of these reactive species.[1]

With the rapid advancement in this and the related technologies of radical detection and radical trapping during the past 20 years, the role of free radicals in physiological and pathological processes has been extensively studied.

Free radicals are thought to be important mediators of oncogenesis and tumor promotion,[2,3] inflammatory disease, lung damage in the adult respiratory distress syndrome,[4] renal damage in acute tubular necrosis, transplant rejection, drug-induced hepatic damage, and equally impor-

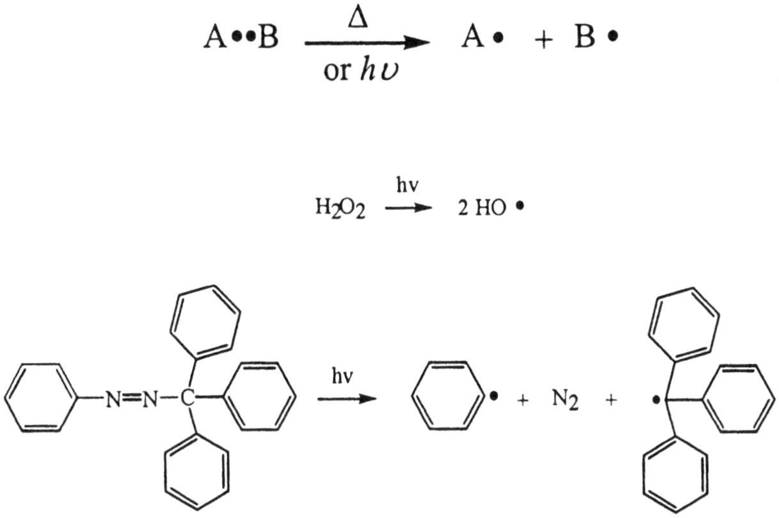

$$A \bullet\bullet B \xrightarrow[\text{or } h\upsilon]{\Delta} A \bullet + B \bullet$$

$$H_2O_2 \xrightarrow{h\nu} 2 \, HO \bullet$$

Scheme 1.

tant in ischemic and postischemic reperfusion cell damage.[5] Drugs such as Adriamycin produce myocardial damage through the generation of free radicals.[6–8] As discussed below, there is an ever-increasing body of evidence that demonstrates the role of free radicals during ischemic and postischemic reperfusion damage in the heart.[9–11] In addition, over

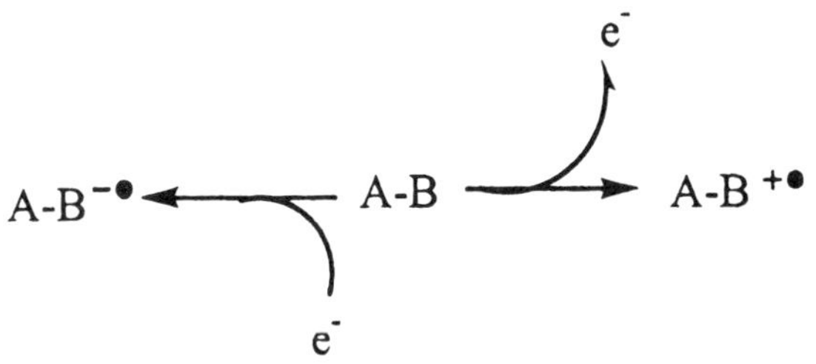

$$2H_2O \longrightarrow H_2O^{+\bullet} + e^- + H_2O^*$$

$$H_2O^* \longrightarrow H\bullet + HO\bullet$$

$$H_2O^{+\bullet} + H_2O \longrightarrow H_3O^+ + HO \bullet$$

Scheme 2.

$$O_2^{-}\bullet \; + \; Fe^{3+} \; \rightarrow \; O_2 \; + \; Fe^{2+}$$
$$H_2O_2 \; + \; Fe^{2+} \; \rightarrow \; HO\bullet \; + \; HO^{-} \; + \; Fe^{3+}$$

net reaction: $O_2^{-}\bullet \; + \; H_2O_2 \; \rightarrow \; HO\bullet \; + \; HO^{-} \; + \; O_2$

Scheme 3.

the last several years, it has been reported that free radicals have a critical role in the pathogenesis of arteriosclerosis, hypertension, and heart failure.

Radicals can be generated through homolytic cleavage of a covalent bond either by thermolysis or photolysis (Scheme 1). Examples are the generation of the hydroxyl radical, $HO\bullet$, from H_2O_2, or phenyl ($Ph\bullet$) and trityl ($Ph_3C\bullet$) radicals from phenylazotriphenylmethane (PAT) in the presence of ultraviolet (UV) light or heat in the case of PAT.

Radicals can also be generated by ionizing radiation that causes loss or capture of an electron. In the case of pulse radiolysis (Scheme 2), use of high-energy radiation such as gamma rays can yield the excited state water molecule H_2O^{*} that can subsequently decompose to $HO\bullet$ and radical cations $H_2O^{-}\bullet$. This radical cation was also found to generate $HO\bullet$.[12]

The $HO\bullet$ radical is one of the most reactive free radicals produced in biological systems with rate constants ranging from 10^7 to 10^{11} $M^{-1} s^{-1}$ at biological pH and rates of reaction with most organic compounds approaching the diffusion limit.[13] In biological systems, the hydroxyl radical is typically generated by reaction of superoxide, $O_2^{-}\bullet$, and hydrogen peroxide, H_2O_2, catalyzed by transition metals such as Fe^{3+} or Cu^{2+} (Scheme 3). This reaction is usually referred to as the superoxide-driven

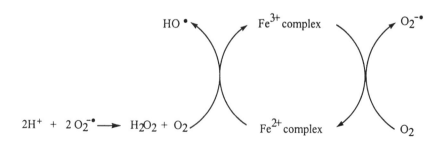

Figure 2. A superoxide-driven Fenton reaction as an iron cycle.

$$O_2 \xrightarrow{\text{1e-}} O_2^{-\bullet} \xrightarrow{\text{1e-}} H_2O_2 \xrightarrow{\text{1e-}} HO\bullet \xrightarrow{\text{1e-}} H_2O$$

Scheme 4.

Fenton reaction or the iron-catalyzed Haber-Weiss reaction. It can be visualized as a simple iron redox cycle as shown in Figure 2. Iron is ubiquitous in biological systems, and low molecular weight chelates, hematin, or protein-bound iron such as hemoglobin, myoglobin, or ferritin can potentially catalyze the formation of $HO\bullet$.[14,15]

In normal oxidative phosphorylation involving cytochrome oxidase catalysis, O_2 is reduced by four electrons to form H_2O. Energy is produced from this process and serves the energy demand of the cell. Incomplete 1-, 2-, and 3-electron reduction of O_2 lead to the generation of reactive oxygen species (Scheme 4).

Radical stability depends on the extent of delocalization of the unpaired electron within the molecule. For example, nitroxides $R_2NO\bullet$ (Figure 3) or trityl radicals $Ph_3C\bullet$ are relatively stable with half-lives ranging from minutes to hours while most other radicals such as the oxygen-derived superoxide and hydroxyl radicals are short-lived with half-lives of only nanoseconds to milliseconds.

Oxygen-centered radicals are difficult to detect unless they are trapped to form more stable adducts such as nitroxides. The stability of nitroxides is due to the delocalization of the unpaired electron between the nitrogen and oxygen atoms. The strong 3-electron N-O bond has high delocalization energy (ca. 32 kcal/mol) that contributes to its thermodynamic stability. It should be noted, however, that persistent radicals are not necessarily stable.

Radical trapping, commonly termed spin trapping, is the most conventional method for detecting most carbon, sulfur, or oxygen-centered radicals. Nitrones are a class of compounds that have an ability to react with radicals to form more stable and persistent radicals called nitroxides or spin adducts (Figure 4). These radicals are stable enough to be detected

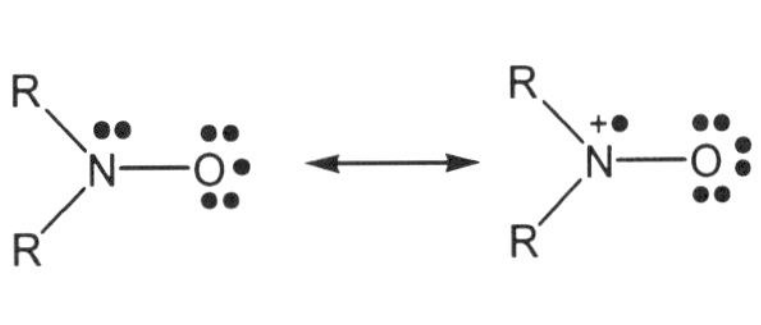

Figure 3. Resonance structure of a nitroxyl group.

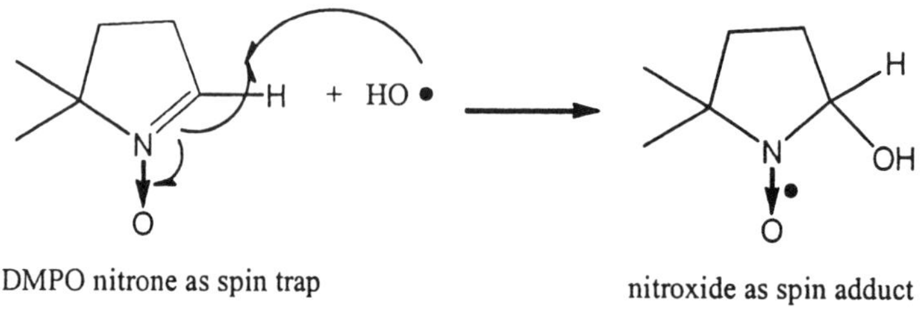

DMPO nitrone as spin trap   nitroxide as spin adduct

Figure 4. Hydroxyl radical trapping by DMPO giving a hydroxyl spin adduct.

by EPR, thus providing a wealth of information into the nature of radicals generated in biological samples. The most commonly used nitrone is PBN or DMPO, while improved more stable nitrones such as DEPMPO[16] and BMPO[17] now are also utilized.

Sites and Mechanisms of Radical Generation in Disease

Radicals and active oxygen species derived from molecular oxygen (superoxide, hydrogen peroxide, and hydroxyl radical) are of critical importance in a broad range of cardiovascular diseases. These oxidants were first intensively studied and their role characterized in the pathogenesis of the tissue injury that accompanies myocardial ischemia and reperfusion, although in recent years much effort has also focused on their role in a variety of cardiovascular diseases from hypertension to atherosclerosis. In this context, several pathways of radical generation have been identified. These include the enzyme xanthine oxidase (XO) primarily within endothelial cells, radical leakage from mitochondrial respiratory chain primarily from myocytes, nicotinamide adenine dinucleotide phosphate (NADPH) oxidase from neutrophils and macrophages, a vascular NAD(P)H oxidase, as well as from byproducts of arachidonic acid metabolism, and oxidation of catecholamines.[18] Most recently it has also been shown that nitric oxide synthase (NOS) is also a source of oxygen radicals, with this process modulated by the levels of the substrate l-arginine or the cofactor tetrahydrobiopterin.[19,20]

Xanthine Oxidase

It was first proposed by McCord et al.[21–23] that the primary source of superoxide in reperfused reoxygenated tissues is the enzyme XO. The mechanism of radical generation as initially proposed for the feline intestine[24] depends on the conversion of the native enzyme xanthine dehydrogenase to XO released during ischemia by a calcium-triggered proteolytic attack on xanthine dehydrogenase. The XO formed catalyzes the reaction of xanthine or hypoxanthine and O_2 (Figure 5). During ischemia, ATP is metabolized to adenosine, which is converted to inosine by adenosine deaminase. Inosine further decomposes to hypoxanthine and upon reaction with O_2 via catalysis by XO, $O_2^-\cdot$, xanthine, urate, and H_2O_2 are produced. This reaction occurs at only a very low rate when O_2[20] is not abundant. Once O_2 is introduced in large quantities during reperfusion, the reaction is greatly accelerated. It has also been shown[25] that XO can also generate $HO\cdot$ radical particularly under hypoxic conditions via the further reduction of its product H_2O_2.

The burst of XO-mediated free radical generation in the postischemic heart is triggered by a large increase in substrate formation, specifically

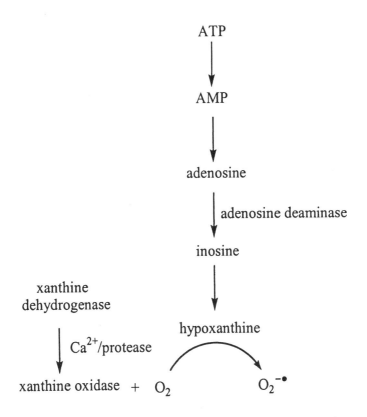

Figure 5. Xanthine oxidase as a mechanism of radical generation.

xanthine and hypoxanthine, whose formation occurs secondary to the degradation of adenine nucleotides during ischemia. However, this XO substrate formation could be blocked by inhibiting adenosine deaminase or blocking nucleotide transport (NT) from the myocytes to endothelium. Experiments were performed on isolated rat hearts where substrate formation was blocked with the adenosine deaminase inhibitor erythro-9-(2-hydroxy-3-nonyl)adenine (EHNA). Chromatographic measurements of the intracellular adenine nucleotide pool showed that preischemic administration of EHNA blocked postischemic hypoxanthine, xanthine, and inosine formation, while electron paramagnetic resonance spin trapping measurements of radicals generated showed that inhibition of adenosine deaminase with EHNA blocked the free radical generation pathway and that it also increased the recovery of contractile function by more than 2-fold. Exogenous infusion of hypoxanthine and xanthine totally reversed the protective effects of EHNA. These results demonstrated that blockade of XO substrate formation by adenosine deaminase inhibition can prevent free radical generation and contractile dysfunction in the postischemic heart.[26]

Xanthine oxidase has been observed in a variety of ischemic tissue homogenates, while the presence and importance of radical generation by the enzyme in intact tissues have also been investigated.[27,28] It has been demonstrated to be a major source of oxidative injury in the reperfused rat heart. The oxidase content in the heart muscle doubles from 10% to 20% of the total in about 8 minutes following coronary occlusion.[21] This enzyme conversion is believed to be activated by a Ca^{2+} protease. Evidence shows that cytosolic Ca^{2+} concentration increases rapidly during severe ischemia and that this process occurs on the same time scale as the conversion of xanthine dehydrogenase to XO. Proteases have been implicated by the fact that oxidase formation is irreversible, and its activity is dependent on Ca^{2+} influx to the cell. It was also suggested that cytosolic Ca^{2+} influx is provoked by xanthine/XO and is responsible for $HO\cdot$-mediated cytotoxicity.[29]

In spite of the relatively low amounts of xanthine dehydrogenase/oxidase present in human and rabbit muscles, free radical scavenging still appears beneficial as particularly demonstrated in rabbits. One alternative explanation is that radicals may have been generated through another mechanism but a more plausible explanation is that radical production may be most injurious in vascular endothelial cells that have a relatively high concentration of the enzyme. Spin trapping and EPR spectroscopy show that prominent oxygen radical production occurs in endothelial cells. The observed EPR signal is quenched by superoxide dismutase (SOD) or catalase, and XO blocker oxypurinol decreases radical generation by 60%. This further explains the effectiveness of exogenously administering radical scavengers such as SOD, considering its high molecular weight and low membrane permeability. Endothelial cell free radical generation may be a central mechanism of cellular injury in postischemic tissues.[30,31] Furthermore, these cells have interrelationship with other radical-producing mechanisms and/or cell injury.[32–34]

Mitochondrial Respiratory Chain

Mitochondria isolated from myocardium can be observed to form $O_2^-\cdot$ as perhaps a product from a side reaction that is believed to be a leakage in the complex electron transport activities within the inner mitochondrial membrane.[35–38] In view of the high concentration of mitochondria in cardiac muscle, it is particularly important to understand the contribution of mitochondrial respiration to radical generation. It is estimated that under normal conditions, 1–2% of oxygen consumed by mitochondria are converted to superoxide.[39] This "leak" of radical generation can be inactivated by endogenous scavenging mechanisms present within the cell,[40] while radical generation can be enhanced in vitro when mitochondrial respiration is stimulated by altered redox state and decreased availability of ADP.[41–46] Furthermore, radical generation from mitochondria would be expected to increase under conditions of hyperoxia and hyperbaric oxygen exposure as well following postischemic reperfusion. In fact, H_2O_2 production has been shown to be increased under hyperoxic conditions.[47,48] In addition, decreased activity of radical scavenging enzymes can greatly alter the delicate balance between radical generation and detoxification.[49] Although most of the radical generation reported occurs in the mitochondrial matrix, the outer mitochondrial membrane is known to be a large source of H_2O_2 through catalytic oxidative deamination of primary aromatic amines along with other long chain diamines and cyclic tertiary amines by monoamine oxidase.[50] The H_2O_2 produced could further decompose to $HO\cdot$. This could be involved in neurodegenerative diseases such as Parkinson's and Alzheimer's diseases by oxidative damage to mitochondrial membrane.

Studies of isolated mitochondria show that 1-electron reduction of O_2 occurs with the production of $O_2^-\cdot$ and subsequently H_2O_2. The major sources of this radical generation within the mitochondria have been identified to be the NADH dehydrogenase and ubiquinone. Figure 6 shows the ubiquinone cycle in which ubiquinone (Q) reduces cytochrome *b* through multiple processes that also lead to the oxidation of NADH dehydrogenase. The cycle is coupled to the electron transfer process that occurs between ubiquinol (QH_2) and cytochrome *c1* via proteins containing Fe-S clusters. At the site of this electron transfer process, an electron is "leaked" to the O_2 molecule to give $O_2^-\cdot$ then subsequently H_2O_2. Amytal and KCN can be employed as blockers for NADH dehydrogenase

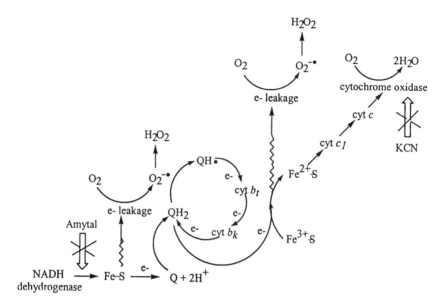

Figure 6. Schematic representation of the mitochondrial respiratory chain and the sources of oxygen radical formation.

and cytochrome oxidase, respectively. Studies of heart and nonsynaptic brain mitochondria of mammals and birds show that oxygen radicals are generated at complex I in heart and brain mitochondria in States 4 and 3, while complex III (ubiquinone cytochrome c reductase) generates radicals only in heart mitochondria and only in State 4.[51]

NADPH Oxidase- and Leukocyte-Derived Radicals

Leukocytes, including neutrophils, other granulocytes, and macrophages, are known to have bacterial killing properties due to their ability to generate oxygen radicals.[52–61] The antibacterial character of activated leukocytes has been viewed as one of the benefits arising from free-radical generation. Leukocyte activation leads to assembly of membrane and cytosolic subunits of the NADPH oxidase with oxidation of O_2 to $O_2^- \cdot$ and H_2O_2 (Figure 7). Release of these oxidants into the extracellular milieu leads to oxidative damage of neighboring leukocytes and may lead to a chain reaction causing activation of the rest of these cells.

Other important sources of reactive oxygen species in granulocytes and phagocytes include the myeloperoxidase (MPO)-H_2O_2-halogen system that is also triggered by leukocyte stimulation.

There are a large number of chemical mediators that act as "activa-

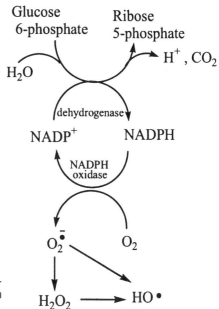

Figure 7. Radical production from NADPH-dependent electron transport chain in phagocytes.

tors" of the neutrophil functions, including radical production, adhesion, and chemotaxis. The most extensively studied activators of neutrophils include leukotriene B_4, chemotactic factors, and phorbol esters,[62] all acting via a pathway involving protein kinase C, and mechanical disturbance of cell membrane. Adhesion of neutrophils to vascular endothelium could be enhanced during ischemia and/or inflammatory conditions by hypercarbic acidosis (20% CO_2) despite a decrease in intercellular adhesion molecule-1 (ICAM-1) expression.[63] Adhesion of neutrophils also may be regulated by endothelial cytosolic free Ca^{2+}.[29] Endothelial intracellular Ca^{2+} stores are released upon initial contact leading to subsequent adhesion of human leukocytes to human aortic endothelial cells. This may be mediated by specific adhesion proteins and in turn may regulate the affinity of surface adhesion molecules or facilitate transendothelial migration of leukocytes.[64]

It has been demonstrated that oxidants such as hydrogen peroxide (H_2O_2) and superoxide (O_2^-·) from endothelial sources could trigger further injury due to subsequent leukocyte adhesion and adhesion molecule expression during reperfusion of ischemic tissues. EPR spin trapping measurements demonstrated that the antioxidative actions of both SOD and catalase could decrease PMN adhesion and CD18 expression, resulting in marked suppression of PMN-mediated injury in the postischemic heart. Thus, endothelial-derived H_2O_2 and O_2^-· further amplify postischemic injury by triggering CD18 expression on the surface of PMNs, leading to increased PMN adhesion within the heart.[65] In a similar study,[66] O_2^-·, HO·, and H_2O_2 oxidants could modulate the expression of leukocyte adhesion molecules such as integrins and selectins on the surface of human PMNs, thereby triggering PMN activation. Plasma factors, from the complement cascade, are also reported to be required for neutrophil activation,[67] and certain PMN inhibitors such as the soluble complement receptor type 1 (sCR1) have been found to be effective in preventing postischemic myocardial contractile dysfunction and enhancing the recovery of coronary flow.

Inflammatory cells are present in the myocardium in many human disease states. Neutrophils are drawn to the interface of the ischemic zone and throughout reperfused heart muscle. Complement factors[57] as well as leukotrienes appear to be responsible for attracting leukocytes during ischemia. Inhibitors of the lipoxygenase pathway of arachidonic acid metabolism[68,69] appear strikingly effective in reducing both the leukocyte content of ischemic and reperfused myocardium and the extent of myocardial necrosis. In fact, the stimulus to production of free radicals by leukocytes can be provided by a brief period of exposure to anoxia followed by reoxygenation, as shown in cell suspensions.[70,71] With periods of myocardial ischemia of 60–90 minutes in the dog, the localization of neutrophils is principally intravascular, resulting in intense interaction between the vascular endothelium of small arterioles, capillaries, and venules, and adherent white cells. When reperfusion is carried out after 60–90 minutes of ischemia, neutrophils in both the intravascular and the extravascular compartments are activated and free radicals are generated at both sides. Thus, during postischemic reperfusion, adhesion of white cells to the endothelium with resultant capillary plugging may play a major role in their accumulation, which could result in microvascular injury and the no-flow phenomenon.

Over the last decade, it has also become clear that there is a nonleukocyte NAD(P)H oxidase that is of critical importance in the regulation of vascular tone and function. While this was initially thought to be identical to the leukocyte oxidase, there is increasing evidence that the vascular oxidase is a unique enzyme or enzymes distinct from leukocyte oxidase.[72,73]

Arachidonic Acid Metabolism

Arachidonic acid conversion to its metabolites, which include prostaglandins, thromboxane, prostacyclin, and leukotrienes, can mediate several important cellular processes such as chemotaxis, inflammation, and muscle tone. However, this metabolite formation concurrently generates ROS that can lead to various types of oxidative damage such as DNA

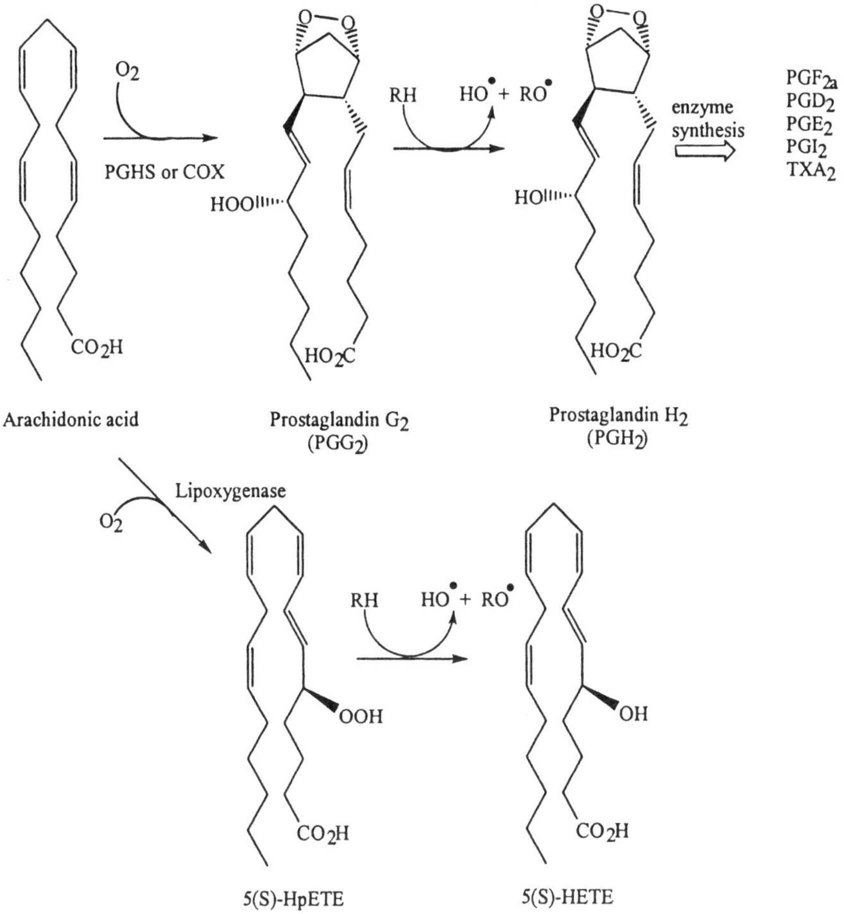

Figure 8. Radical generation from the COX and LPO pathways of arachidonic acid metabolism.

breakage or lipid oxidation. Two common arachidonic metabolism pathways involve oxidative catalysis by the enzymes, cyclooxygenase (COX), also known as prostaglandin synthase (PGHS), and lipoxygenase (LPO). COX and LPO pathways give products PGG_2 and HpETEs, respectively (see Figure 8). These hydroperoxides are relatively unstable and are reduced to PGH_2 and HETEs by the same enzymes in a typical peroxidase reaction in which radicals are known to be also generated as byproducts. These two-step reactions are similar for both known isoforms of COX, COX-1, and COX-2. Recent studies showed that oxygen radical-induced genetic damage may be mediated by products of lipid peroxidation, in particular, arachidonic acid. HETEs are found to be more potent in DNA breakage than HPTEs.[74] Chronic exposure to linoleic acid and arachidonic acid could induce genetic damage through oxygen radical production.[75]

A wide variety of stimuli lead to the increased synthesis of prostaglandins and leukotrienes from arachidonic acid.[55,76–79] It has been proposed that $O_2^-\cdot$ generation comes from the LPO pathway and not the COX pathway and is linked to the glutathione cycle.[80] Hydroxyl radicals can stimulate arachidonic acid metabolite PGF_2 formation, which indicates that the mechanism of metabolite formation is mediated by $HO\cdot$.[81] In contrast, results from epidermal 12-lipoxygenase inhibition by ROS show that ROS such as H_2O_2, $O_2^-\cdot$, and $HO\cdot$ radicals can inhibit enzyme activity.[82] Whether the radicals produced from the conversion of PGG_2 to PGH_2 are direct byproducts of the reaction itself or result from the reaction of the hydroperoxidase with one of a variety of other substrates initially stimulated by increased cyclooxygenase activity is still unclear. In a number of in vitro studies, cellular and subcellular injury that can be inhibited by free radicals has been documented to result from this metabolic source. Thus, free radical byproducts resulting from enhanced prostaglandin and leukotriene synthesis may play an important role in the radical production.

Catecholamine Oxidation and Synthesis

Catecholamines are ring compounds containing two OH groups and an amino group. They can be oxidized to $O_2^-\cdot$ and H_2O_2 to form semi-

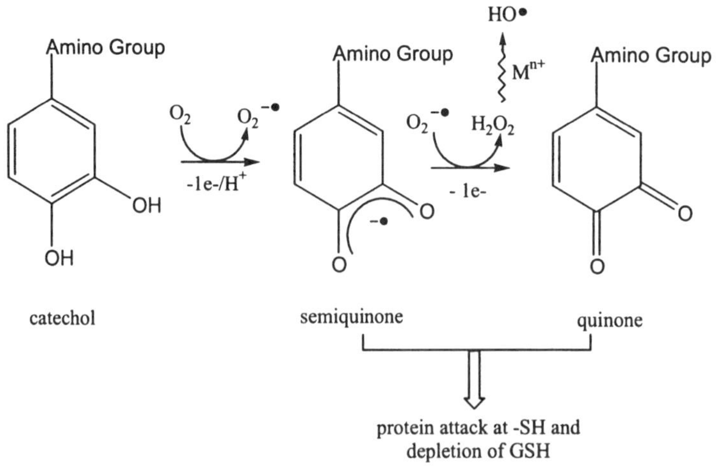

Figure 9. Radical generation from oxidation of catecholamine.

quinones and quinones. One example is the oxidation of the neurotransmitter dopamine to l-dopa that also produces $O_2^- \cdot$ and H_2O_2. The presence of transition metals, or Fe-proteins/hemes, can catalyze the formation $HO\cdot$ (Figure 9).

Administration of catecholamines in both animals and humans is known to induce patchy myocardial necrosis similar to that observed in reperfusion following ischemia. It has been proposed by Dhalla and coworkers[83] that this catecholamine-induced myocardial injury could be a direct cause of oxygen-derived radicals as evidenced by a significant reduction of such types of injuries when free radical scavengers are introduced.[84]

The burst of norepinephrine during ischemia can lead to progression of cell injury.[85,86] Excessive accumulation of norepinephrine occurs during the early stages of ischemia. After complete ischemia in isolated rat hearts, the amount of norepinephrine becomes disproportionately larger than the epinephrine and dopamine. It has been suggested[87] that the release of norepinephrine involves two pathways: first, escaping from its intracellular storage vesicles and then accumulating in the cytoplasma of the neuron; and second, norepinephrine is transported across the plasma membrane. Formation of $HO\cdot$ [88] is induced by iron release from ferritin during ischemia and then subsequently reacting with XO. Moreover, catecholamine oxidation is more favored at lower pH accompanied by release of Fe^{2+} to the cytosol. Catecholamine production is effectively inhibited by the amine-uptake-blocking agent, propranolol, which prevents catecholamine binding to receptors, thus providing protection from oxidative damage.

Nitric Oxide Synthase (NOS)

Endothelial cells produce an endothelium-derived relaxing factor (EDRF) which is a vascular muscle relaxant.[89,90] This EDRF was later identified as the free radical nitric oxide ($NO\cdot$),[91,92] a colorless gas with moderate solubility in water similar to O_2. Some of the important reactions of $NO\cdot$ are shown in Figure 10, depicting how reactive nitrogen species are formed. Contrary to popular belief, $NO\cdot$ is relatively unreactive and is neither a strong oxidant nor reductant. In fact, the reduction potential for $NO\cdot$ is about 0.39 V compared to $HO\cdot$ of 2.31 V. The enzyme nitric oxide synthase (NOS) synthesizes $NO\cdot$ [93,94] based on the following reaction[95]:

$$\text{L-Arg} + 2O_2 + 1.5\text{NADPH} + 2H^+ \rightarrow \text{L-citrulline} + NO\cdot + 2H_2O + 1.5\text{NADP}^+$$

There are three major types of mammalian NOS isoforms that exist and can catalyze $NO\cdot$ production: the neuronal NOS (nNOS, NOS1), inducible NOS (iNOS, NOS2), and endothelial NOS (eNOS, NOS3). All of

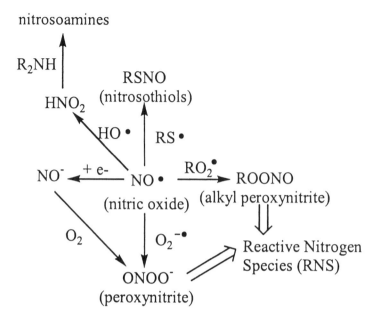

Figure 10. Chemical reactions of nitric oxide.

these isoforms catalyze NO• via the same two-step process because of similarities in their modular architecture. This mechanism was supported by Poulos et al.[96] with their crystallographic structure of the eNOS heme domain complexed with NO•. It should also be remembered that NO• also can be produced nonenzymatically through either direct disproportionation or reduction of nitrite to NO• under acidic and highly reduced conditions—conditions common during ischemia.[97,98]

Immunocytochemical studies have demonstrated the presence of NOS in the mitochondria.[99,100] Most enzymes that generate O_2^-• and its derivatives contain Fe-S clusters that can bind efficiently to NO•.[101,102] Evidence suggests that NO• can mediate Fe-S degradation and can result in protein nitrosation and formation of dinitrosyl-Fe(I) complex.[103,104] These metalloproteins have heme structures in both Fe^{3+} and Fe^{2+} states that can provide broad enzymatic specificity. This leads us to conclude that NO• can have an inhibitive effect on most mitochondrial metabolism that involves Fe redox reactions.

Nitric oxide is known to inhibit electron transfer and could increase superoxide production in mitochondria.[105] Respiratory rates and adenosine triphosphate (ATP) synthesis of intact mitochondria in State 4 can decrease by 40% in the presence of NO•-generating substrates. Competitive and reversible inhibition by NO• of cytochrome oxidase with O_2

does occur, suggesting the role of NO$\cdot$ as a modulator of cytochrome oxidase.[106,107] Catabolism of NO$\cdot$ by cytochrome c oxidase in submitochondrial particles yields NO_3^- and NO_2^- anions.[106,108] Perhaps one important role of NO is its ability to regulate oxygen uptake and hydrogen peroxide release. Results from isolated beating rat hearts suggest that NO$\cdot$ released by the endothelium not only exhibits coronary vasodilatation but also lowers O_2 uptake with increased $O_2^-\cdot$.[109]

Regulation of oxygen radical production by NO$\cdot$ is consistent with studies done on mitochondria showing the inverse proportionality of H_2O_2 production with respiratory rates.[105,110] The mechanism for this increased O_2 uptake involves redox reactions between NO$\cdot$ and ubiquinol and peroxynitrite formation.[111] Reversibility of NO$\cdot$ inhibition of mitochondrial components is dose-dependent, while peroxynitrite causes much of the irreversible damage and inhibition, particularly on complex I,[112] complex II, aconitase,[113] cytochrome c^{3+},[114] NADH,[115] creatine kinase, and ATP synthase.[107] It was also reported[116] that ONOO- from mitochondrial NOS could promote mitochondrial Ca^{2+} release by stimulation of thiol crosslinks and hydrolysis of NAD^+.

Nitric oxide can be trapped by metal coordinate complexes such as Fe^{2+}-N-methyl-D-glucamine dithiocarbamate (Fe-MGD), forming an adduct that is detectable by EPR.[117] EPR spectra of Fe proteins with bound NO$\cdot$ have also provided insights into the mechanistic aspects of NO$\cdot$ generation by NOS.[118] Recently developed EPR imaging techniques have allowed direct visualization of NO formation following the onset of ischemia and spatial mapping of its distribution in isolated hearts and in small animals.[119–122]

Molecular Mechanisms of Free Radical Injury

Oxygen radical reaction with biomolecules has been demonstrated to cause oxidative damage. Of particular importance is the oxidative modification caused by $\cdot$OH radicals on lipid membranes,[123,124] proteins,[50,125–127] and DNA.[50,126]

Polyunsaturated fatty acids are more susceptible to hydrogen abstraction than the polysaturated fatty acids due to the presence of allylic hydrogen (CH_2 groups that are next to a doubly bonded carbon). The mechanism for lipid peroxidation is shown in (Figure 11).

Hydroxyl radicals can initiate peroxidation by hydrogen atom abstraction at the allylic position of the fatty acid to form water and lipid alkyl radicals (L$\cdot$). The radical L$\cdot$ can react with molecular oxygen, forming the lipid peroxyl radical (L-OO$\cdot$). This L-OO$\cdot$ radical can abstract hydrogen from adjacent membrane lipid, thus achieving a propagation cycle in which the L$\cdot$ radicals are regenerated and in which lipid hydroperox-

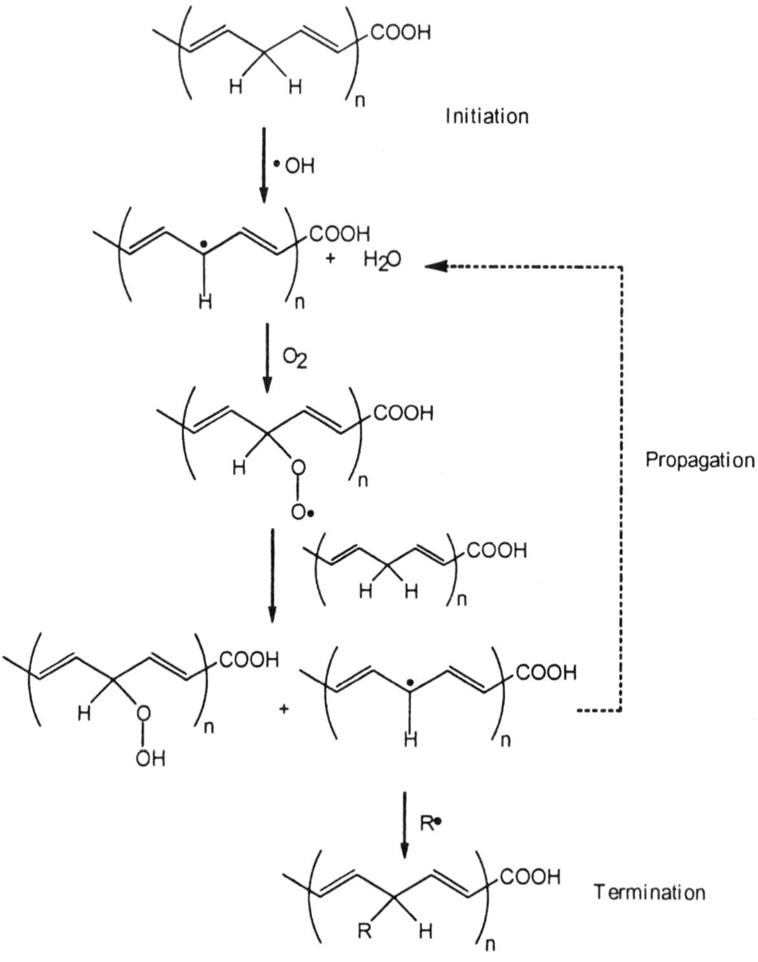

Figure 11. Mechanism of hydroxyl radical initiated lipid peroxidation.

ide (L-OOH) is formed. Lipid hydroperoxides decompose in the presence of certain Fe^{II} complexes to form alkoxy radicals (LO·) and subsequently to L-OO·, which could lead to a similar propagation mechanism for lipid peroxidation as mentioned above. Cyclic peroxides are also formed from L-OOH that upon further oxidation by O_2 and hydrolysis gives malondialdehyde (MDA) that is commonly used to measure the degree of oxygen radical-induced membrane peroxidation. Species such as L-OO· and LO· with sufficient reactivity for hydrogen abstraction can initiate lipid peroxidation, while O_2^-· and H_2O_2 do not.[123] However, O_2^-· and H_2O_2 can react via the Fenton reaction to generate $\cdot$OH, which in turn can initiate lipid peroxidation.

Oxidative stress and ROS can cause either inactivation or activation of enzymes. Damage to enzymes or proteins could occur via direct attack of the radical or by some indirect mechanism involving radicals generated as end-products from lipid peroxidation. Hydroxyl radical reaction with amino acid residues containing phenyl rings results in the formation of hydroxylated aromatic rings, or in the case of –SH groups that can be easily oxidized by H_2O_2 and $O_2^-\cdot$ to form disulfides. Since –SH groups for the most part support the native structure of proteins or their functions, enzymes rich in cysteine such as ribonuclease inhibitor or sulfhydryl repair enzymes such as thioltransferase/glutathione disulfide reductase[125] can significantly be affected by this oxidative modification. Nitric oxide inhibits cytochrome oxidase activity, which may be involved in physiological regulation of respiration rate in cellular systems,[107] while addition of peroxynitrites ($ONOO^-$) to isolated mitochondria results in oxidative damage to respiratory enzymes complexes I (NADH dehydrogenase) and III (cytochrome c reductase).[128]

The mutagenic and carcinogenic nature of ionizing radiation originates from the generation of HO$\cdot$ in cellular systems via homolysis of water. These radicals are also said to be responsible for several diseases and in the aging process.[129] The chemistry of DNA damage mostly occurs on the purine and pyrimidine bases, resulting in the formation of modified DNA bases structures[130] through oxidation or ring opening (Figure 12). The addition of HO$\cdot$ radical to guanine at C-8 yields 8-hydroxyguanine (8-OHdG) and is commonly used as a measure of oxidative DNA damage. 8-Hydroxyguanine could also be generated from peroxynitrite as demonstrated by Spencer et al.[131]

Radicals also react with the sugar moiety of DNA to yield a variety of degradation products resulting in eventual cleavage of the DNA strand. This process has been proposed to be the mechanism of action of the antineoplastic activity of Adriamycin and daunorubicin, both of which chelate iron and subsequently generate HO$\cdot$.[7,132] However, transfer of damage also can occur from a base to a sugar. Oxidative stress on mitochondrial DNA has been suggested to be higher than in nuclear DNA due to its proximity to the different radical-generating systems present in mitochon-

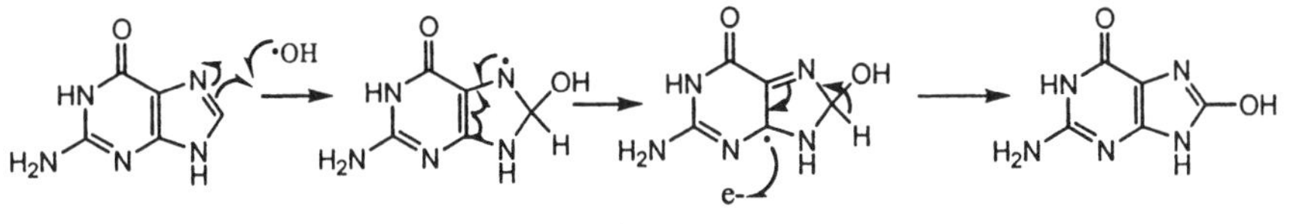

Figure 12. Chemistry of oxidative damage on guanine base.

drial membranes or electron transport chain complexes.[129] Benzoyl peroxide (BzPO) although not mutagenic has been observed to generate strand scissions in a cell-free system using phi X-174 plasmid DNA. These actions are presumed to be mediated by free radical derivatives of BzPO. Previous studies suggested that the metabolism of BzPO in keratinocytes proceeds via the initial cleavage of the peroxide bond, yielding benzoyloxy radicals, which in turn can either fragment to form phenyl radicals and carbon dioxide or abstract H atoms from biomolecules to yield benzoic acid.[133] There are several reactive oxygen species known to react with DNA bases (e.g., $ROO\cdot$, $RO\cdot$, $ONOO^-$, O_3), but there are few reported that are nonreactive (e.g., $O_2^-\cdot$ and H_2O_2).

Antioxidant, as a general term, applies to biomolecules or small molecules that significantly protect cells from potentially harmful effects of ROS when present in low concentration compared to the concentration of oxidizable substrates. Free radical scavenging is commonly used to describe antioxidants since they catalytically remove radicals. Most common among these scavengers are the enzymes superoxide dismutase (SOD),[134] catalase, and glutathione peroxidases.

SOD exists in two major forms: as a CuZnSOD (copper- and zinc-containing SOD) that is primarily present in cytosol while MnSOD (manganese-containing SOD) is located in the mitonchondria. There is also an FeSOD (iron-containing SOD) that has chemical similarities with MnSOD such as deactivation at high pH and resistance to CN^- inactivation. CuZnSOD catalyzes the dismutation of $O_2^-\cdot$ to yield H_2O_2 and O_2 with a rate constant of $2 \times 10^9\ M^{-1}\ s^{-1}$.[135] The overall dismutation reaction of metal SOD involves an alternate redox reaction (Scheme 5).

CuZnSOD (SOD1) is mostly located in the cytosol and in some species could exist in the lysosome, nucleus, and in mitochondrial intermembrane space, while MnSOD and FeSOD are both found in mitochondria and in *E. coli*. In addition to the cytosolic CuZnSOD, there is a distinct extracellular isoform, ECSOD, that associates with the outer surface of the endothelial plasma membrane.

Peroxisome, the hemeprotein catalase mostly located in subcellular organelles, contains ferric ion bound to each of four protein subunits, and acts in liaison with SOD in eliminating H_2O_2 generated either directly

$$M_a^n\text{-SOD} + O_2^-\cdot \rightarrow M_b^{(n-1)}\text{-SOD} + O_2$$
$$M_b^{(n-1)}\text{-SOD} + O_2^-\cdot + 2H^+ \rightarrow M_a^n\text{-SOD} + H_2O_2$$

net reaction:
$$2O_2^-\cdot + 2H^+ \rightarrow H_2O_2 + O_2$$
$$(\text{where } M_a/M_b = Cu^{2+}/Cu^{1+};\ Mn^{3+}/Mn^{2+};\ Fe^{3+}/Fe^{2+})$$

Scheme 5.

from 2 electron reduction of O_2 or the dismutation of $O_2^-\cdot$. The catalase reaction involves a two-step reaction in which Fe^{3+} reduces H_2O_2 to H_2O and formation of a compound whose structure is believed to contain an Fe^{4+} oxidation bound to an oxo-porphyrin cation radical. This compound then reacts with another H_2O_2 to form the reduced Fe^{3+} catalase, H_2O and O_2. The net reaction is given as:

$$2H_2O_2 \rightarrow O_2 + 2H_2O$$

While catalase is specific for H_2O_2 and not for hydroperoxides, glutathione peroxidase (GPX) catalyses both the decomposition of H_2O_2 and organic peroxides. GPX consist of four protein subunits, each containing a selenium atom at the active site that catalyzes the decomposition of peroxides though the oxidation of glutathione (GSH) to GSSG (two GSH molecules in which the –SH groups of cysteine moieties are bridged by a disulfide bond). Hydrogen peroxides are reduced to H_2O and alkyl hydroperoxides are reduced to alcohol and water.

$$LOOH + 2GSH \rightarrow GSSG + LOH + H_2O$$

In addition to these antioxidant enzymes, nonenzymatic molecules such as alpha-tocopherol, carotenoids, vitamin A, ascorbate, spermine,[136] and certain sulfhydryl and thioether compounds,[137] for example, have been proven to function as a second line of defense against oxidative damage when radicals escape decomposition by antioxidant enzymes. It is important to note that antioxidant property is not limited to direct interaction of antioxidants with the substrate of interest. There are proteins such as transferrins that can indirectly limit the radical concentration in cells by sequestering certain metal ions such as iron or copper that are directly responsible for the catalytic production of radicals. Metal chelators such as deferoxamine[138] are known to improve postischemic myocardial function and metabolism. Recently manganese(II) complexes, with a bis(cyclohexylpyridine)-substituted macrocyclic ligand (M40403), have been developed with high catalytic SOD activity and demonstrated to cross cell membranes and to be chemically and biologically stable in vivo. Injection of M40403 into rat models of inflammation and ischemia-reperfusion injury protected the animals against tissue damage. Such SOD mimetics may provide potent clinical therapies for diseases mediated by superoxide radicals.[139]

Conclusion

Over the last decade, it has become clear that free radicals are critical mediators of cardiovascular function and disease. It is clear that while free radicals at low concentrations play critical roles in modulating cell function, signaling, and immune response, at high levels they are central mediators of cellular injury. There are a series of specific pathways responsible for the production of oxygen radicals and nitric oxide. Enzyme deactivation, DNA breakage, and lipid peroxidation are caused by reactive oxygen and/or nitrogen species. Defense mechanisms including antioxidants and antioxidant enzymes exist in cells primarily to eliminate or modulate the destructive action of radicals; however, under some pathological conditions, these defenses are overwhelmed. In recent years techniques including EPR spectroscopy and imaging as well as spin trapping have allowed unambiguous determination of the presence of radicals, their quantitation, and in vivo detection and mapping in biological tissues. The challenge in the future is to characterize the specific molecular and cellular pathways involved in cardiovascular disease and to develop genetic, molecular, and pharmacological approaches to prevent or ameliorate free radical-mediated cardiovascular disease.

References

1. Steacie EWR. Atomic and free radical reactions. In: The Kinetics of Gas-Phase Reactions Involving Atoms and Organic Radicals. Rheinhold Pub. Co., NY, 1946.
2. Fitzpatrick FA. Inflammation, carcinogenesis and cancer. Int Immunopharmacol 2001;1:1651–1667.
3. Valko M, Morris H, Mazur M, et al. Oxygen free radical generating mechanisms in the colon: do the semiquinones of vitamin K play a role in the aetiology of colon cancer? Biochim Biophys Acta 2001;1527:161–166.
4. Sanders SP, Bassett DJ, Harrison SJ, et al. Measurements of free radicals in isolated, ischemic lungs and lung mitochondria. Lung 2000;178:105–118.
5. Bilenko MV. Ischemia and Reperfusion of Various Organs: Injury, Mechanisms, Methods of Prevention and Treatment. Nova Science Pub. Inc., Huntington, NY, 2001.
6. Zweier JL. Reduction of O_2 by iron-Adriamycin. J Biol Chem 1984;259:6056–6058.
7. Gianni L, Zweier JL, Levy A, et al. Characterization of the cycle of iron-mediated electron transfer from Adriamycin to molecular oxygen. J Biol Chem 1985;260:6820–6826.
8. Zweier JL. Iron-mediated formation of an oxidized Adriamycin free radical. Biochim Biophys Acta 1985;839:209–213.
9. Zweier JL, Flaherty JT, Weisfeldt ML. Direct measurement of free radical generation following reperfusion of ischemic myocardium. Proc Natl Acad Sci USA 1987;84:1404–1407.
10. Zweier JL, Kuppusamy P, Williams R, et al. Measurement and characterization of postischemic free radical generation in the isolated perfused heart. J Biol Chem 1989;264:18890–18895.
11. Ambrosio G, Zweier JL, Duilio C, et al. Evidence that mitochondrial respiration is a source of potentially toxic oxygen free radicals in intact rabbit hearts subjected to ischemia and reflow. J Biol Chem 1993;268:18532–18541.
12. Weiss J. Radiochemistry of aqueous solutions. Nature 1944;153:748–750.

13. Grisham MB, McCord JM. Chemistry and cytotoxicity of reactive oxygen metabolites. In: Taylor AE, Metalon S, Ward PA, eds. Physiology of Oxygen Free Radicals. Williams & Wilkins, Baltimore, 1986; 1–18.
14. Floyd RA. Direct demonstration that ferrous ion complexes of di- and triphosphate nucleotides catalyze hydroxyl free radical formation from hydrogen peroxide. Arch Biochem Biophys 1983;225:263–270.
15. Floyd RA, Lewis CA. Hydroxyl free radical formation from hydrogen peroxide by ferrous iron-nucleotide complexes. Biochemistry 1983;22:2645–2649.
16. Roubaud V, Sankarapandi S, Kuppusamy P, et al. Quantitative measurement of superoxide generation using the spin trap 5-(diethoxyphosphoryl)-5-methyl-1-pyrroline-N-oxide. Anal Biochem 1997;247:404–411.
17. Zhao H, Joseph J, Zhang H, et al. Synthesis and biochemical applications of a solid cyclic nitrone spin trap: a relatively superior trap for detecting superoxide anions and glutathiyl radicals. Free Radic Biol Med 2001;31:599–606.
18. Hearse DJ, Manning AS, Downey JM, et al. Xanthine oxidase: a critical mediator of myocardial injury during ischemia and reperfusion? Acta Physiol Scand(Suppl)1986;548:65–78.
19. Xia Y, Dawson VL, Dawson TM, et al. Nitric oxide synthase generates superoxide and nitric oxide in arginine-depleted cells leading to peroxynitrite-mediated cellular injury. Proc Nat Acad Sci USA 1996;93:6770–6774.
20. Xia Y, Tsai AL, Berka V, et al. Superoxide generation from endothelial nitric oxide synthase: a Ca^{2+}/calmodulin-dependent and tetrahydrobiopterin regulatory process. J Biol Chem 1998;273:25804–25808.
21. McCord JM. Oxygen-derived free radicals in postischemic tissue injury. N Engl J Med 1985;312:159–163.
22. McCord JM. Free radicals and myocardial ischemia: overview and outlook. Free Radic Biol Med 1988;4:9–14.
23. Chambers DE, Parks DA, Patterson G, et al. Xanthine oxidase as a source of free radical damage in myocardial ischemia. J Mol Cell Cardiol 1985;17:145–152.
24. Granger DN, Rutili G, McCord JM. Superoxide radicals in feline intestinal ischemia. Gastroenterology 1981;81:22–29.
25. Kuppusamy P, Zweier JL. Characterization of free radical generation by xanthine oxidase: evidence for hydroxyl radical generation. J Biol Chem 1989;264:9880–9884.
26. Xia Y, Khatchikian G, Zweier JL. Adenosine deaminase inhibition prevents free radical-mediated injury in the postischemic heart. J Biol Chem 1996;271:10096–10192.
27. Thompson-Gorman SL, Zweier JL. Evaluation of the role of xanthine oxidase in myocardial reperfusion injury. J Biol Chem 1990;265:6656–6663.
28. Xia Y, Zweier JL. Substrate control of free radical generation from xanthine oxidase in the postischemic heart. J Biol Chem 1995;270:18797–18803.
29. Az-ma T, Saeki N, Yuge O. Cytosolic Ca2+ movements of endothelial cells exposed to reactive oxygen intermediates: role of hydroxyl radical-mediated redox alteration of cell-membrane Ca^{2+} channels. Br J Pharmacol 1999;126:1462–1470.
30. Zweier JL, Kuppusamy P, Thompson-Gorman S, et al. Measurement and characterization of free radical generation in reoxygenated human endothelial cells. Am J Physiol 1994;266:C700–708.
31. Zweier JL, Kuppusamy P, Lutty GA. Measurement of endothelial cell free radical generation: evidence for a central mechanism of free radical injury in postischemic tissues. Proc Natl Acad Sci USA 1988;85:4046–4050.

32. Rosen GM, Freeman BA. Detection of superoxide generated by endothelial cells. Proc Natl Acad Sci USA 1984;81:7269–7273.
33. Jarasch ED, Grund C, Bruder G, et al. Localization of xanthine oxidase in mammary-gland epithelium and capillary endothelium. Cell 1981;25:67–82.
34. Jarasch ED, Bruder G, Heid HW. Significance of xanthine oxidase in capillary endothelial cells. Acta Physiol Scand (Suppl)1986;548:39–46.
35. Boveris A. Mitochondrial production of superoxide radical and hydrogen peroxide. Adv Exp Med Biol 1977;78:67–82.
36. Nohl H, Breuninger V, Hegner D. Influence of mitochondrial radical formation on energy-linked respiration. Eur J Biochem 1978;90:385–390.
37. Otani H, Tanaka H, Inoue T, et al. In vitro study on contribution of oxidative metabolism of isolated rabbit heart mitochondria to myocardial reperfusion injury. Circ Res 1984;55:168–175.
38. Turrens JF. Superoxide production by the mitochondrial respiratory chain. Biosci Rep 1997;17:3–8.
39. Turrens JF, McCord JM. Mechanisms and consequences of tissue injury. In: Zelenock GB, D'Alecy LG, Fantone JC, et al., eds. Clinical Ischemic Syndromes. C.V. Mosby Co., St. Louis, MO, 1990; 203–212.
40. Hess ML, Manson NH. Molecular oxygen: friend and foe. The role of the oxygen free radical system in the calcium paradox, the oxygen paradox and ischemia/reperfusion injury. J Mol Cell Cardiol 1984;16:969–985.
41. Chance B, Sies H, Boveris A. Hydroperoxide metabolism in mammalian organs. Physiol Rev 1979;59:527–605.
42. Boveris A, Chance B. The mitochondrial generation of hydrogen peroxide: general properties and effect of hyperbaric oxygen. Biochem J 1973;134:707–716.
43. Loschen G, Azzi A, Richter C, et al. Superoxide radicals as precursors of mitochondrial hydrogen peroxide. FEBS Lett 1974;42:68–72.
44. Cadenas E, Boveris A, Ragan CI, et al. Production of superoxide radicals and hydrogen peroxide by NADH-ubiquinone reductase and ubiquinol-cytochrome c reductase from beef-heart mitochondria. Arch Biochem Biophys 1977;180:248–257.
45. Turrens JF, Boveris A. Generation of superoxide anion by the NADH dehydrogenase of bovine heart mitochondria. Biochem J 1980;191:421–427.
46. Turrens JF, Alexandre A, Lehninger AL. Ubisemiquinone is the electron donor for superoxide formation by complex III of heart mitochondria. Arch Biochem Biophys 1985;237:408–414.
47. Turrens JF, Freeman BA, Crapo JD. Hyperoxia increases H_2O_2 release by lung mitochondria and microsomes. Arch Biochem Biophys 1982;217:411–421.
48. Turrens JF, Freeman BA, Levitt JG, et al. The effect of hyperoxia on superoxide production by lung submitochondrial particles. Arch Biochem Biophys 1982;217:401–410.
49. Arduini A, Mezzetti A, Porreca E, et al. Effect of ischemia and reperfusion on antioxidant enzymes and mitochondrial inner membrane proteins in perfused rat heart. Biochim Biophys Acta 1988;970:113–121.
50. Cadenas E, Davies KJ. Mitochondrial free radical generation, oxidative stress, and aging. Free Radic Biol Med 2000;29:222–230.
51. Barja G. Mitochondrial oxygen radical generation and leak: sites of production in states 4 and 3, organ specificity, and relation to aging and longevity. J Bioenerg Biomembr 1999;31:347–366.
52. Zhao BL, Duan SJ, Xin WJ. Lymphocytes can produce respiratory burst and

oxygen radicals as polymorphonuclear leukocytes. Cell Biophys 1990; 17: 205–211

53. Hansen PR. Role of neutrophils in myocardial ischemia and reperfusion. Circulation 1995;91:1872–1885.
54. Dahm LJ, Schultze AE, Roth RA. Activated neutrophils injure the isolated, perfused rat liver by an oxygen radical-dependent mechanism. Am J Pathol 1991;139:1009–1020.
55. Rowe GT, Manson NH, Caplan M, et al. Hydrogen peroxide and hydroxyl radical mediation of activated leukocyte depression of cardiac sarcoplasmic reticulum: participation of the cyclooxygenase pathway. Circ Res 1983;53:584–591.
56. Hess ML, Rowe GT, Caplan M, et al. Identification of hydrogen peroxide and hydroxyl radicals as mediators of leukocyte-induced myocardial dysfunction: limitation of infarct size with neutrophil inhibition and depletion. Adv Myocardiol 1985;5:159–175.
57. Rowe GT, Eaton LR, Hess ML. Neutrophil-derived, oxygen free radical-mediated cardiovascular dysfunction. J Mol Cell Cardiol 1984;16:1075–1079.
58. Johnston RB Jr, Keele BB Jr, Misra HP, et al. The role of superoxide anion generation in phagocytic bactericidal activity: studies with normal and chronic granulomatous disease leukocytes. J Clin Invest 1975;55:1357–1372.
59. Root RK, Metcalf JA. H_2O_2 release from human granulocytes during phagocytosis: relationship to superoxide anion formation and cellular catabolism of H_2O_2: studies with normal and cytochalasin B-treated cells. J Clin Invest 1977;60:1266–1279.
60. Schmid-Schonbein GW, Engler RL. Granulocytes as active participants in acute myocardial ischemia and infarction. Am J Cardiovasc Pathol 1987;1:15–30.
61. Romson JL, Hook BG, Kunkel SL, et al. Reduction of the extent of ischemic myocardial injury by neutrophil depletion in the dog. Circulation 1983;67:1016–1023.
62. Gabrielson EW, Kuppusamy P, Povey AC, et al. Measurement of neutrophil activation and epidermal cell toxicity by palytoxin and 12-O-tetradecanoylphorbol-13-acetate. Carcinogenesis 1992;13:1671–1674.
63. Serrano CV Jr., Fraticelli A, Paniccia R, et al. pH dependence of neutrophil-endothelial cell adhesion and adhesion molecule expression. Am J Physiol 1996;271:C962–970.
64. Ziegelstein RC, Corda S, Pili R, et al. Initial contact and subsequent adhesion of human neutrophils or monocytes to human aortic endothelial cells releases an endothelial intracellular calcium store. Circulation 1994;90:1899–1907.
65. Serrano CV Jr., Mikhail EA, Wang P, et al. Superoxide and hydrogen peroxide induce CD18-mediated adhesion in the postischemic heart. Biochim Biophys Acta 1996;1316:191–202.
66. Fraticelli A, Serrano CV Jr, Bochner BS, et al. Hydrogen peroxide and superoxide modulate leukocyte adhesion molecule expression and leukocyte endothelial adhesion. Biochim Biophys Acta 1996;1310:251–259.
67. Shandelya SM, Kuppusamy P, Weisfeldt ML, et al. Evaluation of the role of polymorphonuclear leukocytes on contractile function in myocardial reperfusion injury: evidence for plasma-mediated leukocyte activation. Circulation 1993;87:536–546.
68. Mullane KM, Moncada S. The salvage of ischemic myocardium by BW755C in anesthetized dogs. Prostaglandins 1982;24:255–266.

69. Jolly SR, Lucchesi BR. Effect of BW755C in an occlusion-reperfusion model of ischemic myocardial injury. Am Heart J 1983;106:8–13.
70. Mullane KM, Salmon JA, Kraemer R. Leukocyte-derived metabolites of arachidonic acid in ischemia-induced myocardial injury. Fed Proc 1987;46: 2422–2433.
71. McCord JM. Oxygen-derived radicals: a link between reperfusion injury and inflammation. Fed Proc 1987;46:2402–2406.
72. de Souza H, Laurindo F, Ziegelstein R, et al. Vascular NAD(P)H oxidase is different from the phagocytic enzyme and is involved in vascular reactivity control. Am J Physiol 2001;280:H658–H667.
73. Suh YA, Arnold RS, Lassegue B, et al. Cell transformation by the superoxide-generating oxidase Mox1. Nature 1999;401:79–82.
74. Weitberg AB, Corvese D. Hydroxy- and hydroperoxy-6,8,11,14-eicosatetraenoic acids induce DNA strand breaks in human lymphocytes. Carcinogenesis 1989;10:1029–1031.
75. de Kok TM, ten Vaarwerk F, Zwingman I, et al. Peroxidation of linoleic, arachidonic and oleic acid in relation to the induction of oxidative DNA damage and cytogenetic effects. Carcinogenesis 1994;15:1399–1404.
76. Marnett LJ, Dix TA, Sachs RJ, et al. Oxidations by fatty acid hydroperoxides and prostaglandin synthase. Adv Prostaglandin Thromboxane Leukot Res 1983;11:79–86.
77. Siedlik PH, Marnett LJ. Oxidizing radical generation by prostaglandin H synthase. Methods Enzymol 1984;105:412–416.
78. Kontos HA, Wei EP, Povlishock JT, et al. Cerebral arteriolar damage by arachidonic acid and prostaglandin G2. Science 1980;209:1242–1245.
79. Okabe E, Kato Y, Kohno H, et al. Inhibition by free radical scavengers and by cyclooxygenase inhibitors of the effect of acidosis on calcium transport by masseter muscle sarcoplasmic reticulum. Biochem Pharmacol 1985;34:961–968.
80. Jahn B, Hansch GM. Oxygen radical generation in human platelets: dependence on 12-lipoxygenase activity and on the glutathione cycle. Int Arch Allergy Appl Immunol 1990; 93:73–79.
81. Liu D, Li L. Prostaglandin F2 alpha rises in response to hydroxyl radical generated in vivo. Free Radic Biol Med 1995;18:571–576.
82. Muller K, Gawlik I. Effects of reactive oxygen species on the biosynthesis of 12 (S)-hydroxyeicosatetraenoic acid in mouse epidermal homogenate. Free Radic Biol Med 1997;23:321–330.
83. Yates JC, Taam GM, Singal PK, et al. Protection against adrenochrome-induced myocardial damage by various pharmacological interventions. Br J Exp Pathol 1980;61:242–255.
84. Wolin MS, Belloni FL. Superoxide anion selectively attenuates catecholamine-induced contractile tension in isolated rabbit aorta. Am J Physiol 1985;249: H1127–1133.
85. Wheatley AM, Thandroyen FT, Opie LH. Catecholamine-induced myocardial cell damage: catecholamines or adrenochrome. J Mol Cell Cardiol 1985;17: 349–359.
86. Kalyanaraman B, Felix CC, Sealy RC. Peroxidatic oxidation of catecholamines: a kinetic electron spin resonance investigation using the spin stabilization approach. J Biol Chem 1984;259:7584–7589.
87. Schomig A, Richardt G. The role of catecholamines in ischemia. J Cardiovasc Pharmacol 1990;16(Suppl 5):S105–112.
88. Allen DR, Wallis GL, McCay PB. Catechol adrenergic agents enhance hy-

droxyl radical generation in xanthine oxidase systems containing ferritin: implications for ischemia/reperfusion. Arch Biochem Biophys 1994;315: 235–243.

89. Furchgott RF, Zawadzki JV. The obligatory role of endothelial cells in the relaxation of arterial smooth muscle by acetylcholine. Nature 1980;288:3 73–376.

90. Furchgott RF, Vanhoutte PM. Endothelium-derived relaxing and contracting factors. Faseb J 1989;3:2007–2018.

91. Palmer RM, Ferrige AG, Moncada S. Nitric oxide release accounts for the biological activity of endothelium-derived relaxing factor. Nature 1987;327: 524–526.

92. Ignarro LJ, Byrns RE, Buga GM, et al. Endothelium-derived relaxing factor from pulmonary artery and vein possesses pharmacologic and chemical properties identical to those of nitric oxide radical. Circ Res 1987;61:866–879.

93. Moncada S, Palmer RM, Higgs EA. Biosynthesis of nitric oxide from L-arginine: a pathway for the regulation of cell function and communication. Biochem Pharmacol 1989;38:1709–1715.

94. Bredt DS, Hwang PM, Glatt CE, et al. Cloned and expressed nitric oxide synthase structurally resembles cytochrome P-450 reductase. Nature 1991;351: 714–718.

95. Dinerman JL, Lowenstein CJ, Snyder SH. Molecular mechanisms of nitric oxide regulation: potential relevance to cardiovascular disease. Circ Res 1993; 73:217–222.

96. Li H, Raman CS, Martasek P, et al. Crystallographic studies on endothelial nitric oxide synthase complexed with nitric oxide and mechanism-based inhibitors. Biochemistry 2001;40:5399–406.

97. Zweier JL, Samouilov A, Kuppusamy P. Non-enzymatic nitric oxide synthesis in biological systems. Biochim Biophys Acta 1999;1411:250–262.

98. Zweier JL, Wang P, Samouilov A, et al. Enzyme-independent formation of nitric oxide in biological tissues. Nat Med 1995;1:804–809.

99. Giulivi C, Poderoso JJ, Boveris A. Production of nitric oxide by mitochondria. J Biol Chem 1998;273:11038–11043.

100. Lopez-Figueroa MO, Caamano C, Morano MI, et al. Direct evidence of nitric oxide presence within mitochondria. Biochem Biophys Res Commun 2000; 272:129–133.

101. Henry Y, Guissani A. Interactions of nitric oxide with hemoproteins: roles of nitric oxide in mitochondria. Cell Mol Life Sci 1999;55:1003–1014.

102. Henry Y. Cross regulation of metalloenzymes triggered by nitric oxide. In: Ducastel B, ed. Nitric Oxide Research from Chemistry to Biology. R.G. Landes Co., Austin, TX, 1997.

103. Foster MW, Bian S, Surerus KK, et al. Elucidation of a [4Fe-4S] cluster degradation pathway: rapid kinetic studies of the degradation of chromatium vinosum HiPIP. J Biol Inorg Chem 2001;6:266–274.

104. Foster MW, Cowan JA. Chemistry of nitric oxide with protein-bound iron sulfur centers: insights on physiological reactivity. J Am Chem Soc 1999; 121:4093–4100.

105. Poderoso JJ, Carreras MC, Lisdero C, et al. Nitric oxide inhibits electron transfer and increases superoxide radical production in rat heart mitochondria and submitochondrial particles. Arch Biochem Biophys 1996;328:85–92.

106. Giulivi C. Functional implications of nitric oxide produced by mitochondria in mitochondrial metabolism. Biochem J 1998;332(Pt 3):673–679.

94 · Oxidative Stress and Cardiac Failure

107. Brown GC. Nitric oxide and mitrochondrial respiration. Biochem Biophys Acta 1999;1411:351–369.
108. Brudvig GW, Stevens TH, Chan SI. Reactions of nitric oxide with cytochrome c oxidase. Biochemistry 1980;19:5275–5285.
109. Poderoso JJ, Peralta JG, Lisdero CL, et al. Nitric oxide regulates oxygen uptake and hydrogen peroxide release by the isolated beating rat heart. Am J Physiol 1998;274:C112–119.
110. Sarkela TM, Berthiaume J, Elfering S, et al. The modulation of oxygen radical production by nitric oxide in mitochondria. J Biol Chem 2001;276:6945–6949.
111. Poderoso JJ, Lisdero C, Schopfer F, et al. The regulation of mitochondrial oxygen uptake by redox reactions involving nitric oxide and ubiquinol. J Biol Chem 1999;274:37709–37716.
112. Riobo NA, Clementi E, Melani M, et al. Nitric oxide inhibits mitochondrial NADH:ubiquinone reductase activity through peroxynitrite formation. Biochem J 2001;359:139–145.
113. Grune T, Blasig IE, Sitte N, et al. Peroxynitrite increases the degradation of aconitase and other cellular proteins by proteasome. J Biol Chem 1998;273:10857–10862.
114. Cassina AM, Hodara R, Souza JM, et al. Cytochrome c nitration by peroxynitrite. J Biol Chem 2000;275:21409–21415.
115. Valdez LB, Alvarez S, Arnaiz SL, et al. Reactions of peroxynitrite in the mitochondial matrix. Free Radic Biol Med 2000;29:349–356.
116. Bringold U, Ghafourifar P, Richter C. Peroxynitrite formed by mitochondrial NO synthase promotes mitochondrial Ca^{2+} release. Free Radic Biol Med 2000;29:343–348.
117. Wang P, Zweier JL. Measurement of nitric oxide and peroxynitrite generation in the postischemic heart: evidence for peroxynitrite-mediated reperfusion injury. J Biol Chem 1996;271:29223–29330.
118. Migita CT, Salerno JC, Masters BS, et al. Substrate binding-induced changes in the EPR spectra of the ferrous nitric oxide complexes of neuronal nitric oxide synthase. Biochemistry 1997;36:10987–10992.
119. Kuppusamy P, Chzhan M, Wang P, et al. Three-dimensional gated EPR imaging of the beating heart: time-resolved measurements of free radical distribution during the cardiac contractile cycle. Magn Reson Med 1996;35:323–328.
120. Kuppusamy P, Chzhan M, Zweier JL. Development and optimization of three-dimensional spatial EPR imaging for biological organs and tissues. J Magn Reson B 1995;106:122–130.
121. Kuppusamy P, Wang P, Samouilov A, et al. Spatial mapping of nitric oxide generation in the ischemic heart using electron paramagnetic resonance imaging. Magn Reson Med 1996;36:212–218.
122. Kuppusamy P, Wang P, Zweier JL. Three-dimensional spatial EPR imaging of the rat heart. Magn Reson Med 1995;34:99–105.
123. Gutteridge JMC, Westermarck T, Halliwell B. Oxygen radical damage in biological systems. In: Free Radicals, Aging, and Degenerative Diseases. Alan R. Liss, Inc., NY, 1985; 99–139.
124. Halliwell B, Gutteridge JMC. Oxidative stress: adaptation, damage and death. In: Free Radicals in Biology and Medicine. Oxford University Press, Oxford, 1999.
125. Starke DW, Chen Y, Bapna CP, et al. Sensitivity of protein sulfhydryl repair enzyme to oxidative stress. Free Rad Biol Med 1997;23:373–384.

126. Floyd RA, Carney JM. Free radical damage to protein and DNA: mechanisms involved and relevant observations on brain undergoing oxidative stress. Ann Neurol 1992;32:S22–27.
127. Tabatabaie T, Potts JD, Floyd RA. Reactive oxygen species-mediated inactivation of pyruvate dehydrogenase. Arch Biochem Biophys 1996;336:290–296.
128. Pearce LL, Epperly MW, Greenberger JS, et al. Identification of respiratory complexes I and II as mitochondrial sites of damage following exposure to ionizing radiation and nitric oxide. Nitric Oxide Biol Chem 2001;5:128–136.
129. Wiseman H, Halliwell B. Damage to DNA by reactive oxygen and nitrogen species: role in inflammatory disease and progression to cancer. Biochem J 1996;313:17–29.
130. Croteau DL, Bohr VA. Repair of oxidative damage to nuclear and mitochondrial DNA in mammalian cells. J Biol Chem 1997;272:25409–25412.
131. Spencer JP, Wong J, Jenner A, et al. Base modification and strand breakage in isolated calf thymus DNA and in DNA from human skin epidermal keratinocytes exposed to peroxynitrite or 3-morpholinosydnonimine. Chem Res Toxicol 1996;9:1152–1158.
132. Zweier JL, Gianni L, Muindi J, et al. Differences in O_2 reduction by the iron complexes of Adriamycin and daunomycin: the importance of the sidechain hydroxyl group. Biochim Biophys Acta 1986;884:326–336.
133. Swauger JE, Dolan PM, Zweier JL, et al. Role of the benzoyloxyl radical in DNA damage mediated by benzoyl peroxide. Chem Res Toxicol 1991;4:223–228.
134. Wang P, Chen H, Qin H, et al. Overexpression of human copper, zinc-superoxide dismutase (SOD1) prevents postischemic injury. Proc Natl Acad Sci USA 1998;95:4556–4560.
135. Fridovich I. Oxygen radicals, hydrogen peroxide, and oxygen toxicity. In: Pryor WA, ed. Free Radicals in Biology. Academic Press, NY, 1976; 239.
136. Ha HC, Sirisoma NS, Kuppusamy P, et al. The natural polyamine spermine functions directly as a free radical scavenger. Proc Natl Acad Sci USA 1998; 95:11140–11145.
137. Shankar RA, Hideg K, Zweier JL, et al. Targeted antioxidant properties of N-[(tetramethyl-3-pyrroline-3-carboxamido)propyl]phthalimide and its nitroxide metabolite in preventing postischemic myocardial injury. J Pharmacol Exp Ther 2000;292:838–845.
138. Ambrosio G, Zweier JL, Jacobus WE, et al. Improvement of postischemic myocardial function and metabolism induced by administration of deferoxamine at the time of reflow: the role of iron in the pathogenesis of reperfusion injury. Circulation 1987;76:906–915.
139. Salvemini D, Wang ZQ, Zweier JL, et al. A nonpeptidyl mimic of superoxide dismutase with therapeutic activity in rats. Science 1999;286:304–306.

• 4 •

Evidence of Oxidative Stress in Heart Failure

Kenneth Y.K. Wong, MA (Oxon), BM BCh (Oxon),
Allan D. Struthers, MD, and Jill J.F. Belch, MD

Introduction

Heart failure is a common condition that causes much mortality and morbidity. Congestive heart failure (CHF) can be thought of as a syndrome in which the pump function of the heart is unable to meet its workload. As a result, there is increased sympathetic activity, which leads to increased heart rate, and hence, further increase in the workload of the heart. Myocardial contractility is impaired by loss of muscle, for example, secondary to myocardial infarction or by pressure or volume overload.[1] This pressure or volume overload causes myocardial ischemia, which can generate free radicals.[2,3]

Support for this hypothesis comes from work in animal models of heart failure where doxorubicin toxicity may result from myocardial injury induced by oxidative damage.[4] Oxidative stress has been demonstrated in different animal models of heart failure: volume overload, pressure overload, and myocardial infarction.

Over the past decade, clinical evidence has begun to emerge that confirms the experimental evidence from animal models that heart failure is associated with increased oxidative stress; we are also beginning to understand the pathophysiological mechanisms of damage caused by free radicals. In particular, there is now strong evidence to suggest that oxidative stress in heart failure increases endothelial dysfunction. Impor-

From: Kukin ML, Fuster V (eds). *Oxidative Stress and Cardiac Failure.* Armonk, NY: Futura Publishing Co., Inc. ©2003.

tantly, it appears that angiotensin may be a key player contributing to endothelial dysfunction, and that it mediates, at least in part, its harmful effects via oxidative stress. Further, it is now known that therapies that benefit patients with heart failure, such as beta-blockers[5,6] and captopril,[7,8] also have beneficial effects on myocardial oxidative metabolism. Clearly, the therapeutic implications are enormous, but in this chapter, the focus is on the evidence that links oxidative stress to heart failure.

Is There Evidence of Increased Oxidative Stress in Heart Failure?

Much experimental evidence in animal models has suggested that there is increased oxidative stress in heart failure. In the 1990s, clinical evidence began to emerge in favor of this hypothesis. In 1991, Belch et al. measured plasma lipid peroxides (malondialdehyde) and thiols in 45 patients with CHF and in 45 controls. The greater the amount of oxidative stress, the higher the concentration of malondialdehyde and the lower the concentration of thiol. Malondialdehyde concentrations were significantly higher in the patients with CHF (median 9.0 nmol/mL) than in the controls (median 7.7 nmol/mL). Plasma thiols were significantly lower in CHF (median 420 μmol/L) than in the controls (median 463 μmol/L). There was a significant but weak negative correlation between malondialdehyde and left ventricular ejection fraction (LVEF) (r=−0.35) and a positive correlation between plasma thiols and LVEF (r=0.39). This study provides clinical support for experimental data indicating that free radicals may be important in heart failure.[9] It also suggests that the degree of free radical production may be linked to the severity of the disease.

Recently, further evidence supporting the hypothesis that free radical production is linked to the severity of heart failure has been obtained. Isoprostaglandin $F_{2\alpha}$ is a member of the prostanoid family called F_2 isoprostanes. These are produced as a result of cell membrane lipid peroxidation mediated by free radicals. Cracowski et al.[10] reported that urinary excretion of isoprostaglandin $F_{2\alpha}$ could be used to assess the extent of oxidative stress in heart failure patients and that urinary concentrations correlated with the functional severity of disease, in that patients with New York Heart Association (NYHA) functional class IV had significantly higher concentrations of isoprostaglandin $F_{2\alpha}$ than those in NYHA classes II and III. However, the authors did not find a significant correlation between urinary concentrations of isoprostaglandin $F_{2\alpha}$ and LVEF per se.[10] Nevertheless, if the results of this study involving 25 patients and 25 healthy controls can be replicated in a larger study, the technique may have potential for development as a noninvasive quantitative tool for monitoring response to treatment in patients with heart failure.

How Do Free Radicals Worsen Myocardial Function?

In animal models, free radicals cause impairment of myocyte metabolism and contraction.[11] Mitochondrial, sarcoplasmic reticular, and enzymatic function may be deranged.[11,12] Oxidative stress impairs the function of sarcoplasmic reticulum by oxidation of sulfhydryl groups in Ca^{2+}-ATPase.[13] As a result, there is reduced calcium efflux and calcium overload, an important mechanism of myocyte dysfunction. In addition, free radicals themselves depress calcium binding and uptake into the sarcoplasmic reticulum;[14] this leads to a decrease in cardiac contractility.

Free radicals induce dysrhythmias.[15] Lipid peroxidation may cause disruption of membrane-bound enzymes and increase membrane permeability,[16] thus increasing the predisposition to cardiac dysrhythmias. Cardiac dysrhythmias can, of course, worsen left ventricular function. Sadly, a substantial proportion of deaths in patients with CHF occur suddenly (7 out of 19 in a series of 44 patients with class 3 and 4 symptomatic left ventricular systolic dysfunction secondary to ischemic heart disease, followed up for 3 years).[17] It was found that the group of patients who died suddenly had a significantly higher interlead variability of QT intervals (QT dispersion). QT dispersion is now recognized to be associated with ventricular tachycardia.[18]

Free radicals may be involved in the genesis of certain types of acute myocardial dysfunction (reperfusion injury and myocardial stunning).[19,20] Underlying coronary artery disease may predispose to stunning. Repeated episodes of stunning may lead to permanent myocardial dysfunction.[21]

Adrenergic activity is increased in CHF.[22] Catecholamines may augment free radical generation by at least two mechanisms: increasing mitochondrial respiration and undergoing auto-oxidation themselves.[23,24]

Further, in patients with heart failure, many other organs such as the kidneys undergo hypoperfusion/reperfusion cycles. Lactic acidosis may enhance hyperoxia in these tissues,[25] hence increasing free radical generation. A vicious cycle is thus established.

Finally, it has been shown that free radicals cause endothelial dysfunction.[26]

Oxidative Stress and Endothelial Dysfunction in Heart Failure (Figure 1)

Chronic heart failure is associated with endothelial dysfunction, including impaired endothelium-mediated, flow-dependent dilation. Endothelial-derived vasodilatation is now thought to be due, at least in part, to nitric

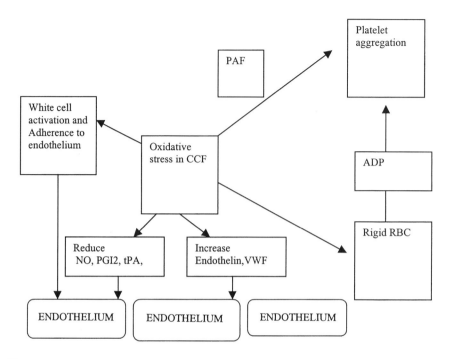

Figure 1. The mechanism whereby oxidative stress with heart failure promotes cardiovascular disease. NO = nitric oxide; PGI2 = prostacyclin; tPA = tissue plasminogen activator; VWF = Von Willebrand factor; ADP = adenosine diphosphate; PAF = platelet activating factor; CCF = congestive cardiac failure.

oxide (NO). Nitric oxide provides a common final pathway explaining the mechanism of vasodilating action of drugs such as nitrates, which not only reduce the workload of the heart by dilating arterioles and venules, but also cause vasodilation in the coronary arteries. That explains why nitrates have such an important role in the management of coronary artery disease and also in the acute management of heart failure. It was hypothesized that NO was inactivated by free radicals. To test this hypothesis, Hornig et al.[27] determined the effect of the antioxidant vitamin C on flow-dependent dilatation in patients with CHF. High-resolution ultrasound and Doppler were used to measure radial artery diameter and blood flow in 15 patients with CHF and in 8 healthy volunteers. Vascular effects of vitamin C (25 mg/min IA) and placebo were determined at rest and during reactive hyperemia (causing endothelium-mediated dilation) before and after intra-arterial infusion of N-monomethyl-L-arginine (L-NMMA) to inhibit endothelial synthesis of NO. Vitamin C restored flow-dependent dilatation in patients with heart failure after acute intra-arterial administration (13.2 ± 1.7% versus 8.2 ± 1.0%;

$P<0.01$) and after 4 weeks of oral therapy (11.9 ± 0.9% versus 8.2 ± 1.0%; $P<0.05$). In particular, the portion of flow-dependent dilatation mediated by NO (i.e., inhibited by L-NMMA) was increased after acute as well as after chronic treatment (CHF baseline: 4.2 ± 0.7%; acute: 9.1 ± 1.3%; chronic: 7.3 ± 1.2%; normal subjects: 8.9 ± 0.8%; $P<0.01$). In other words, vitamin C improves endothelial-mediated flow-dependent dilatation in patients with CHF as the result of increased availability of NO. This observation is important as it supports the concept that endothelial dysfunction in patients with CHF is, at least in part, due to accelerated degradation of NO by radicals.[27]

Angiotensin May Worsen Endothelial Dysfunction by Increasing Oxidative Stress

Angiotensin II is formed from its precursor angiotensin I by the angiotensin-converting enzyme (ACE). It has a number of deleterious actions that account for mortality and morbidity in heart failure. It is well known that angiotensin II increases the formation of aldosterone. Aldosterone promotes sodium and water absorption, thereby increasing blood pressure and workload of the heart. In addition, angiotensin II increases the workload of the heart by other mechanisms such as increasing extracellular fluid volume by increasing the sensation of thirst, and importantly, angiotensin II leads to vasoconstriction. It is now believed that the vasoconstriction effects of angiotensin II are mediated, at least in part, by increasing oxidative stress,[28] formation of free radicals, and endothelial dysfunction.

Evidence for the hypothesis that angiotensin II stimulates superoxide anion formation comes from work done by Griendling et al. in 1994.[29] They found that treatment of vascular smooth muscle cells with angiotensin II for 4 to 6 hours caused a 2.7-fold increase in intracellular superoxide anion formation. This superoxide appeared to result from activation of both the nicotinamide adenine dinucleotide phosphate (NADPH) and nicotinamide adenine dinucleotide (NADH) oxidases. More recently, it was demonstrated in a rabbit model that hypercholesterolemia was associated with AT_1-receptor upregulation, endothelial dysfunction, and increased NADH-dependent vascular $O_2 \cdot^-$ production. Treatment of cholesterol-fed animals with an AT_1-receptor antagonist improved endothelial dysfunction, normalized vascular $O_2 \cdot^-$ and NADH-oxidase activity, decreased macrophage infiltration, and reduced early plaque formation. Therefore, it appears that angiotensin II-mediated $O_2 \cdot^-$ production plays a crucial role in the early stage of atherosclerosis.[29]

Work from the Mayo Clinic[30] demonstrated the possibility that small increments in angiotensin II are responsible for an increase in blood pressure and maintenance of hypertension through the stimulation of oxidative stress. A low dose of angiotensin II (2–10 ng/kg/min, which does not elicit an immediate pressor response), when given for 7 to 30 days by continuous intravenous infusion, can increase mean arterial pressure by 30 to 40 mm Hg. This slow pressor response to angiotensin is accompanied by the stimulation of oxidative stress, as measured by a significant increase in levels of 8-iso-prostaglandin $F_{2\alpha}$ (F_2-isoprostane). Superoxide radicals and NO can combine chemically to form peroxynitrites, which can then oxidize arachidonic acid to form F_2-isoprostanes. F_2-isoprostanes exert potent vasoconstrictor and antinatriuretic effects. Peroxynitrites themselves then react with iron to produce the very toxic hydroxyl radical. Furthermore, angiotensin II can stimulate endothelin production, which also has been shown to stimulate oxidative stress. In this way, a reduction in the concentration of NO (which is quenched by superoxide), along with the formation of F_2-isoprostanes and endothelin, could potentiate the vasoconstrictor effects of angiotensin II. It would be interesting to know if these mechanisms, which underlie the development of the slow pressor response to angiotensin II, also participate in the production of hypertension when circulating angiotensin II levels appear normal, as occurs in many cases of essential and renovascular hypertension.

Free Radicals, Endothelial Dysfunction, and Thrombosis (Figure 1)

Free radicals also promote thrombosis, both directly and indirectly. Free radicals directly activate platelets. Lipid peroxidation of red blood cells (RBCs) increases RBC rigidity and allows cellular leak of adenosine diphosphate and further platelet aggregation. Free radicals stimulate platelet activating factor release from white cells, augmenting, once again, platelet aggregation. Enhanced platelet aggregation has been linked to cardiovascular events.

In addition to increasing thrombotic tendency within the blood, free radicals also encourage thrombus formation through endothelial damage. Prostacyclin (PGI_2) is another endothelial-produced vasodilator. It is produced through metabolism of arachidonic acid, in equal proportion to thromboxane A_2, a prostanoid from platelets that promotes vasoconstriction and platelet aggregation. Oxidative stress speeds up arachidonic acid metabolism but lipid peroxides selectively impair PGI_2 synthase function in the endothelium. Thus, free radical generation selectively impairs PGI_2 formation from the endothelium, promoting adherence and aggregation of platelets. The platelet plug is fixed to the endothelium by fibrin formation, and free radicals thereafter impair fibrinolysis by decreasing the endothelium's ability to produce tissue-type plasminogen activator (tPA).

Clinical Implications and Future Work

If angiotensin does indeed generate oxidative stress leading to endothelial dysfunction, then blocking the formation of angiotensin is likely to improve cardiovascular prognosis not only in patients with symptomatic heart failure, but also in patients with asymptomatic left ventricular impairment and indeed in arteriopaths who do not yet have evidence of left ventricular impairment. The effectiveness of ACE inhibitors in both symptomatic and asymptomatic heart failure has long been known. More recently, the HOPE Study[31] elegantly demonstrated that ramipril 10 mg od significantly reduced death from cardiovascular causes, myocardial infarction, and stroke, in addition to death from all causes, in patients with evidence of vascular disease or diabetes plus one other cardiac risk factor. There is ongoing debate about whether the mortality benefit seen in HOPE can be explained entirely by the blood pressure-lowering effect of ramipril or whether it is true that blood pressure lowering accounts for only part of the benefits of ramipril. Its additional benefits could be reduction of angiotensin's deleterious effects on oxidative stress and endothelial dysfunction. The group receiving ramipril had on average a lower blood pressure than the placebo group by approximately 3 mm Hg systolic and 1 mm Hg diastolic. It can be extrapolated from the results of studies such as SHEP,[32] Syst-Eur,[33] and HDFP,[34,35] that a 3-mm Hg reduction of systolic blood pressure can result in 20% reduction in heart failure, 20% reduction in cerebrovascular accident risk, and 12% reduction in angina. In the blood pressure limb of UKPDS, there is no difference in efficacy between beta-blockers and ACE inhibitors in reducing mortality.[36] One might even argue that in the CAPP trial,[37] there is an increased risk of stroke in the ACE inhibitor group. However, it should be noted that the blood pressure of the group treated with ACE inhibitors in the CAPP trial was actually higher. On the other hand, data from the Glasgow Blood Pressure Clinic suggest that patients on ACE inhibitors have a better prognosis compared with those on other agents such as calcium antagonists.

The Glasgow Blood Pressure Clinic finding is interesting albeit limited because of the observational nature of the study. It has nevertheless generated an important hypothesis that has yet to be validated in a randomized controlled trial that has an adequate number of patients and endpoint events.

In the absence of well-conducted prospective double-blinded randomized controlled trials, using an adequate sample size, the existing mortality evidence is at least weakly in support of the notion that angiotensin II not only does harm by increasing blood pressure, but also through other deleterious mechanisms. We have provided evidence in this chapter to support the hypothesis that these deleterious effects of angiotensin II may be mediated, at least in part, by endothelial dysfunction due to oxidative stress inactivating endogenous NO.

Conclusions (Figure 2)

Oxidative stress is indeed present in CHF. Congestive heart failure can generate oxidative stress, which in turn may exacerbate heart failure via a variety of mechanisms, including, for example, cardiac dysrhythmias and endothelial dysfunction.

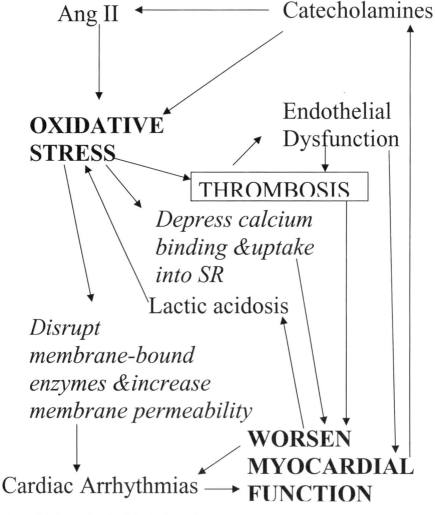

Figure 2. The pathophysiological mechanisms linking oxidative stress and heart failure (see text for explanations). Ang II = angiotensin II; SR = sarcoplasmic reticulum inside cardiac myocytes.

References

1. Parmley WW. Pathophysiology of congestive heart failure. Am J Cardiol 1985; 55:9A–14A.
2. McCord JM. Oxygen-derived free radicals in postischemic tissue injury. N Engl J Med 1985;312:159–163.
3. Belch JJ, Chopra M, Hutchison S, et al. Free radical pathology in chronic arterial disease. Free Radical Biol Med 1989;6:375–378.
4. Goodman J, Hochstein P. Generation of free radicals and lipid peroxidation by redox cycling of Adriamycin and daunomycin. Biochem Biophys Res Commun 1977;77:797–803.
5. Andersson B, Blomstrom-Lundqvist C, Hedner T, et al. Exercise hemodynamics and myocardial metabolism during long-term beta-adrenergic blockade in severe heart failure. J Am Coll Cardiol 1991;18:1059–1066.
6. Beanlands RS, Nahmias C, Gordon E, et al. The effects of beta(1)-blockade on oxidative metabolism and the metabolic cost of ventricular work in patients with left ventricular dysfunction: a double-blind, placebo-controlled, positron-emission tomography study. Circulation 2000;102:2070–2075.
7. Chopra M, Scott N, McMurray J, et al. Captopril: a free radical scavenger. Br J Clin Pharmacol 1989;27:396–399.
8. Chopra M, McMurray J, McLay J, et al. Oxidative damage in chronic heart failure: protection by captopril through free radical scavenging? Adv Exp Med Biol 1990;264:251–255.
9. Belch JJ, Bridges AB, Scott N, et al. Oxygen free radicals and congestive heart failure. Br Heart J 1991;65:245–248.
10. Cracowski JL, Tremel F, Marpeau C, et al. Increased formation of F(2)-isoprostanes in patients with severe heart failure. Heart 2000;84:439–440.
11. Goldhaber JI, Ji S, Lamp ST, et al. Effects of exogenous free radicals on electromechanical function and metabolism in isolated rabbit and guinea pig ventricle: implications for ischemia and reperfusion injury. J Clin Invest 1989; 83:1800–1809.
12. Kim MS, Akera T. O_2 free radicals: cause of ischemia-reperfusion injury to cardiac Na^+- K^+-ATPase. Am J Physiol 1987;252:H252–H257.
13. Scherer NM, Deamer DW. Oxidative stress impairs the function of sarcoplasmic reticulum by oxidation of sulfhydryl groups in the Ca^{2+}-ATPase. Arch Biochem Biophys 1986;246:589–601.
14. Hess ML, Okabe E, Kontos HA. Proton and free oxygen radical interaction with the calcium transport system of cardiac sarcoplasmic reticulum. J Mol Cell Cardiol 1981;13:767–772.
15. Pallandi RT, Perry MA, Campbell TJ. Proarrhythmic effects of an oxygen-derived free radical generating system on action potentials recorded from guinea pig ventricular myocardium: a possible cause of reperfusion-induced arrhythmias. Circ Res 1987;61:50–54.
16. Halliwell B, Gutteridge JM. Free radicals and antioxidant protection: mechanisms and significance in toxicology and disease. Hum Toxicol 1988;7:7–13.
17. Barr CS, Naas A, Freeman M, et al. QT dispersion and sudden unexpected death in chronic heart failure. Lancet 1994;343:327–329.
18. Pye M, Quinn AC, Cobbe SM. QT interval dispersion: a non-invasive marker of susceptibility to arrhythmia in patients with sustained ventricular arrhythmias? Br Heart J 1994;71:511–514.
19. Myers ML, Bolli R, Lekich RF, et al. Enhancement of recovery of myocardial function by oxygen free-radical scavengers after reversible regional ischemia. Circulation 1985;72:915–921.

20. Kloner RA, Przyklenk K, Whittaker P. Deleterious effects of oxygen radicals in ischemia/reperfusion: resolved and unresolved issues. Circulation 1989;80: 1115–1127.
21. Figueras J, Cinca J, Senador G, et al. Progressive mechanical impairment associated with progressive but reversible electrocardiographic ischemic changes during repeated brief coronary artery occlusion in pigs. Cardiovasc Res 1986; 20:797–806.
22. Chidsey CA, Harrison DC, Braunwald E. Augmentation of the plasma norepinephrine response to exercise in patients with congestive heart failure. N Engl J Med 1962;267:650–654.
23. McCord JM. Free radicals and myocardial ischemia: overview and outlook. Free Radic Biol Med 1988;4:9–14.
24. Graham DG, Tiffany SM, Bell WR Jr, et al. Autoxidation versus covalent binding of quinones as the mechanism of toxicity of dopamine, 6-hydroxydopamine, and related compounds toward C1300 neuroblastoma cells in vitro. Mol Pharmacol 1978;14:644–653.
25. Wolbarsht ML, Fridovich I. Hyperoxia during reperfusion is a factor in reperfusion injury. Free Radic Biol Med 1989;6:61–62.
26. Stewart DJ, Pohl U, Bassenge E. Free radicals inhibit endothelium-dependent dilation in the coronary resistance bed. Am J Physiol 1988;255:H765–H769.
27. Hornig B, Arakawa N, Kohler C, et al. Vitamin C improves endothelial function of conduit arteries in patients with chronic heart failure. Circulation 1998; 97:363–368.
28. Oskarsson HJ, Heistad DD. Oxidative stress produced by angiotensin II: implications for hypertension and vascular injury. Circulation 1997;95:557–559.
29. Griendling KK, Minieri CA, Ollerenshaw JD, Alexander RW. Angiotensin II stimulates NADH and NADPH activity in cultured vascular smooth muscle cells. Circ Res 1994;74:1141–1148.
30. Romero JC, Reckelhoff JF. State-of-the-art lecture. Role of angiotensin and oxidative stress in essential hypertension. Hypertension 1999;34:943–949.
31. Yusuf S, Sleight P, Pogue J, et al. Effects of an angiotensin-converting-enzyme inhibitor, ramipril, on cardiovascular events in high-risk patients. The Heart Outcomes Prevention Evaluation Study Investigators [published errata appear in N Engl J Med 2000;342(10):748 and 2000;342(18):1376]. N Engl J Med 2000;342:145–153.
32. SHEP Cooperative Research Group. Prevention of stroke by antihypertensive drug treatment in older persons with isolated systolic hypertension: final results of the Systolic Hypertension in the Elderly Program (SHEP). JAMA 1991; 265:3255–3264.
33. Staessen JA, Fagard R, Thijs L, et al. Randomised double-blind comparison of placebo and active treatment for older patients with isolated systolic hypertension. The Systolic Hypertension in Europe (Syst-Eur) Trial Investigators. Lancet 1997;350:757–764.
34. Daugherty SA. Mortality findings beyond five years in the Hypertension Detection and Follow-Up Program (HDFP). J Hypertens 1988;6:S597–S601.
35. The Hypertension Detection and Follow-up Program Cooperative Research Group. The effect of antihypertensive drug treatment on mortality in the presence of resting electrocardiographic abnormalities at baseline: the HDFP experience. Circulation 1984;70:996–1003.
36. UK Prospective Diabetes Study Group. Efficacy of atenolol and captopril in

reducing risk of macrovascular and microvascular complications in type 2 diabetes: UKPDS 39. Br Med J 1998;317:713–720.

37. Hansson L, Lindholm LH, Niskanen L, et al. Effect of angiotensin-converting-enzyme inhibition compared with conventional therapy on cardiovascular morbidity and mortality in hypertension: the Captopril Prevention Project (CAPPP) randomised trial. Lancet 1999;353:611–616.

• 5 •

Animal Models:
Apoptosis and Oxidative Stress

Hani N. Sabbah, PhD,
and Elaine J. Tanhehco, PhD

Introduction

Left ventricular (LV) dysfunction, once established as a result of a primary insult to the myocardium such as an acute MI, can deteriorate over a period of months or years, despite the absence of clinically apparent intercurrent adverse events.[1–3] This progressive functional deterioration frequently culminates in the syndrome of congestive heart failure. The mechanism or mechanisms responsible for the progressive hemodynamic worsening are not fully understood but have been partly attributed to entry into a so-called vicious circle whereby compensatory mechanisms intended to maintain homeostasis, such as compensatory LV hypertrophy, dilation,[4,5] and enhanced sympathoadrenergic activity and renin-angiotensin activity,[6,7] themselves become factors that accelerate the process of progressive LV dysfunction. A working hypothesis advanced by us as well as others is that activation of these compensatory mechanisms can lead to ongoing progressive intrinsic contractile dysfunction of cardiomyocytes or to ongoing loss of viable cardiomyocytes or both. Structural alterations of cardiomyocyte and interstitium occur in the hypertrophied and failing heart, which, acting individually or in concert, can adversely impact global LV performance. Aside from cardiomyocyte hypertrophy, these abnormalities include myofibrillar disruption and disarray,[8] abnormalities of mitochondria with disruption of the internal membrane and organelle hyperplasia,[9] and car-

Supported, in part, by a grant from the National Heart, Lung and Blood Institute HL49090-07. From: Kukin ML, Fuster V (eds). *Oxidative Stress and Cardiac Failure.* Armonk, NY: Futura Publishing Co., Inc. ©2003.

diac interstitial abnormalities characterized by reactive interstitial fibrosis.[10,11] Electron microscopic studies of failed human hearts[12–17] and hearts of dogs with experimentally induced heart failure[8,9] have clearly demonstrated the existence of cardiomyocyte degeneration. These observations support the concept that ongoing myocyte loss may indeed occur in the failing heart. Recent studies from our laboratory in dogs and in patients with heart failure[18–20] have shown that cardiomyocyte death through apoptosis occurs in end-stage heart failure. What follows is a review of current evidence that supports the occurrence of cardiomyocyte apoptosis in ischemia and reperfusion, acute MI, cardiac hypertrophy and dilation, and chronic congestive heart failure. In addition, the discussion will focus on oxidative stress as a mediator of cardiomyocyte apoptosis.

Cell Death by Apoptosis Versus Death by Necrosis

Although considerable knowledge exists with respect to our understanding of the processes that govern cell proliferation, less is known about processes that control cell death. We have come to realize, and not by mere accident, that cardiomyocyte cell death occurs primarily through an evolutionary form of cell self-destruction termed "apoptosis," which was first described in 1972.[21] Apoptosis is an active, precisely regulated, energy-requiring, gene-directed process. Apoptosis plays a critical role in the control of cell populations in adult tissues and a central role in normal tissue development.[22–25] We have finally come to realize that even so-called post-mitotic cells or terminally differentiated cells, such as cardiac myocytes, retain the genetic machinery needed for programmed cell death.[26] Given that in mammals adult cardiac myocytes have, at best, a very limited capacity for self-renewal and are intended to survive and function for the entire life of the organism, death of any substantial number of adult cardiac muscle cells would have a devastating consequence as clearly illustrated in the clinical sequelae of acute MI.

While apoptosis is an active form of cell death dependent on gene-directed machinery,[27–29] necrosis is best described as an accidental death caused by cell injury due to external factors such as ischemia, toxins, and viruses.[25] Key features of necrosis are cell membrane rupture with associated inflammation.[30–32] This is not the case with apoptosis where death occurs in the absence of membrane rupture[33,34] and the cell can remain metabolically active for many hours[25] and perhaps even days. Early ultrastructural manifestations of apoptosis include compaction and segregation of nuclear chromatin into sharply delineated masses that abut the nuclear envelope,[18] cell shrinkage,[18] condensation of the cytoplasm, and mild convolution of the nuclear and cellular outlines. Subsequently, nu-

clear fragmentation occurs and the cell surface develops pediculated pro-
tuberances or "blebbing" and separate into membrane-bound apoptotic
bodies, which are phagocytosed or digested by adjacent cells. In contrast
to necrosis, the apoptotic cell-bound or membrane-bound bodies do not
rupture before being engulfed by macrophages.[34]

Another important feature of apoptosis is that it leads to the recognition, uptake, and degradation of membrane-intact dying cells by phagocytes without the release of cellular cytoplasmic contents and, consequently, without the induction of an inflammatory response, the latter a
characteristic feature of necrosis.[25,35] At the biochemical level, the apoptotic cell, unlike the cell undergoing necrosis, appears to initiate its own
death by the activation of endogenous proteases.[35] Activation of endogenous endonucleases leads to internucleosomal chromatin cleavage so that
extracted DNA runs as a characteristic "ladder" of oligonucleosomal fragments upon electrophoresis.[36,37] This is in contrast to the smear of de-
graded DNA characteristic of necrotic cells.[35] The surest way of confirming
apoptosis, however, remains the identification of characteristic morphological features by transmission electron microscopy. Because the process
of apoptosis runs its course in a short time, identifying and quantitating
cells undergoing apoptosis by this method is extremely difficult. Several
methods are used to identify and/or quantify apoptosis. One is based on
the demonstration of a characteristic ladder of small DNA fragments
(approximately 180 base pairs) on agarose-gel electrophoresis (DNA
ladder assay). Another is based on histochemical visualization of nuclear
DNA fragments by terminal deoxynucleotidyl transferase-mediated de-
oxyuridine triphosphate nick-end labeling (TUNEL method). Other methods include the use of Taq and Pfu polymerase probes, annexin V, and flow
cytometry.

Cardiomyocyte Apoptosis in Animal Models of Ischemia-Reperfusion and Acute Myocardial Infarction

It is well known that prolonged periods of myocardial ischemia lead
to tissue injury and cell death. Early reperfusion, even though vital for
myocardial tissue salvage, can also lead to increased myocyte loss in response to activation of inflammatory processes and the formation of oxygen free radical species.[38–40] It has long been maintained that myocyte loss
secondary to prolonged ischemia and/or ischemia/reperfusion results from
overt necrosis. While this form of cell death remains a primary cause of
tissue injury, recent studies have suggested that myocardial muscle cell
death, in the setting of an acute MI, may also occur through apoptosis.[41–46]
Cardiomyocyte apoptosis has been identified in both the early and the late

stages of acute MI in rats. Studies in rats with acute MI produced by coronary artery ligation showed apoptosis to be involved in muscle cell death within 2 hours of coronary ligation.[41] Furthermore, the number of cardiac myocytes undergoing apoptosis within 2 hours of coronary ligation far exceeded that of necrotic cardiomyocytes.[41] In this rat study, apoptosis continued to represent the major form of myocyte cell death for up to 6 hours after coronary ligation. Studies in rats with acute MI also showed a considerable number of apoptotic cardiac myocytes present for up to 7 days after MI. A study by Cheng et al., also conducted in rats with MI, showed that internucleosomal DNA fragmentation, a characteristic feature of apoptosis, could be detected as early as 3 hours after coronary artery occlusion and was also present for up to 1 month after coronary ligation,[43] suggesting that apoptosis may contribute to delayed myocyte loss following MI.[41,42] Studies in rats and rabbits have also demonstrated cardiomyocyte apoptosis following reperfusion of ischemic myocardium.[42,46] Studies in rats suggested that even though coronary reperfusion lowers the overall number of myocytes undergoing apoptosis in myocardium at risk, it accelerates myocyte apoptosis in nonsalvageable myocardium.[42] Cardiac myocyte apoptosis has also been observed in humans in the setting of acute MI.[44,45] A common theme that emerges from the above animal and human studies of ischemia/reperfusion and MI is the high prevalence of cardiomyocyte apoptosis in the peri-infarct border zone in comparison to myocardial regions remote from the infarction. This finding is also prominent in myocardium both in humans with end-stage heart failure secondary to coronary artery disease and in animal models of chronic heart failure produced by intracoronary microembolizations.[18,47]

Cardiomyocyte Apoptosis in Animal Models of Ventricular Hypertrophy and Dilation

Both ventricular hypertrophy and/or dilation are associated with loss of cardiac myocytes that result in focal sites of replacement fibrosis traditionally attributed to necrosis.[48,49] Recent studies, however, have shown that both hypertrophy and passive myocardial stretch, as in chamber dilation, are associated with myocyte apoptosis.[50–52] Studies by Cheng et al. showed a 21-fold higher incidence of myocyte DNA strand breaks in rat posterior papillary muscles exposed to high tension levels (50 mN/mm^2) as a result of overstretch compared to papillary muscles exposed to lower tension levels (7–8 mN/mm^2).[50] DNA laddering studies using extracts from muscles exposed to high stretch also revealed the presence of DNA fragments consistent with apoptosis, while degradation of DNA was not observed in nonoverstretched papillary muscles.[50] These data suggest that myocardial stretch alone, as can occur under conditions of acute or chronic volume overload, may be associated with myocyte loss through apoptosis. Studies in rats with pressure overload cardiac hypertrophy produced by aortic banding also showed the existence of cardiac myocyte apoptosis.[51] In this model, Teiger et al. identified myocyte apoptosis during the first 7 days after instituting aortic banding.[51] Indeed, cardiocyte apoptosis appeared to peak at 4 days and gradually subsided after 1 month of aortic banding. In contrast, cell growth in this animal model continued to occur up to 1 month after aortic banding. Based on these data, the authors concluded that in cardiac hypertrophy, an initial wave of cardiocyte apoptosis is linked to cell growth,[51] suggesting the possibility that apoptosis may be a prerequisite for cardiac remodeling. Recent studies from other laboratories have suggested that cardiocyte apoptosis may be important in the transition from compensated hypertrophy to failure.[52] In spontaneously hypertensive rats (SHRs) with symptoms of heart failure, Li et al. showed an almost 5-fold increase in the number of cardiac myocytes undergoing apoptosis compared to nonfailing SHRs.[52] These results suggest that the functional deterioration and loss of muscle mass that accompanies the transition from stable compensated hypertrophy to failure may be due, in part, to cardiac muscle cell death through apoptosis.

Cardiomyocyte Apoptosis in Animal Models of Heart Failure

As mentioned earlier, a characteristic feature of heart failure is the progressive worsening of global LV function that occurs despite the absence of any clinically evident adverse cardiac events. While the exact mechanisms that underlie this process are not known, the possibility that progressive LV dysfunction occurs, in part, as a result of ongoing loss of viable cardiomyocytes has been advanced based primarily on evidence of myocyte degeneration observed in hypertrophied and failed human hearts as well as in hearts of dogs with experimentally induced chronic heart failure.[7,8,53,54] Studies in animal models of heart failure have provided strong evidence for the existence of cardiac myocyte apoptosis. The very fact that myocyte apoptosis occurs in chronic heart failure, albeit at a pace yet to be defined and with a magnitude yet uncertain, supports the concept of ongoing loss of functional cardiac units in this disease state.

In our laboratory, cardiac myocyte apoptosis[18] was identified in a dog model of chronic heart failure produced by multiple sequential intracoronary microembolizations.[18,55] The model manifests many of the sequelae of heart failure seen in humans, including marked and sustained depression of LV systolic and diastolic function, LV hypertrophy and dilation, reduced cardiac output, increased systemic vascular resistance, and enhanced activity of the sympathetic nervous system evidenced by marked elevation of plasma norepinephrine concentration.[55] In a study by Sharov et al.,[18] two methods were used to establish the existence of myocyte apoptosis in the failed heart, namely, assessment by transmission electron microscopy for ultrastructural features of apoptosis and by the TUNEL method. To identify cells of myocyte origin, sections were double-stained with a monoclonal mouse ventricular heavy chain muscle antimyosin antibody.[18] The identification of myocytes is an essential step in localizing and estimating the number of cardiomyocytes undergoing apoptosis in the heart, given the considerable number of other interstitial cells that normally undergo apoptosis and are found even in the normal myocardium.[18]

Electron microscopic evidence of cardiomyocytes at various stages of apoptosis were identified in LV tissue obtained from every dog with heart failure but in none of the tissue specimens obtained from the LV of normal dogs.[18] Features of early stages of myocyte apoptosis included evidence of compaction of nuclear chromatin into sharply circumscribed uniformly dense masses that abut on the nuclear envelope. In these cells, the inner organelles were preserved and the sarcolemma was intact. Features of cardiomyocytes in advanced stages of apoptosis included an intact sarcolemma in the presence of highly disorganized inner organelles with only remnants of myofibrils and Z-band material that allowed the recognition of these bodies as cardiac myocytes in origin. Myocytes in advanced stages of apoptosis also manifested sarcolemmal blebbing or severe endocytosis and, in some instances, shrinkage and engulfment of the apoptotic remnant myocyte by macrophages.[18] In heart failure dogs, the majority of myocytes with features consistent with apoptosis were: (1) located in LV regions bordering old infarcts, (2) approximately 10-fold smaller than viable cardiocytes, (3) were frequently encircled by large amounts collagen, and (4) present in the absence of any associated inflammatory response.[18] In LV tissue from normal dogs examined by Sharov et al., none of the apoptotic cells positively labeled for nuclear DNA strand breaks could be ascribed to cardiomyocytes since none could be confirmed to contain myosin based on labeling with antimyosin antibody, suggesting that the process of cardiac myocyte apoptosis is very rare, if at all existent, in the normal myocardium. In contrast, in failed LV tissue apoptotic cardiac myocytes were invariably present and were primarily localized to LV regions bordering scar tissue or old infarcts.[18]

In a recent study, also conducted in our laboratory in dogs with microembolization-induced heart failure, the number of cardiomyocytes undergoing apoptosis was quantified histomorphometrically based on an assessment of the number of myocytes positively labeled for nuclear DNA strand breaks per 1000 cardiomyocytes.[56] Assessments were made in LV regions bordering old infarcts or scar tissue as well as in LV regions remote from any infarcts. In this study, as in previous studies, there was no evidence of nuclear DNA fragmentation in cardiac myocytes of normal dogs, whereas in dogs with heart failure, nuclear DNA fragmentation was identified in cardiomyocytes remote from any infarcts as well as in constituent cardiomyocytes of infarct border regions. As in previous studies,[18] the number of cardiomyocytes undergoing apoptosis was significantly higher in LV regions bordering old infarcts compared to LV regions remote from any infarcts (4.0 ± 0.5 versus 0.5 ± 0.3 nuclear DNA fragmentation events per 1000 cardiomyocytes). This observation further suggests that in the failing heart, the peri-infarct border region may be a primary site of myocyte loss through apoptosis, a finding consistent with the observation of profound ultrastructural cardiomyocyte abnormalities in these LV regions.[18,57]

Programmed cardiomyocyte cell death was also examined by Liu et al. in dogs with heart failure produced by rapid ventricular pacing. In all dogs, DNA laddering was determined and the number of myocyte nuclei showing DNA strand breaks was assessed using the TUNEL method. In addition, the percentage of cardiac myocytes labeled by the cell surface protein Fas, a molecular indicator of apoptotic cell death to be discussed later in this review, was measured by immunocytochemistry. DNA laddering, with stretches of DNA equivalent to 160 bp and 320 bp being most abundant, was detected in myocardium of dogs with heart failure but not in sham-operated control dogs.[18] Also consistent with observations in the microembolization model of heart failure, groups of apoptotic myocytes were frequently found in proximity to small areas of replacement fibrosis (scar tissue).[18]

Cardiomyocyte Apoptosis in Animal Models of the Failing Aged Heart

The aging process in both humans and animals is characterized, in part, by a significant loss of cardiac myocytes and by hypertrophy of the remaining myocytes.[58,59] In a healthy 70-year-old human male, nearly 30% of all of LV myocytes are lost over time as a result of the aging process alone and independent of any other cardiac disease state.[59,60] This cell loss may be partially responsible for the development of ventricular dysfunction and failure in the elderly. In recent years, a few studies have emerged that evoked apoptosis as a modality that contributes to the overall process of myocyte loss in the aging heart.[52,60] Kajstura et al. used Fischer 344 rats of varying age groups to quantify cardiomyocyte necrosis and apoptosis.[60] Groups of rats ages 3, 7, 12, 16, and 24 months were injected with antimyosin antibody to localize necrotic myocytes; they were subsequently killed and the hearts were harvested. The presence of DNA strand breaks in nuclei of cardiomyocytes was used to identify apoptosis and was confirmed by DNA laddering using whole tissue. The results showed that in the LV free wall, the extent of both myocyte necrosis and apoptosis increased with increasing age. In this rat model, the progressive increase in apoptotic and necrotic cell death was associated with the development of ventricular dysfunction and failure, which became apparent between 16 and 24 months of age.[60] An interesting finding of this study was the observation that, in contrast to cell necrosis, which tended to peak early and level off between 12 and 24 months of life, apoptosis tended to increase sharply between 12 and 24 months of life, suggesting perhaps that triggers of both forms of cell death may be different. The role of apoptosis in the transition from compensated cardiac hypertrophy to failure was examined by Li et al. in SHRs of advanced age.[52] The incidence of apoptotic myocyte nuclei in failed SHRs was ~40 cells per 100,000 nuclei compared to ~8 cells per 100,000 nuclei in nonfailed SHR rats. In age-matched WKY rats, the incidence of apoptotic nuclei of myocyte origin was ~2 per cells per 100,000 nuclei.[52]

Triggers of Cardiomyocyte Apoptosis

While our knowledge of the molecular machinery needed to activate this internally encoded genetic suicide program in proliferating cell populations is appreciable, less is known about the exact molecular circuit that controls apoptosis in postmitotic or terminally differentiated cells such as neurons or cardiac myocytes. The best-known factors controlling apoptosis are a multigene family of Bcl-2-like proteins with homologous structure, some of which, such as Bcl-2 itself, inhibits apoptosis and others, such as Bax, promote apoptosis.[61–63] In residual viable myocardium of rats with MI and ventricular failure in which cardiac myocyte apoptosis was present, Cheng et al. reported a decrease in the expression of Bcl-2 and an increase in the expression of Bax, an imbalance that favors apoptosis.[43] In myocardium of SHRs with heart failure, expression of Bcl-2 was unchanged compared to nonfailing SHRs.[52] Another well-known factor involved in apoptosis is the tumor suppressor p53, a ubiquitous DNA-binding protein implicated in cell cycle arrest through upregulation of p21/WAF-1, a cyclin-dependent kinase (Cdk) inhibitor.[63] The p53 protein is believed to induce apoptosis in response to DNA damage[64] and other signals such as increased expression of c-myc in a manner independent of cell cycle arrest.[65] In myocardium of SHRs with heart failure, WAF-1 mRNA levels were significantly increased in comparison to levels in myocardium of nonfailing rats.[52] Increased expression of p53 and expression of c-myc has also been reported from our laboratory in dogs with chronic heart failure.[66] Another factor involved in the regulation of apoptosis is the inteleukin-converting enzyme (ICE) family of cysteine proteases (ICE/CED-3) also known as caspases. Recent studies have suggested that

ICE-like proteases can mediate apoptosis in ventricular myocytes[67] and in rats with acute MI,[68] a suggestion based on the ability of certain pharmacological inhibitors of ICE-like proteases, such as ZVAD-fmk, a peptide caspase inhibitor, to block, at least in part, the apoptosis process.[67,68] Triggering of Fas/APO-1 (CD95) has also been shown to induce activation of stress-activated protein kinases (SAPKs), also known as Jun kinases (JNKs),[69] which are members of the mitogen-activated protein kinases (MAPKs).

Factors other than reentry into the cell cycle may also induce apoptosis in failing cardiomyocytes. It has been suggested that apoptosis accompanies loss of mitochondrial function, which could mean that mitochondria may have an important function in regulating apoptosis. The proto-oncogene Bcl-2, a protein that blocks programmed cell death, is localized to the inner mitochondrial membrane.[61] Furthermore, several intermediaries proposed in the linking of Bcl-2 to caspase activation include mitochondrial release of cytochrome *c* and mitochondrial release of an apoptosis-inducing factor.[35] Mitochondrial abnormalities have been described in patients and in dogs with heart failure that include structural disruption of the inner membrane, hyperplasia, and reduced organelle size.[8] In myocardium of dogs with chronic heart failure, we have also shown a marked decrease in mitochondrial respiratory parameters compared to normal dogs.[70]

While factors that trigger cardiocyte apoptosis in the failing heart are not fully understood, there is some evidence to suggest that certain pathophysiological conditions common to the heart failure state may contribute to, or indeed, may play an important role in promoting cardiac myocyte apoptosis. The possibility exists that apoptosis may be induced by the same agents that produce necrosis, with the type of cell death being dependent on the severity of the insult rather than its qualitative nature.[71] Some evidence exists that suggests that increased cytosolic calcium concentration,[72] formation of oxygen free radicals,[73] and exposure to hypoxia or excess levels of angiotensin II or norepinephrine may each be a trigger for apoptosis. One cannot exclude the possibility that some of these triggers, and perhaps all, may exist in the failing heart. Of these, the formation of oxygen free radicals has received considerable interest in recent years.

Oxidative Stress and Apoptosis

Oxidants, such as superoxide, hydroxyl radicals, hydrogen peroxide (H_2O_2), and peroxynitrite, have been implicated as arbiters of tissue damage in a variety of pathologies, including myocardial ischemia and heart failure. Even though endogenous antioxidants normally maintain intracellular redox levels, these defenses may be overwhelmed under certain physiological situations. Excessive free radical production results in cellular necrosis; however, sublethal levels can trigger apoptosis. Potential intracellular sources of free radicals include mitochondria, xanthine oxidase, and arachidonate metabolism. The heart may be especially susceptible to oxidative stress since its continual activity may contribute to the generation of oxidants, which are byproducts of metabolism.[74] Infiltration of neutrophils into the area at risk and locally produced nitric oxide represent two other sources of oxygen free radicals. The metabolism of certain drugs can generate oxidants to the extent that they elicit tissue damage. The antineoplastic agent, doxorubicin, is a known inducer of congestive heart failure and stimulates apoptosis in rat cardiomyocytes.[75] This effect is reversed by the water soluble antioxidant, trolox, indicating that doxorubicin toxicity occurs via the generation of oxygen free radicals.[75]

Reintroduction of oxygenated blood to previously ischemic or hypoxic tissue may also precipitate the generation of free radicals. Such a situation can occur during the treatment of myocardial ischemia or heart failure. In the failing heart, development of fibrosis impedes oxygen diffusion to the cardiomyocytes. A decrease in capillary density and increase in oxygen diffusion distance between myocytes have also been observed in failing hearts.[76] It has been proposed that hypoxia and reoxygenation trigger apoptosis during heart failure and are partially responsible for the loss of cardiomyocytes in this disease. In cases of ischemic cardiomyopathy, the heart may be subjected to intermittent periods of hypoxia and reoxygenation. Even though cardiomycyte apoptosis can be detected throughout the failing heart, apoptotic cardiomyocyte cells, as alluded to earlier, are particularly dense around the borders of old infarcts, where most fibrosis occurs.

Even though the process by which free radicals induce apoptosis remains to be fully elucidated, it is clear that oxidants upregulate the expression and activation of apoptosis-related proteins. The c-Jun N-terminal/stress-activated protein kinase (JNK/SAPK), and mitogen-activated/extracellular signal-regulated kinase (MAPK/ERK) pathways can be activated by reactive oxygen species (Figure 1).[77,78] Both of these cascades have been shown to be involved in apoptosis. Exposure of cardiomyocytes to H_2O_2 causes caspase-3 cleavage[79] and increases MAPK activity.[78] Hydrogen peroxide also increases ERK activity, which is blocked by genistein, a tyrosine kinase inhibitor.[80] Oxidative stress induced by hypoxia and reoxygenation increases cleavage of caspases[81] and expression of Fas[82] and Raf-1,[83] all of which are associated with the induction of apoptosis. Recently, we also determined that exposure of failing cardiomyocytes to hypoxia/reoxygenation increases p38 MAPK activity and that inhibition of MAPK prevents hypoxia-induced apoptosis.[84]

Mitochondria are thought to be an important organelle in the initia-

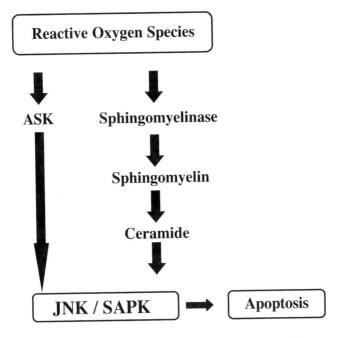

Figure 1. Activation of the JNK/SAPK pathway by oxidants via ASK or ceramide triggers apoptosis.

tion and regulation of apoptosis (Figure 2). In addition to serving as an abundant source of oxidants, they are also physically associated with some apoptotic proteins. Prior to the induction of apoptosis, Bax, a pro-apoptotic protein, translocates to mitochondria and its subsequent dimerization triggers cell death.[85] The mitochondrial membrane potential is also thought to influence the incidence of apoptosis. A loss of mitochondrial membrane potential ensues after exposure of cardiomyocytes to H_2O_2.[79] It has been proposed that Bcl-2 may aid in maintaining the mitochondrial membrane potential, since it can form ion-conducting pores.[79,86] Oxidative stress can also cause cytochrome *c* release from mitochondria.[79] Cook et al. have suggested that H_2O_2 induces the translocation of Bad, which leads to the loss of Bcl-2 from the mitochondrial membrane, thus depolarizing the mitochondria and stimulating cytochrome *c* release, triggering apoptosis.[79] Cytochrome *c* activates caspases, which are essential enzymes for the induction of apoptosis.[87] Another apoptotic protein affected by oxygen free radicals is the aspartic protease, cathepsin D. Oxidative stress causes cathepsin D release from lysosomes to the cytosol and is reversed by alpha tocopherol succinate.[88,89] Although cathepsin D release was not correlated with apoptosis in this study, it has been previously reported that inhibition of cathepsin D release prevents free radical-induced apoptosis.[89,90]

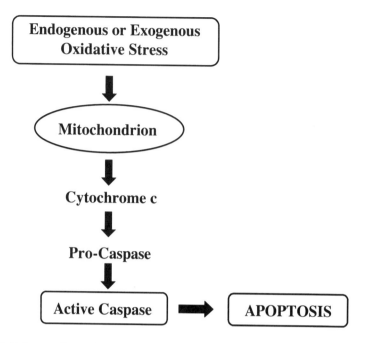

Figure 2. Release of cytochrome *c* from mitochondria into the cytosol by reactive oxygen species induces apoptosis by activating caspases.

Adderley et al. found that cardiomyocytes incubated with H_2O_2 or doxorubicin increase cyclooxygenase (COX-2) as well as ERK 1/2 expression.[91] Inhibition of ERK activation blocks the elevation in COX-2 production.[91] Since COX-2 is essential for prostaglandin synthesis and prostaglandins protect cells from a variety of stresses, expression of COX-2 may be an endogenous protective mechanism against apoptosis and free radical-mediated cell injury.

The ability of reoxygenation to elicit apoptosis may depend on the availability of intracellular antioxidants, namely thiols, to counteract the oxidant load. While only small changes are noted in apoptotic protein expression and activation during hypoxia itself, significant increases occur upon reoxygenation. Laderoute and Webster demonstrated that JNK/SAPK activation was inversely correlated with reductions in intracellular glutathione (GSH).[92] Reoxygenation did not activate JNK/SAPK until a there was a sufficient reduction in GSH levels induced by hypoxia. They also determined that antioxidants inhibit JNK/SAPK activation and that depletion of GSH activates JNK/SAPK upon reoxygenation. In addition, reoxygenation increases c-Jun phosphorylation. Interestingly, these effects were specific to cardiomyocytes, as hypoxia and reoxygenation did not activate kinases in skeletal myotubes or primary cardiac fibroblasts. Another theory implicating the role of endogenous antioxidants in reoxygenation-mediated apoptosis centers around Fas and thioredoxin. It has been proposed that Fas activates apoptosis signal-regulating kinase (ASK1), which then activates MAP kinase kinase (MAPKK). MAPKK can subsequently activate the pro-apoptotic JNK/SAPK and p38 MAP kinases.[77] ASK1 activity is downregulated by binding to thioredoxin, an endogenous antioxidant.[93] Overexpression of ASK1 has been shown to promote apoptosis, indicating its importance to cell death.[94]

Reactive oxygen species have also been shown to mediate cytokine-induced degradation of sphingomyelin to ceramide. Ceramide activates the JNK/SAPK cascade and can trigger apoptosis[95] (Figure 1). Cardiomyocytes treated with TNF-α or interleukin-1β exhibited a reduction in GSH levels, accompanied by hydrolysis of sphingomyelin to ceramide, and apoptosis. The presence of exogenously administered antioxidants blocked all of these effects. In addition, exposure of cardiomyocytes to oxidants also resulted in degradation of sphingomyelin to ceramide, which was inhibited by antioxidants.[96]

Apoptosis is thought to contribute to the tissue injury that occurs during myocardial ischemia and reperfusion. Antioxidants have been shown to be cardioprotective in a variety of ischemia/reperfusion models and it has been proposed that inhibition of apoptosis may be one mechanism by which they exert their beneficial effects.[97,98] Attenuation of reperfusion-induced apoptosis by antioxidants indicates that free radicals mediate this mode of cell death in the ischemic heart.[98] In isolated rabbit hearts subjected to ischemia and reperfusion, treatment with the p38 MAPK inhibitor, SB203580, decreased the incidence of apoptosis, reduced infarct size and creatine kinase loss, and maintained hemodynamic function compared with vehicle-treated controls.[99] Similar to cells exposed to hypoxia and reoxygenation, only small increases in p38 were detected during the ischemic period. However, upon reperfusion, significant elevations in p38 levels occurred. Activation of p38 was highest at 10 minutes after reperfusion and, accordingly, SB203580 was most effective when given before ischemia as opposed to after the initiation of reperfusion. These observations fit well given the short life of free radicals. In contrast, in an in vivo rat model of myocardial ischemia/reperfusion, chronic treatment (7 weeks) with antioxidants started 3 days after infarction also prevented apoptosis, caspase-3 activity, p53, and Bax expression.[100] However, these parameters were not correlated with function or infarct expansion, and therefore the physiological consequences of these effects are not known. These studies emphasize the importance of considering the differences between ischemia/reperfusion models when interpreting data regarding mechanisms of apoptosis.

Conclusions and Future Directions

At present, there appears to be sufficient evidence based on studies in animal models of heart failure and in explanted failed human hearts to support the concept that cardiomyocyte apoptosis takes place in the failing heart. While important, the significance of this finding in the context of the overall pathophysiology of this disease remains uncertain. Two critical questions remain unanswered. First, what pathophysiological factor(s) inherent to heart failure trigger cardiomyocyte apoptosis? While the concept of oxygen free radicals is, at present, appealing, it is by no means established. Lacking is also an answer to a second question, namely, how important is cardiomyocyte apoptosis in the progression of LV dysfunction and the transition to overt failure? An answer to this question requires an accurate determination of the rate at which cardiomyocytes are lost in the failing heart as a result of apoptosis. This is by no means an easy task. While undoubtedly difficult, future studies must be directed toward obtaining answers to these central questions. Only then will the importance of apoptosis in the setting of heart disease be fully appreciated.

References

1. Ertl G, Kochsiek K. Development, early treatment, and prevention of heart failure. Circulation 1993;87:IV1–IV2.
2. Mckee PA, Castelli WP, Mcnamara PM, et al. The natural history of congestive heart failure: the Framingham Study. N Engl J Med 1971;285:1441–1446.
3. Konstam MA, Rousseau MF, Kronenberg MW, et al. Effects of the angiotensin-converting enzyme inhibitor enalapril on long-term progression of left ventricular dysfunction in patients with heart failure. Circulation 1992;86:431–438.
4. Anversa P, Olivetti G, Capasso JM. Cellular basis of ventricular remodeling after myocardial infarction. Am J Cardiol 1991;68:7D–16D.
5. Pfeffer MA, Lamas GA, Vaughan DE, et al. Effect of captopril on progressive ventricular dilatation after anterior myocardial infarction. N Engl J Med 1988;319:80–86.
6. Levine TB, Francis GS, Goldsmith SR, et al. Activity of the sympathetic nervous system assessed by plasma hormone levels and their relation to hemodynamic abnormalities in congestive heart failure. Am J Cardiol 1982;49:1659–1666.
7. Curtiss C, Cohn JN, Vrobel T, et al. Role of the renin-angiotensin system in the systemic vasoconstriction of chronic congestive heart failure. Circulation 1978;58:763–770.
8. Sabbah HN, Sharov VG, Riddle JM, et al. Mitochondrial abnormalities in myocardium of dogs with chronic heart failure. J Mol Cell Cardiol 1992;24:1333–1347.
9. Sharov VG, Sabbah HN, Shimoyama H, et al. Abnormalities of contractile structures in viable myocytes of the failing heart. Intl J Cardiol 1994;43:287–297.

10. Schaper J, Hein S. The structural correlate of reduced cardiac function in human dilated cardiomyopathy. Heart Failure 1993;9:95–111.
11. Sabbah HN, Sharov VG, Lesch M, et al. Progression of heart failure: a role for interstitial fibrosis. Mol Cell Biochem 1995;147:29–34.
12. Perennec J, Hatt PY. Myocardial morphology in cardiac hypertrophy and failure: electron microscopy in man. In: Swynghedauw B, ed. Cardiac Hypertrophy and Failure. John Libbey Eurotext, London, 1988; 267–276.
13. Baandrup U, Florio RA, Roters FF, et al. Electron microscopic investigation of endomyocardial biopsy samples in hypertrophy and cardiomyopathy: a semiquantitative study in 48 patients. Circulation 1981;63;1289–1297.
14. Knieriem HJ. Electron-microscopic findings in congestive cardiomyopathy. In: Kaltenbach M, Loogen F, Olsen EGJ, eds. Cardiomyopathy and Cardiac Biopsy. Springer-Verlag, NY, 1978; 71–86.
15. Kunkel B, Lapp H, Kober G, et al. Ultrastructural evaluations in early and advanced congestive cardiomyopathies. In: Kaltenbach M, Loogen F, Olsen EGJ, eds. Cardiomyopathy and Cardiac Biopsy. Springer-Verlag, NY, 1978; 87–99.
16. Maron BJ, Ferrans VJ, Roberts WC. Ultrastructural features of degenerated cardiac muscle cells in patients with cardiac hypertrophy. Am J Pathol 1975; 79:387–413.
17. Ferrans VJ, Morrow AG, Roberts WC. Myocardial ultrastructure in idiopathic hypertrophic subaortic stenosis: a study of operatively excised left ventricular outflow tract muscle in 14 patients. Circulation 1972;45:769–792.
18. Sharov VG, Sabbah HN, Shimoyama H, et al. Evidence of cardiocyte apoptosis in myocardium of dogs with chronic heart failure. Am J Pathol 1996;148: 141–149.
19. Narula J, Haider N, Virmani R, et al. Apoptosis in myocytes in end-stage heart failure. N Engl J Med 1996;335;1182–1189.
20. Olivetti G, Abbi R, Quaini F, et al. Apoptosis in the failing human heart. N Engl J Med 1996;336:1131–1141.
21. Kerr JFR, Wyllie AH, Curie AR. Apoptosis: a basic biological phenomenon with widespread implication in tissue kinetics. Br J Cancer 1972;26:239–257.
22. Steller H. Mechanisms and genes of cellular suicide. Science 1995;267:1445–1449.
23. Gerschenson LE, Rotello RJ. Apoptosis and cell proliferation are terms of the growth equation. In: Tomei LD, Cope FO, eds. Apoptosis: The Molecular Basis of Cell Death. Cold Spring Harbor Laboratory Press, Plainview, NY, 1991; 3:175–192.
24. Budtz PE. Epidermal homeostasis: a new model that includes apoptosis. In: Tomei LD, Cope FO, eds. Apoptosis II: The Molecular Basis of Apoptosis in Disease. Cold Spring Harbor Laboratory Press, Plainview, NY, 1994; 8:165–183.
25. Savill J. Apoptosis in disease. Eur J Clin Invest 1994;24:715–723.
26. Barr PJ, Tomei LD. Apoptosis and its role in human disease. Bio/Technology 1994;12:487–493.
27. Wyllie AH, Kerr JFR, Currie AR. Cell death: the significance of apoptosis. Int Rev Cytol 1980;68:251–306.
28. Cohen JJ. Programmed cell death in the immune system. Adv Immunol 1991; 50:55–85.
29. Ellis RE, Yuan J, Horvitz HR. Mechanisms and functions of cell death. Ann Rev Cell Biol 1991;7:663–698.
30. Reimer KA, Jennings RB. Ion and water shifts, cellular. In: Cowley RA, Trump BF, eds. Pathophysiology of Shock, Anoxia, and Ischemia. Williams and Wilkins, Baltimore/London, 1992; 132–146.

31. Trump BF, Berezesky IK, Cowley RA. The cellular and subcellular characteristics of acute and chronic injury with emphasis on the role of calcium. In: Cowley RA, Trump BF, eds. Pathophysiology of Shock, Anoxia, and Ischemia. Willams and Wilkins, Baltimore/London, 1982; 6–46.
32. Fleckenstein A, Janke J, Doring HJ, et al. Ca^{++} overload as the determinant factor in the production of catecholamine-induced myocardial lesions. Rec Adv Stud Card Struct Metabol 1973;2:445–466.
33. Kerr JFR. A histochemical study of hypertrophy and ischemic injury of rat liver with special reference to changes in lysosomes. J Pathol Bacteriol 1965; 90:419–455.
34. Kerr JFR. Shrinkage necrosis: a distinct mode of cellular death. J Pathol 1971; 105:13–20.
35. Thompson CB. Apoptosis in the pathogenesis and treatment of disease. Science 1995;267:1456–1462.
36. Wyllie AH. Glucocorticoid-induced thymocyte apoptosis is associated with endogenous endonuclease activation. Nature 1980;284:555–556.
37. Arends MJ, Morris RG, Wyllie AH. Apoptosis: the role of the endonuclease. Am J Pathol 1990;136:593–608.
38. Entman ML, Smith CW. Postreperfusion inflammation: a model for reaction to injury in cardiovascular disease. Cardiovasc Res 1994;28:1301–1311.
39. Jeroudi MO, Hartley CJ, Bolli R. Myocardial reperfusion injury: role of oxygen radicals and potential therapy with antioxidants. Am J Cardiol 1994;73: 2B–7B.
40. Kloner RA, Przyklenk K, Whittacker P. Deleterious effects of oxygen radicals in ischemia/reperfusion: resolved and unresolved issues. Circulation 1989;80: 1115–1127.
41. Kajstura J, Cheng W, Reiss K, et al. Apoptotic and necrotic myocyte cell death are independent contributing variables of infarct size in rats. Lab Invest 1996; 74:86–107.
42. Fliss H, Gattinger D. Apoptosis in ischemic and reperfused myocardium. Circ Res 1996;79:949–956.
43. Cheng W, Kajstura J, Nitahara JA, et al. Programmed myocyte cell death affects the viable myocardium after infarction in rats. Exp Cell Res 1996;226: 316–327.
44. Saraste A, Pulkki K, Kallajoki M, et al. Apoptosis in human acute myocardial infarction. Circulation 1997;95:320–323.
45. Olivetti G, Quaini F, Sala R, et al. Acute myocardial infarction in humans is associated with activation of programmed myocyte cell death in the surviving portion of the heart. J Mol Cell Cardiol 1994;28:2005–2016.
46. Gottlieb RA, Burleson KO, Kloner RA, et al. Reperfusion injury induces apoptosis in rabbit cardiomyocytes. J Clin Invest 1994;94:1621–1628.
47. Sharov VG, Goussev A, Higgins RSD, et al. Higher incidence of cardiocyte apoptosis in failed explanted hearts of patients with ischemic versus idiopathic dilated cardiomyopathy (abstract). Circulation 1997;96:I-17.
48. Capasso JM, Plackai T, Olivetti G, et al. Left ventricular failure induced by long-term hypertension in rats. Circ Res 1990;66:1400–1412.
49. Tomanek RJ, Aydelotte MR. Late onset renal hypertension in old rats alters left ventricular structure and function. Am J Physiol 1992;262:H531–H538.
50. Cheng W, Li B, Kajstura J, et al. Stretch-induced programmed myocyte cell death. J Clin Invest 1995;96:2247–2259.
51. Teiger E, Dam T-V, Richard L, et al. Apoptosis in pressure overload-induced heart hypertrophy in the rat. J Clin Invest 1996;97:2891–2897.

52. Li Z, Bing OHL, Long X, et al. Increased cardiomyocyte apoptosis during the transition to heart failure in the spontaneously hypertensive rat. Am J Physiol 1997;272:H2313–H2319.
53. Perennec J, Hatt PY. Myocardial morphology in cardiac hypertrophy and failure: electron microscopy in man. In: Swynghedauw B, ed. Cardiac Hypertrophy and Failure. John Libbey Eurotext, London, 1988; 267–276.
54. Baandrup U, Florio RA, Roters FF, et al. Electron microscopic investigation of endomyocardial biopsy samples in hypertrophy and cardiomyopathy: a semiquantitative study in 48 patients. Circulation 1981;63:1289–1297.
55. Sabbah HN, Stein PD, Kono T, et al. A canine model of chronic heart failure produced by multiple sequential coronary microembolizations. Am J Physiol 1991;260:H1379–H1384.
56. Sabbah HN, Sharov VG, Goussev A, et al. Evidence for ongoing loss of cardiomyocytes in dogs with progressive left ventricular dysfunction and failure. Circulation 1997;96:I-754.
57. Sharov VG, Sabbah HN, Ali AS, et al. Abnormalities of cardiomyocytes in regions bordering fibrous scars in dogs with chronic heart failure. Int'l J Cardiol 1997;60:273–279.
58. Anversa P, Hiler B, Ricci R, et al. Myocyte cell loss and myocyte hypertrophy in the aging rat heart. J Am Coll Cardiol 1986;8:1441–1448.
59. Olivetti G, Melissari M, Capasso JM, et al. Cardiomyopathy of the aging human heart: myocyte loss and reactive cellular hypertrophy. Circ Res 1991;68:1560–1568.
60. Kajstura J, Cheng W, Sarangarajan R, et al. Necrotic and apoptotic myocyte cell death in the aging heart of Fischer 344 rats. Am J Physiol 1996;271:H1215–H1228.
61. Hockenberg D, Nunez G, Milliman C, et al. Bcl-2 is an inner mitochondrial membrane protein that blocks programmed cell death. Nature 1990;348:334–336.
62. Allsopp TE, Wyatt S, Paterson HF, et al. The proto-oncogene Bcl-2 can selectively rescue neutrophic factor-dependent neurons from apoptosis. Cell 1993;73:295–307.
63. MacLellan WR, Schneider MD. Death by design: programmed cell death in cardiovascular biology and disease. Circ Res 1997;81:137–144.
64. Clarke AR, Purdie CA, Harrison DJ, et al. Thymocyte apoptosis induced by p53-dependent and independent pathways. Nature 1993;362:786–787.
65. Wagner AJ, Kokontis JM, Hay N: Myc-mediated apoptosis requires wild-type p53 in a manner independent of cell cycle arrest and the ability of p53 to induce p21waf1/cipl. Genes Dev 1994;8:2817–2830.
66. Sharov VG, Sabbah HN, Goussev A, et al. Apoptosis associated proteins c-myc and p53 are expressed in cardiomyocytes isolated from dogs with chronic heart failure (abstract). Circulation 1996;94:I-471.
67. Pabla R, Rees SA, Know KA, et al. Apoptosis is mediated by ICE-like proteases in ventricular myocytes (abstract). Circulation 1986;94:I-282.
68. Bialik S, Geenen DL, Sasson IE, et al. The caspase family of cysteine proteases mediate cardiac myocyte apoptosis during myocardial infarction (abstract). Circulation 1997;96:I552.
69. Cahill MA, Peter ME, Kischkel FC, et al. CD95 (APO-1/Fas) induces activation of SAP kinases downstream of ICE-like proteases. Oncogene 1996;13:2087–2096.
70. Sharov VG, Cook JM, Lesch M, et al. Transmural dysfunction of mitochondrial respiration in the failing canine left ventricle (abstract). J Mol Cell Cardiol 1996;28:A142.

71. Kerr JFR, Harmon BV. Definition and incidence of apoptosis: an historical perspective. In: Tomei LD, Cope FO, eds. Apoptosis: The Molecular Basis of Cell Death. Cold Spring Harbor Laboratory Press, Plainview, NY, 1991; 5–29.

72. Orrenius S, McConkey DJ, Bellomo G, et al. Role of Ca^{2+} in toxic cell killing. Trends Pharmacol Sci 1989;10:281–285.

73. Gottlieb RA, Burleson KO, Kloner RA, et al. Reperfusion injury induces apoptosis in rabbit cardiomyocytes. J Clinic Invest 1994;94:1621–1628.

74. Feuerstein G, Yue TL, Ma X, et al. Novel mechanisms in the treatment of heart failure: inhibition of oxygen radicals and apoptosis by carvedilol. Progr Cardiovasc Dis 1998;41(Suppl 1):17–24.

75. Kumar D, Kirshenbaum L, Li T, et al. Apoptosis in isolated adult cardiomyocytes exposed to Adriamycin. Ann NY Acad Sci 1999;874:156–168.

76. Sabbah HN, Sharov VG, Lesch M, et al. Progression of heart failure: a role for interstitial fibrosis. Mol Cell Biochem 1995;147:29–34.

77. Davis W Jr, Ronai Z, Tew KD. Cellular thiols and reactive oxygen species in drug induced apoptosis. J Pharmacol Exp Therap 2001;296:1–6.

78. Guyton KZ, Liu Y, Gorospe M, et al. Activation of mitogen-activated protein kinase by H_2O_2. J Biol Chem 1996;271:4138–4142.

79. Cook SA, Sugden PH, Clerk A. Regulation of Bcl-2 family proteins during development and in response to oxidative stress in cardiac myocytes: association with changes in mitochondrial membrane potential. Circ Res 1999;85:940–949.

80. Aikawa R, Komuro I, Yamazaki T, et al. Oxidative stress activates extracellular signal-regulated kinases through Src and Ras in cultured cardiac myocytes of neonatal rats. J Clin Invest 1997;100:1813–1821.

81. Hampton MB, Fadeel B, Orrenius S. Redox regulation of the caspases during apoptosis. Ann NY Acad Sci 1998;854:328–335.

82. Tanaka M, Ito H, Adachi S, et al. Hypoxia induces apoptosis with enhanced expression of Fas antigen messenger RNA in cultured neonatal rat cardiomyocytes. Circ Res 1994;75:426–433.

83. Seko Y, Tobe K, Ueki K, et al. Hypoxia and hypoxia/reoxygenation activate Raf-1, mitogen-activated protein kinase kinase, mitogen-activated protein kinases, and S6 kinase in cultured rat cardiac myocytes. Circ Res 1996;78:82–90.

84. Sharov VG, Todor A, Mishima T, et al. Hypoxia, angiotensin-II, and norepinephrine-mediated apoptosis is stimulus-specific in canine failed cardiomyocytes: a role for p38 MAPK, fas-L, and cyclin D_1. In preparation.

85. Gross A, Jockel J, Wei MC, et al. Enforced dimerization of BAX results in its translocation, mitochondrial dysfunction and apoptosis. EMBO J 1998;17:3878–3885.

86. Schlesinger PH, Gross A, Yin XM, et al. Comparison of the ion channel characteristics of proapoptotic Bax and antiapoptotic Bcl-2. Proc Natl Acad Sci 1997;94:11357–11362.

87. Liu X, Kim CN, Yang J, et al. Induction of apoptotic program in cell-free extracts: requirement for dATP and cytochrome c. Cell 1996;86:147–157.

88. Roberg K, Ollinger K. Oxidative stress causes relocation of the lysosomal enzyme cathepsin D with ensuing apoptosis in neonatal rat cardiomyocytes. Am J Pathol 1998;152:1151–1156.

89. Kagedal K, Johansson U, Ollinger K. The lysosomal protease cathepsin D mediates apoptosis induced by oxidative stress. FASEB J 2001;15:1592–1594.

90. Ollinger K. Inhibition of cathepsin D prevents free radical-induced apoptosis in rat cardiomyocytes. Arch Biochem Biophys 2000;373:346–351.

91. Adderley SR, Fitzgerald DJ. Oxidative damage of cardiomyocytes is limited by extracellular regulated kinases 1/2-mediated induction of cyclooxygenase-2. J Biol Chem 1999;274:5038–5046.
92. Laderoute KR, Webster KA. Hypoxia/reoxygenation stimulates Jun kinase activity through redox signaling in cardiac myocytes. Circ Res 1997;80:335–344.
93. Saitoh M, Nishitoh H, Fujii M, et al. Mammalian thioredoxin is a direct inhibitor of apoptosis signal-regulating kinase (ASK) 1. EMBO J 1998;17:2596–2606.
94. Ichijo H, Nishida E, Irie K, et al. Induction of apoptosis by ASK1, a mammalian MAPKKK that activates SAPK/JNK and p38 signaling pathways. Science 1997;275:90–94.
95. Verheij M, Bose R, Lin XH, et al. Requirement for ceramide-initiated SAPK/JNK signaling in stress-induced apoptosis. Nature 1996;380:75–79.
96. Singh I, Pahan K, Khan M, et al. Cytokine-mediated induction of ceramide production is redox sensitive: implications to proinflammatory cytokine-mediated apoptosis in demyelinating diseases. J Biol Chem 1998;273:20354–20362.
97. Dobsak P, Courderot-Masuyer C, Zeller M, et al. Antioxidative properties of pyruvate and protection of the ischemic rat heart during cardioplegia. J Cardiovasc Pharmacol 1999;34:651–659.
98. Maulik N, Yoshida T, Das DK. Oxidative stress developed during the reperfusion of ischemic myocardium induces apoptosis. Free Rad Biol Med 1998;24:869–875.
99. Ma XL, Kumar S, Gao F, et al. Inhibition of p38 mitogen-activated protein kinase decreases cardiomyocyte apoptosis and improves cardiac function after myocardial ischemia and reperfusion. Circulation 1999;99:1685–1691.
100. Oskarsson HJ, Coppey L, Weiss RM, et al. Antioxidants attenuate myocyte apoptosis in the remote non-infarcted myocardium following large myocardial infarction. Cardiovasc Res 2000;45:679–687.

• 6 •

Oxygen Free Radicals, Iron, and Cytokines in Heart Failure:
From Bench to Bedside

Mona Shawky, MD, Neelam Khaper, PhD,
and Peter Liu, MD

Introduction

Heart Failure Is a State of Increased Oxidative Stress

Heart failure is a disease complex that initiates with cardiac injury, followed by a series of adaptations that include genomic, biochemical, structural, and functional adaptations. When the intrinsic adaptive capacity is exceeded, we observe the progressive ventricular dysfunction and adverse remodeling associated with worsening clinical symptoms and compromised survival.[1] One of the pathways that is stimulated in this process is oxidative stress.

Previously it was difficult to demonstrate oxidative stress in the setting of heart failure. With the advent of techniques measuring markers of oxidative stress, there has been accumulating evidence that heart failure is a state of free radical excess. Initial studies by Diaz-Velez documented in 53 patients that malondialdehyde levels are linearly correlated with the duration of heart failure, and inversely related to left ventricular ejection fraction.[2] McMurray has also documented multiple parameters of oxidative stress to be elevated in patients with heart failure of either ischemic or nonischemic etiology, as compared to normals.[3]

Supported in part by grants from the Heart and Stroke Foundation of Ontario, and the Canadian Institutes of Health Research.
From: Kukin ML, Fuster V (eds). *Oxidative Stress and Cardiac Failure*. Armonk, NY: Futura Publishing Co., Inc. ©2003.

More recently, Keith et al. have has also documented the increase of lipid peroxides in the serum of patients with heart failure, and this directly correlated with the severity of heart failure.[4] Furthermore, the levels correlated with the concentration of soluble TNF receptors, indicating an association of oxidative stress with cytokines and inflammatory markers. Therefore, we have consistent evidence to suggest that markers of oxidative stress correlate with the severity of heart failure from multiple studies involving multiple populations.

Clinical Importance of Increased Oxidative Stress

To date the majority of the data on oxidative stress have suggested an important link between markers of free radical activation in association with heart failure. Whether they actually contribute to disease progression is more challenging to prove amidst the multitude of activated pathways. However, there are increasing data to suggest that oxidative stress is an important prognostic factor in heart failure. In the PROFILE trial, in which the patients were randomized to either the vasodilator-inotrope flosequinon or placebo, on the background of standard heart failure treatment medications, many patients reached the final endpoint of death. Interestingly, of the various neurohumoral markers of prognosis, the best predictor of the group was the adrenochromes, which are the oxidation products of catecholamines. This suggests that the oxidation process in concert with neurohumoral activation may be a particularly potent prognosticator.

From a mechanistic point of view, there is a plethora of evidence that oxidative stress is an important facilitator of heart failure progression. Dhalla and Singal have shown that in a guinea pig aortic banding model, initial hypertrophy at 10 weeks was associated with a high redox state but few peroxidation products. However, at 20 weeks when there is heart failure, there was marked escalation of peroxidation.[5] They have also demonstrated that the administration of vitamin E significantly decreased the myofibrillar disorganization and improved the ventricular function with time following injury. This has also been replicated in a rat model of myocardial infarction, with reduction in catalase and reduced glutathione and concomitant increase in lipid peroxidation.[6] These mechanisms are also the dominant determinants in the outcomes in the setting of adriamycin cardiomyopathy.[7]

Potential Biological Role of Oxidative Stress

Oxygen free radicals indeed have wide-ranging biological and pathological effects that include the induction of gene expression, promotion of cell proliferation and hypertrophy, apoptosis, anoikis,[8] modulation of endothelial function, decreased EDRF (NO), increased predisposition to thrombosis, expression of a proinflammatory phenotype, and modification of the extracellular matrix.[9,10] A potential mechanism of oxidative damage that is less appreciated is the nitration of tyrosine residues of proteins, peroxidation of lipids, and degradation of DNA and oligonucleotide fragments.

In view of potent biological effects of free radicals, even though they are the normal byproducts of oxidative metabolism, several mechanisms have evolved to protect the cells from potential cytotoxic damage. Cells have developed various enzymatic (such as superoxide dismutase, catalase, and glutathione peroxidase) and nonenzymatic defense systems to control excited oxygen species. The importance of the antioxidant mechanisms such as manganese superoxide dismutase (MnSOD) in the regulation of oxidative stress in the myocardium was demonstrated when homozygous knockout mice deficient in MnSOD developed normally in utero but died soon after birth with dilated cardiomyopathy.[11]

However, despite the elaborate antioxidant systems in the cells, a certain fraction still will escape the cellular defense and may cause permanent or transient damage to nucleic acids within the cells, leading to such events as DNA strand breakage and disruption of calcium metabolism. The rate of residual oxidative damage is directly related to the metabolic rate and inversely related to the life span of the organism. This may explain the association of heart failure with ageing.

Modeling of Heart Failure with Diastolic Iron Overload and Systolic Inflammation-Associated Failure

This chapter focuses particularly on two paradigms of heart failure that are clinically relevant. The first is a model of iron overload that causes diastolic heart failure, particularly in young patients, which has now been found to be directly attributable to free radical excess. The second is a model of systolic dysfunction following cardiac injury that involves cytokine excess, which leads to progressive remodeling and cell deaths, and also involves intrinsically free radical excess.

Iron Overload as a Model of Oxidative Stress Leading to Diastolic Heart Failure

The Clinical Problem of Iron Overload

Primary Hemochromatosis

Iron overload cardiomyopathy can result from both primary and secondary hemochromatosis, and is now increasingly recognized as a potentially treatable form of heart failure. The recent cloning of the candidate gene for primary hemochromatosis, hemochromatosis associated (HFE) gene, identified a common Cys282Tyr mutation on the major intracellular histocompatibility-like protein responsible for heterodimeric protein formation in the endoplasmic reticulum.[12,13] This results in the inability to provide feedback inhibition of iron uptake in the gut wall. Primary hemochromatosis is an autosomal recessive disorder, with a gene frequency higher than any other condition at 1/10 in the North American white population.[14–16] This high gene frequency is likely due to a survival advantage conferred to the host during reproductive years, as females with the HFE mutation are better protected from the threat of iron deficiency. Unfortunately, outside the reproductive setting, the individual with the gene mutation is at a higher risk of iron overload. Long-standing hemochromatosis can lead to increased complications of heart failure (relative risk or rr=306), liver cancer (rr=219), and cirrhosis (rr=13) when compared to a normal population.[17] Interestingly, even individuals heterozygous for the mutation may be at increased risk for myocardial infarction and cerebrovascular disease with attributable risk about twice normal.[18,19]

The importance of screening the general population for primary hemochromatosis and treating the complications cannot be overemphasized. In fact, in the post-Human Genome Project era, the US NIH is initiating efforts to perform population-wide screening of genetic diseases, and the first target gene to be screened population-wide is the primary hemochromatosis gene.[20]

Secondary Hemochromatosis

In the non-Northern European population, the risk of iron overload is even higher due to secondary hemochromatosis from chronic transfusions for hemoglobinopathies. A prime example is β-thalassemia, the most common monogenic disorder worldwide, involving mutations of hemoglobin.[21,22] The homozygous or compound heterozygous individuals with the β-thalassemias are characterized by profound anemia, and survival depends on regular blood transfusion and the lifelong use of chelation agents to prevent iron accumulation.

Unfortunately, despite chelation, these patients are still at risk for iron overload. If the patient is noncompliant or fails to achieve a net negative iron balance with chelation, complications such as heart failure, diabetes, and pituitary insufficiency and cirrhosis will ensue, as well as deaths from heart failure in the third decade.[17,23–25] Recent data suggest that additional risk factors such as cardiac inflammation[26,27] and ApoE polymorphism (indicator of increased oxidative stress)[28] may also contribute to the early onset of heart failure. Many of the countries in which the β-thalassemias occur at a high frequency are having a major demographic transition following improvements in hygiene, diet, and the avail-ability of medical treatment.[29] Even developed nations face similar uphill battles with their thalassemic populations. For example, a recent report from the United Kingdom Thalassemia Registry confirms that more than 50% of UK patients with β-thalassemia die before 35 years of age from heart failure.[30]

The traditional thalassemic patients are now joined by patients with sickle cell disease. Chronic transfusion has been demonstrated to be ef-fective in preventing stroke and as such has led to a rapid increase in giv-ing chronic transfusions for this population and the documented increase in risk of iron overload.[31,32] In addition, anemia is a common and serious problem in patients with end-stage renal disease (ESRD). Parenteral iron is now the treatment of choice in hemodialysis with either absolute or functional iron deficiency. Several studies have now suggested an in-creased risk of cardiac death associated with repetitive parenteral iron administration in this population as well.[33] Iron overload cardiomyopa-thy thus represents a new threat to survival in several new populations at risk.[34]

Clinical Phenotype of Iron Overload Cardiomyopathy and Outcomes

Heart failure is a well-described complication of patients with iron overload; however, early diagnosis of cardiac dysfunction is often not done due to the lack of general awareness. Interestingly, clinical iron overload also is an archetypical example of a restrictive cardiomyopathy, with early presence of severe diastolic dysfunction, but preserved sys-tolic function.[21,26] The initial diastolic dysfunction is characterized by myocardial iron overload, without overt inflammation. However, as time progresses, there is increased fibrosis, often accompanied by inflamma-tion, leading to a more permanent form of cardiomyopathy. The patients ultimately succumb to their heart failure and die of arrhythmias, such as severe heart block or electromechanical dissociation. Early forms of this condition are reversible, in that if the patient is treated aggressively with intravenous chelation, the ventricular dysfunction will reverse and the prognosis will change.[21,35–38] However, if it is left too late, there is a rapidly progressive downhill course, unresponsive to traditional heart failure treatment.

Long-term follow-up studies of patients with β-thalassemia, includ-ing our own series, indicated that in adult patients born before 1976, 37% of the patients had serious clinical cardiac disease, most commonly clini-cal heart failure. Furthermore, 20% have died before reaching age 30, al-most all from heart failure.[23,39] All of the remaining patients have evi-dence of diastolic dysfunction, often accompanied by arrhythmias.

Mechanism of Iron Overload Cardiomyopathy: Generation of Oxidative Stress via Fenton Reaction

A key role that iron plays in biological systems during evolution is its critical role in almost all redox reactions involving oxygen. The examples include hemoglobin, all the cytochromes in the respiratory chain, nitric oxide (NO) synthases and other oxidoreductases (Figure 1). Therefore the iron levels in the tissues are extremely tightly regulated. In addition, the actions of many intracellular reactions involving oxygen species are also regulated by hemoproteins. An example is NO, which reacts with hemoproteins to produce NO-heme adduct. It is this NO-iron complex that can upregulate the activities of other enzymes, such as guanylate cyclase, which is itself a hemoprotein containing 1 mole heme/mole holoenzyme dimer.[40]

Because of the key role that iron plays in redox reaction, it does not come as a surprise that when iron is present in large quantities in the myocardium, for example, it can also play an important catalytic role in the generation of free radicals. Iron can readily catalyze oxygen to produce the free radical superoxide anion ($O_2^-\cdot$):

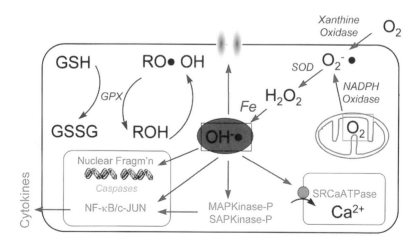

Figure 1. Pathways of free radical activation in iron overload. The presence of increased iron (Fe) facilitates the production of free radicals such as the hydroxyl radicals through the Fenton reaction. The radicals can then target the SRCaATPase to cause relaxation abnormalities, or directly target the nuclear DNA leading to apoptosis. Furthermore, activation of a number of intracellular signaling targets such as the tyrosine kinases can also lead to cell phenotype transition, including the production of cytokines. Meanwhile, the intrinsic antioxidants, including superoxide dismutase (SOD), catalase and, most importantly, glutathione peroxidase (GPX), are critical to limit the extent of free radical formation.

$O_2 + Fe^{2+}$ (water soluble) $\rightarrow O_2^- \cdot + Fe^{3+}$ (insoluble)   [*Equation 1*]

Ordinarily, the superoxide anion can convert to the much more damaging hydroxyl free radical ($\cdot OH$) by the slow Haber-Weiss reaction. However, in the presence of iron, this reaction can be rapidly facilitated by the Fenton reaction:

$$O_2^- \cdot + Fe^{3+} \rightarrow O_2 + Fe^{2+}$$

$$H_2O_2 + Fe^{2+} \rightarrow OH^- + \cdot OH + Fe^{3+} \qquad [\textit{Equation 2}]$$

The resulting hydroxyl free radicals are the most potent reactive oxygen species known.[41,42] The targets for the free radical reaction include structural membranes, enzymes, mitochondria, and chromosomal DNA. Eventually the cells will die from necrosis or apoptosis.[43] The reaction of lipid membranes with free radicals proceeds as follows:

$$LH + R \cdot \rightarrow RH + L \cdot \qquad [\textit{Equation 3}]$$

$$L \cdot + O_2 \rightarrow LOO \cdot$$

$$LOO \cdot + L'H \rightarrow L'O \cdot + LOO \cdot + \text{Aldehydes of different lengths}$$

where LH = unsaturated lipid, R = radical; the aldehydes can be assayed now with a novel technique using GC-mass spectrometry.[44]

A Novel Murine Model of Cardiac Iron Overload to Explore Iron, Free Radicals, and Cardiomyopathy

To study more in depth the pathophysiology of iron overload in the heart, we have created a novel murine iron overload model with specific cardiac dysfunction by intraperitoneally instilling iron in inbred B6D2F1 mice that have a genetic hemoglobinopathy with chronic anemia.[45,46] Through this model, we have learned that there is indeed a dose-related increase in tissue free radical production according to the amount of iron loaded and also iron present in the tissues (Figure 2).[47] Interestingly, the iron appears to be localized to mitochondria and can directly cause mitochondrial damage in the myocytes (Figure 3). This in turn can lead to myocyte death and, in late stages, it can lead to fibrosis.

The free radical load was assayed by the tissue aldehyde level, which is not only a measure of lipid peroxidation, but also the oxidative potential, since these radicals are directly capable of reacting with other lipid species to propagate the free radical reaction.[44] There was also a significant increase in mortality at higher doses of iron load in concert with correspondingly increasing aldehyde levels (Figure 4). Similar to observations made clinically in patients with iron overload cardiomyopathies, the animals also had a dose-related decrease in $-dP/dt$, suggesting difficulties with ventricular relaxation. Furthermore, the left ventricular work done

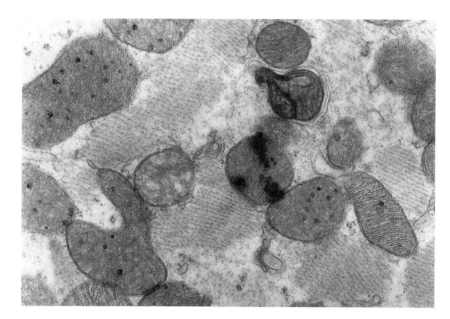

Figure 2. Electronic micrographs of cardiac myocytes subjected to iron overload. The mitochondria are swollen, accompanied by a loss of normal structure including cristae but a gain of electron-dense particles. The latter are thought to be ferritin or other iron-containing protein complexes, which may directly cause localized oxidative stress.

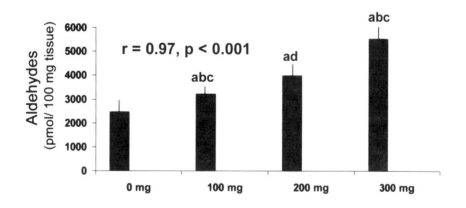

*a = p < 0.001 compared to 0 mg, b = p < 0.001 compared to iron loaded,
c = p < 0.05 compared to iron loaded*

Figure 3. Myocardial aldehyde levels measured by GC-mass spectrometry in murine models of chronic iron overload with the total iron administered listed in the abscissa. There is a dose-related increase in oxidative stress directly within the myocardium as a result of iron loading.

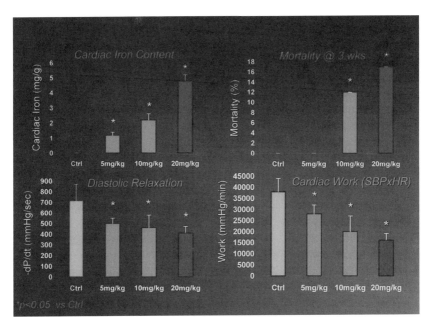

Figure 4. In a group of animals that underwent iron loading at different dose regimen, one can observe the relationship between iron levels, diastolic relaxation, and mortality. There was a dose-related increase in cardiac iron content (with increase in oxidative stress as illustrated in Figure 3), accompanied by a stepwise increase in mortality once a threshold is exceeded. Interestingly, this is particularly associated with a prominent diastolic relaxation abnormality, illustrated here with −dP/dt, and is relevant to the clinical response. Finally, the total cardiac work achieved also progressively diminishes, as the animals develop more heart failure at higher doses. SBP = systolic blood pressure; HR = heart rate).

was also progressively diminished with increasing doses of iron load. As expected, the intrinsic myocardial antioxidants, such as glutathione peroxidase (GPx), show an initial rise after iron load, but then rapidly decline as iron load continues, resulting in prominent tissue injury.[46]

To prove that the elevations in free radicals and aldehydes were fundamentally important in the disease process, aggressive antioxidation experiments were conducted in the models of iron overload. In these studies, the effect of oral feeding of selenium, vitamin E, or morin hydrate, or a combination, was examined in the murine model of iron overload cardiomyopathy.[48,49] When the antioxidants were administered to these iron-loaded animals, there was indeed a significant reduction in both aldehyde and free radical levels accompanied by an improvement in ventricular function. The animals showed significant reductions in aldehyde and free radical levels with antioxidant treatment, and the combination was especially potent when compared to either agent alone. This set of observations also underscores the importance of the intrinsic antioxidant system as a counter-regulatory mechanism in host protection in the face of increasing free radical load.

The Role of Aldehydes in Heart Failure Progression

The preliminary data thus support the free radical hypothesis as the basis for iron-induced cardiac damage in our basic iron overload model, and the elevation of aldehydes in this condition further supports the concept. This is also validated in clinical cases of heart failure, both in iron overload conditions[50,51] as well as in those with dilated cardiomyopathy of other etiology.[52] Previously, aldehydes were thought to be inert byproducts of oxidation, and to have little biological activity. However, recent data suggest that aldehydes may be major contributors to disease pathology, including liver cirrhosis and cancer.[53] Aldehydes, in contrast to transient and locally produced free radicals such as superoxide and hydroxyl radicals, are stable adducts present in the serum and tissue at millimolar concentrations, and can translocate in the blood stream from one organ to another. As a corollary to these observations, aldehydes may indeed evolve to be a therapeutic target, not only in iron overload heart failure, but in heart failure from diverse etiology.

Clinical Evidence of Oxidative Stress in Patients with Iron Overload Cardiomyopathy

To explore these novel themes in the *clinical* setting, we studied patients with iron overload in terms of their aldehyde levels when compared to normals. Indeed, we have confirmed that they have at least a 20% increase in plasma aldehyde levels compared to controls, and a >50% reduction in intrinsic antioxidant glutathione peroxidase (GPx) levels, and this is clearly associated with diastolic dysfunction observed in these patients.[50] The patients who are aggressively chelated for iron have much better protection, but their aldehyde levels are still significantly different from controls.

Nevertheless, even in the presence of iron chelation, the patients continue to require blood transfusions to maintain survival. Each unit of red cell transfusion contains 100 mg of iron, which represents an acute source of excess free radical load. In another study, the patient had blood sampled before and after transfusion in the presence of early iron overload cardiomyopathy on chelation. To our surprise, the free radicals increased, as evidenced by elevations in lipid peroxides and aldehydes, within minutes of the transfusion start, and persisted for hours after transfusion. This shows the potent impact of even a small amount of parenteral iron on tissue membrane oxidation; and despite the fact that they are on chronic chelation therapy, there was still an acute elevation of cytotoxic aldehydes with each episode of transfusion.[51]

These observations establish the tight linkage between *iron loading* and *oxidative stress* in patients with iron overload. These novel observations help to define the critical role that the oxidative stress process plays in the development of iron overload cardiomyopathy, and serves as an archetypal example of the consequences of excess intrinsic radical formation via the Fenton pathway catalyzed by iron in the tissues.

Impact of Free Radicals in Clinical Ventricular Dysfunction

To expand the link between oxidative stress and congestive heart failure (CHF) in general beyond those with iron overload alone, we also conducted a clinical hemodynamic study in patients with various degrees of dilated cardiomyopathy. This study recruited eight CHF patients and eight age-matched controls with normal left ventricular (LV) function to undergo simultaneous ventricular function studies as well as free radical evaluation. The results showed that CHF patients had higher levels of total aldehydes (9311 ± 835 versus 6594 ± 344 nmol/L, $P<.01$), as well as multiple unsaturated aldehydes (t-2-alkenals and 4-OH-alkenals, including 4-hydroxynonenal).[52] In the CHF group, a strong relationship was observed between total aldehyde concentration and both +dP/dt (correlation coefficient = -0.76, $P<.05$) and diastolic relaxation constant tau (correlation coefficient = 0.78, $P<.05$). Thus, we made the novel observation that unsaturated aldehyde levels, as a functional marker of active oxidative stress load, were consistently elevated in CHF patients and were associated with impairment of LV contractility and, more importantly, relaxation.

Lessons Learned From Oxidative Stress in Iron Overload Cardiomyopathy and Clinical Implications

Results from the aforementioned bench-to-bedside investigations in iron load cardiomyopathy have established several important concepts in terms of the relationship between iron, free radicals, and cardiomyopathy. The free radicals that are produced in patients through the iron-catalyzed Fenton reaction are indeed biologically important, and there is a stoichiometrically significant relationship between iron load, free radical production, ventricular dysfunction, and ultimately deaths from cardiomyopathy. The fact that much of the iron-related cardiomyopathy could be ameliorated by antioxidants in the murine models suggests the fundamental role of oxidative stress in contributing to this myopathy.

In addition, apart from the traditional species of radicals such as superoxide and hydroxyl radicals from oxidation reactions, we have also established that tissue aldehydes are not only markers of oxidative stress, but can also participate in the disease process, and directly affect both systolic function and diastolic relaxation. The latter is indeed the predominant form of heart failure in the setting of iron overload, and offers an important insight into the mechanisms of diastolic heart failure, which is an epidemic in the population at large today.

Finally, the ultimate culprit in iron overload cardiomyopathy is the presence of excessive iron, which plays an important catalytic role in the production of free radicals via the Fenton reaction. Therefore, for the patient with iron overload cardiomyopathy, the key to prevention of cardiomyopathy is aggressive chelation and removal of iron accumulation. Interestingly, the mechanism by which current chelation therapy such as desferrioxamine exerts its benefit is at least partially also due to its ability to decrease the production of free radical load in addition to iron removal. This further underscores the importance of chelation and explains the impact of compliance with chelation with survival in this condition. In the future, antioxidants may also become part of the treatment strategy in addition to chelation. Even the oxidation load during acute transfusion is likely important to target as a source for free radicals.

Cytokine Increase in Systolic Dysfunction Associated With Inflammation

TNF Is Upregulated in Systolic Heart Failure: Is This Clinically Important?

Cytokines are another potent mediator of free radical production that is directly related to the progression in heart failure. The prototype cytokine is tumor necrosis factor (TNF-α) or cachexin. Interestingly, TNF is also found in advanced stages of iron overload cardiomyopathy, as outlined above.

TNF-α is a master cytokine with pleotropic properties important for cell-cell signaling. TNF-α binds to either of the tumor necrosis factor receptors TNF-R1 (55kD) or TNF-R2 (75kD) to effect an intracellular signaling cascade for its biological actions. All cells including the myocytes express both TNF-R1 and TNF-R2,[54–56] including the settings of heart failure. TNF-R1 and TNF-R2 are the prototypic receptors of the TNF-R superfamily of receptors that include the nerve growth factor receptor (NGF-R), Fas (CD95), the Hodgkin's lymphoma antigen/receptor CD30, and death receptors designated death receptor 3 (DR3), DR4, and DR5,[57]

Elevations of circulating cytokines such as TNF in heart failure have been well documented. Levine et al. first demonstrated elevated circulating levels of TNF- α in patients with heart failure of diverse etiologies, and the patients with TNF-α elevation had more cachexia and renin-angiotensin activation.[58] Since then, there has been a plethora of studies that consistently documented that *circulating or myocardial TNF levels correlate with the severity of heart failure, and either the circulating levels of TNF or its soluble receptors are the best prognosticators of mortality in heart failure, exceeding the traditional catecholamines or atrial natriuretic peptides.*[56,59–63] Indeed, TNF-α elevation has been associated with a worse degree of cachexia, a general increase in neurohumoral activation, and higher levels of oxidative stress in patients with heart failure.[4,58,59,64] Questions remain as to how and when the TNF becomes activated in the heart after injury, and what is the biological rationale for TNF activation. We propose that at least a significant component of its induction and action is closely linked with the production of oxygen free radicals.

TNF Is Intrinsically Produced in the Myocardium: Timing and Mechanisms

We and others now have strong evidence to suggest that TNF elevation is intrinsic to the myocardium following injury, and that it may be paradoxically "protective" in the infarct zone in the short term but "detrimental" during chronic activation in the remote myocardium. This paradox is now better understood with the elucidation of the human genome, where there are only 30,000 distinct candidate genes. Therefore, the organisms use the same gene/molecule for a completely different function under different conditions (the economy of genes principle). Torre-Amione et al. first demonstrated that the failing human myocardium intrinsically expresses elevated TNF-α and its receptors.[65] More recently, our laboratory demonstrated that in a rat model of myocardial infarction, myocardial TNF-α increased within hours post injury in the infarct and periinfarct zones, which is sustained for 5–7 days (early phase I induction). However, from day 5 onward, the contralateral unaffected noninfarct zone also expressed robust TNF gene expression accompanied by protein production, peaking between 10 and 30 days, without downregulation of the TNF receptors (late phase II). This is associated with increased apoptosis, ventricular dysfunction, and progressive ventricular dilatation in the contralateral wall, setting the stage for progression toward heart failure.[54]

This concept is further confirmed by our recent canine pacing model of heart failure (in collaboration with Dr. Gordon Moe), where, after 3 weeks of pacing, there was intrinsic myocyte production in the failing hearts associated with ventricular dilatation and decreased contractility.[66] The trigger for intrinsic myocardial TNF production is still unknown. Our recent publications on the pathogenesis of inflammatory heart disease have identified that cell membrane-associated receptors and their tyrosine kinases (e.g., p56^{lck}) are the key triggers for intracellular signaling and cytokine production. We have preliminary data to suggest that cytoskeletal anchors such as integrins may act as one of the adaptors of mechanical stretch, which in turn activate cellular signals, including tyrosine kinases and free radicals, to coordinate downstream cytokine activation through redox-sensitive transcription factors such as NF-κB.[55,67–69]

Indeed, mechanical strain and membrane stretch can increase the formation of free radicals in the myocardium by their direct regulation of electron transport activity and oxygen wastage.[70] Regulatory elements of the NF-κB complex such as IκB are exquisitely redox-sensitive, and can in turn dissociate from NF-κB following oxidative phosphorylation, thus permitting nuclear translocation of NF-κB to initiate cytokine transcription.

Once cytokines are present, the presence of free radicals further amplifies their potency. Oxidation reactions are normally used in enzymatic pathways to form intracellular messengers such as the prostaglandins, leukotrienes, and the simplest local signaling molecule, NO. In the setting of increased inflammatory potential with the presence of cytokines such as TNF, nonenzymatic oxidation appears to produce compounds that compete with or inhibit the mediators derived from endogenous enzymatic oxidative processes and in turn can modulate signal transduction events within the cell.[71]

TNF and Cardiac Remodeling

The initial proof that TNF-α production alone is sufficient to induce cardiac remodeling and heart failure came from transgenic models of TNF^{ctg+} overexpression, with human TNF gene targeted to the myocardium using an α-myosin promoter. In this model, the myocardium shows progressive dilatation and increased apoptosis, leading to early death of the host from heart failure.[72,73] Treating these transgenic animals with soluble TNF receptor blockade improves their ventricular function, suggesting that the heart failure phenotype observed is due largely to the myocardial increases in TNF.[74]

TNF and Myocyte Apoptosis and Survival: Interaction With Oxidative Stress

In terms of direct myocyte injury and survival, TNF has pleotropic effects, dependent on the conditions. It has been shown that TNF can induce myocyte apoptosis through sphingolipid or death domain-mediated mechanisms outlined above.[75] However, other investigators have found that cytokines such as TNF may be protective against apoptosis through NF-κB activation pathways, also outlined earlier.[76,77] Our own laboratory data suggest that this difference may be due to the concentration of TNF in the local environment, and particularly the ambient level of free radicals. It is interesting that when adult myocytes in culture were exposed to TNF alone at concentrations found in serum of patients with heart failure, there was no evidence of apoptosis by DNA ladder formation or in situ labeling (Figure 5). However, in the presence of low levels of free radicals, such as H_2O_2, there was a significant increase in detectable apoptosis, suggesting an important synergy between cytokines and free radicals in mediating adverse biological effects.

This observation concurs with Li et al., whose team found that superoxide stimulation induces cardiac myocyte apoptosis. In contrast, cardiac fibroblasts were stimulated to proliferate as demonstrated by the increase in DNA synthesis and cell number. In addition to that, transforming growth factor-β, a key factor responsible for myocardial fibrosis, was upregulated in cardiac fibroblasts in response to superoxide stimulation.[78]

For the myocyte itself, different free radical species may use distinct

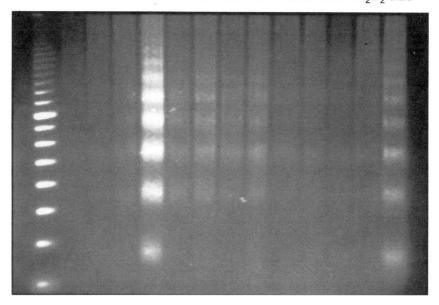

Ctrl   **TNF (µg/l)**   **H_2O_2 (µM)**   **TNF 100**   **TNF 30**
30 100 300   5   10   25   50 + SOD/Vit E   +H_2O_2 5/25

Figure 5. Myocyte apoptosis at different concentrations of cytokine and oxidative stress, showing synergistic effects of the two stress pathways on stable myocyte cultures withdrawn from serum. Tumor necrosis factor (TNF) induced DNA ladder formation only at extremely high levels of 300 mg/L, compatible with patients with severe heart failure or sepsis. However, oxidation agents such as H2O2 can induce a low level of apoptosis. TNF in the presence of antioxidants is protected from the effect of apoptosis, but the combination of TNF with low dose of H2O2 showed significant degree of apoptosis not seen with either agent alone.

apoptotic pathways. Induction of p53 may directly induce apoptosis by the activation of the Bax gene, which encodes an apoptosis-inducing factor. H_2O_2 triggers the release of cytochrome c and the activation of caspase (CPP32) while O_2^- triggered the activation of Mch2α (a different caspase pathway) to promote the apoptotic pathway involving the cleavage of lamin A.[79]

On the other hand, it was demonstrated that heart failure myocytes may be more susceptible to oxidative stress-induced injury, which is not due to decreased antioxidant defense but to the intrinsic properties of cells.[80] Recently metallothionein—a highly conserved, low molecular weight, thiol-rich protein existing in heart tissue—was found to attenuate hypoxia/reoxygenation-induced apoptosis in cardiomyocytes. This is putatively accomplished by inhibiting mitochondrial cytochrome c release and subsequent caspase activation as a result of oxidative stress. Therefore, it is now one of the novel therapeutic approaches to ameliorate ischemic-reperfusion heart injury.[81]

TNF and the Matrix: Contribution of Oxidative Stress

TNF may also have direct effects on the matrix and collagen framework to contribute to the cardiac remodeling.[82] We have recently published that in the setting of repetitive low-level viral infection in the myocardium, even though clear myocarditis is absent, there is progressive ventricular dilation in the heart through a TNF-mediated mechanism.[83]

The cytokine-mediated matrix changes are also enhanced by reactive oxygen species through activation of a number of matrix metalloproteinases (MMPs). Pro-MMPs are produced by myocytes and fibroblasts, and some MMPs are upregulated by proinflammatory cytokines and growth factors such as TNF-α, interleukin-1β, and transforming growth factor-β1, leading to tissue injury. All MMPs are produced as inactive precursors (pro-MMPs), and their activation is particularly triggered by external agents such as oxygen free radicals. Free radicals such as peroxynitrite are reported to activate pro-MMP, possibly through oxidative modification (S-glutathiolation) of the autoinhibitory domain via formation of stable disulfide S-oxide.[84] In addition, peroxynitrite is effective in inactivating the tissue inhibitor of metalloproteinase, thus preserving the activity of MMP after it is generated.

TNF and Cardiac Contractility: "Radical" Thoughts

Cytokines can depress cardiac function directly, or indirectly via NO-dependent mechanisms. We and others have demonstrated that TNF-α can directly decrease the calcium release within the myocytes, possibly influenced by sphingomyelin pathways.[85,86] Indirect myocardial depression via upregulation of the inducible form of NO synthase[87–90] can in turn modulate the contractile response to adrenergic stimulation.[91,92]

The induction of NO by cytokines such as TNF has prompted a debate as to whether it plays a deleterious or protective role in tissue injury. Under high local concentration, it reacts with O_2 to form a number of reactive nitrogen oxide species such as N_2O_3 and peroxynitrite (ONOO-). Schulz and others have demonstrated that the latter can directly cause depression of contractility, and accounts for the majority of cardiac depression associated with cytokine induction.[87,93,94] NO combines readily with superoxide to form peroxynitrite with a rapid reaction constant. They have found that cytokines induced both NO and superoxide formation, and that blockade of either NO production with nitroarginine, or superoxide formation with tiron, all reversed the depression of myocardial contractility.[94]

However, NO at physiological concentrations can also abate the oxidation chemistry mediated by reactive oxygen species such as H_2O_2 and O_2^-. In addition to the antioxidant chemistry, NO protects against cell death mediated by H_2O_2, alkylhydroxyperoxidases, and xanthine oxidase. The attenuation of metal/peroxide oxidative chemistry, as well as lipid peroxidation, seem to be the major chemical mechanisms by which NO may limit oxidative injury to mammalian cells. Therefore, NO may be very protective at the physiological levels of concentration. This role duality is very much central to the modulatory role of NO in biology.[89]

Overview: Potential Therapeutic Opportunities

In this chapter, we have discussed the role of oxidative stress in the setting of heart failure, particularly from the point of view of iron-mediated diastolic heart failure and cytokine-promoted progression of systolic heart failure. However, the question remains if primary blockade of the oxidation pathways and products would be primarily beneficial in heart failure. We certainly have observed in the iron overload model that antioxidant strategies are very beneficial.[48,49] Indeed, the currently employed chelation therapy may be operating precisely through this mechanism as well.[50]

However, clinical trials with antioxidants have been more limited in their impact. Keith et al. conducted a trial in 56 patients with advanced heart failure, and randomized them to vitamin E or placebo in addition to standard therapy for heart failure. Vitamin E therapy significantly increased plasma levels of alpha-tocopheral, but failed to improve other markers of oxidative stress, such as malondialdehyde, isoprostanes, or breath pentane levels. Quality-of-life parameters as well as reflectors of ventricular function such as cytokines or atrial natriuretic peptides did not change between the groups. This study may be underpowered to detect a major change in functional capacity, but was disappointing in failing to show any early indicators of improvement. This suggests that the oxidative stress levels are too high in pathological states such as heart failure, and that a single antioxidant such as vitamin E is inadequate to decrease the free radical load.[95]

An alternative approach to the treatment strategy, in the face of the lack of a major set of antioxidants that are effective in blocking the oxidative damage, is to modify the underlying biology of the disease. Currently, both ACE inhibitors and beta-blockers are standard forms of treatment that have withstood the rigors of clinical trials. Interestingly, both agents will also significantly decrease oxidative stress in patients with cardiovascular disease. Specifically, ACE inhibitors act to decrease levels of angiotensin II, which work through the free radicals generated by the NADPH oxidase pathway to cause vasoconstriction.[96] Removal of the free radical component by either angiotensin blockade or antioxidants negates the biological actions of angiotensin.

Interestingly, beta-blockade also induced a significant and persistent decrease in oxidative stress measured in terms of TBARS over time.[97] This is accompanied by improvement in LV ejection fraction, which is usually accompanied by the reduction in end-diastolic volume in the reverse remodeling step. Therefore, in the absence of a potent directed antioxidant to modify the various molecular pathways, it is very important to search means to modify the underlying disease process. In the future, when there are more effective and targeted antioxidants available, we may be able to treat and prevent heart failure, as we are able to accomplish with iron overload cardiomyopathies today.

References

1. Liu P. The path to cardiomyopathy: cycles of injury, repair and maladaptation. Curr Opinion Cardiol 1996;11:291–292.
2. Diaz-Velez CR, Garcia-Castineiras S, Mendoza-Ramos E, et al. Increased malondialdehyde in peripheral blood of patients with congestive heart failure. Am Heart J 1996;131:146–152.
3. McMurray J, Chopra M, Abdullah I, et al. Evidence of oxidative stress in chronic heart failure in humans. Eur Heart J 1993;14:1493–1498.
4. Keith M, Geranmayegan A, Sole MJ, et al. Increased oxidative stress in patients with congestive heart failure. J Am Coll Cardiol 1998;31:1352–1356.
5. Dhalla AK, Hill MF, Singal PK. Role of oxidative stress in transition of hypertrophy to heart failure. J Am Coll Cardiol 1996;28:506–514.
6. Hill MF, Singal PK. Right and left myocardial antioxidant responses during heart failure subsequent to myocardial infarction. Circulation 1997;96:2414–2420.

7. Singal PK, Iliskovic N. Doxorubicin-induced cardiomyopathy. N Engl J Med 1998;339:900–905.
8. Cahilly C, Ballantyne CM, Lim D-S, et al. A variant of p22phox, involved in generation of reactive oxygen species in the vessel wall, is associated with progression of coronary atherosclerosis. Circ Res 2000;88:391–395.
9. Griendling KK, Sorescu D, Lassègue B, et al. Modulation of protein kinase activity and gene expression by reactive oxygen species and their role in vascular physiology and pathophysiology. Arterioscler Thromb Vasc Biol 2000;20: 2175–2183.
10. Ellis GR, Anderson RA, Lang D, et al. Neutrophil superoxide anion-generating capacity, endothelial function and oxidative stress in chronic heart failure: effects of short- and long-term vitamin C therapy. J Am Coll Cardiol 2000; 36: 1474–1482.
11. Li Y, Huang TT, Carlson EJ, et al. Dilated cardiomyopathy and neonatal lethality in mutant mice lacking managanese superoxide dismutase. Nature Genet 1995;11:376–381.
12. Andrews NC. Disorders of iron metabolism. N Engl J Med 1999;341:1986–1995.
13. Barton JC, Bertoli LF. Hemochromatosis: the genetic disorder of the twenty-first century. Nature Med 1996;2:394–395.
14. Bulaj ZJ, Griffen LM, Jorde LB, et al. Clinical and biochemical abnormalities in people heterozygous for hemochromatosis. N Engl J Med 1996;335:1799–1805.
15. Feder JN, Gnirke A, Thomas W, et al. A novel MHC class I-like gene is mutated in patients with hereditary hemochromatosis. Nature Genet 1996;13: 399–408.
16. Parkkila S, Waheed A, Britton RS, et al. Immunohistochemistry of HLA-H, the protein defective in patients with hereditary hemochromatosis, reveals unique pattern of expression in gastrointestinal tract. Proceed Natl Acad Sci USA 1997;94:2534–2539.
17. Niederau C, Fischer R, Sonnenberg A, et al. Survival and causes of death in cirrhotic and noncirrhotic patients with primary hemochromatosis. N Engl J Med 1985;313:1256–1262.
18. Tuomainen TP, Kontula K, Nyyssonen K, et al. Increased risk of acute myocardial infarction in carriers of the hemochromatosis gene Cys282Tyr mutation: a prospective cohort study in men in eastern Finland. Circulation 1999; 100:1274–1279.
19. Roest M, van der Schouw YT, de Valk B, et al. Heterozygosity for a hereditary hemochromatosis gene is associated with cardiovascular death in women. Circulation 1999;100:1268–1273.
20. Collins FS. Shattuck lecture. Medical and societal consequences of the Human Genome Project. N Engl J Med 1999;341:28–37.
21. Liu P, Olivieri N. Iron overload cardiomyopathies: new insights into an old disease. Cardiovasc Drugs Therap 1994;8:101–110.
22. Olivieri NF. The beta-thalassemias. N Engl J Med 1999;341:99–109.
23. Olivieri NF, Nathan DG, MacMillan JH, et al. Survival in medically treated patients with homozygous beta-thalassemia. N Engl J Med 1994;331:574–578.
24. Schafer AI, Cheron RG, Dluhy R, et al. Clinical consequences of acquired transfusional iron overload in adults. N Engl J Med 1981;304:319–324.
25. Engle MA, Erlandson M, Smith CH. Late cardiac complications of chronic, severe, refractory anemia with hemochromatosis. Circulation 1964;30:698–705.

26. Kremastinos DT, Tiniakos G, Theodorakis GN, et al. Myocarditis in beta-thalassemia major: a cause of heart failure. Circulation 1995;91:66–71.
27. Kremastinos DT, Flevari P, Spyropoulou M, et al. Association of heart failure in homozygous beta-thalassemia with the major histocompatibility complex. Circulation 1999;100:2074–2078.
28. Economou-Petersen E, Aessopos A, Kladi A, et al. Apolipoprotein E epsilon4 allele as a genetic risk factor for left ventricular failure in homozygous beta-thalassemia. Blood 1998;92:3455–3459.
29. Weatherall DJ, Clegg JB. Thalassemia: a global public health problem. Nature Med 1996;2:847–849.
30. Modell B, Khan M, Darlison M. Survival in beta-thalassemia major in the UK: data from the UK thalassemia register. Lancet 2000;355:2051–2052.
31. Adams RJ, McKie VC, Hsu L, et al. Prevention of a first stroke by transfusion in children with sickle cell anemia and abnormal results on transcranial Doppler ultrasonography. N Engl J Med 1998;339:5–11.
32. Harmatz P, Butensky E, Quirolo K, et al. Severity of iron overload in patients with sickle cell disease receiving chronic red blood cell transfusion therapy. Blood 2000;96:76–79.
33. Besarab A, Bolton WK, Browne JK, et al. The effects of normal as compared with low hematocrit values in patients with cardiac disease who are receiving hemodialysis and epoetin. N Engl J Med 1998;339:584–590.
34. Chan PCK, Liu P, Cronin C, et al. The use of nuclear magnetic resonance imaging in monitoring total body iron in hemodialysis patients with hemosiderosis treated with erythropoietin and phlebotomy. Am J Kidney Dis 1992; 19:484–489.
35. Olivieri NF, Berriman AM, Tyler BJ, et al. Reduction in tissue iron stores with a new regimen of continuous ambulatory intravenous deferoxamine. Am J Hematol 1992;41:61–63.
36. Rahko PS, Salerni R, Uretsky BF. Successful reversal by chelation therapy of congestive cardiomyopathy due to iron overload. J Am Coll Cardiol 1986;8: 436–440.
37. Madani TAA, Bormanis J. Reversible severe hereditary hemochromatotic cardiomyopathy. Can J Cardiol 1997;13:391–394.
38. Cutler DJ, Isner JM, Bracey AW, et al. Hemochromatosis heart disease: an unemphasized cause of potentially reversible restrictive cardiomyopathy. Am J Med 1980;69:923–928.
39. Olivieri N, McGee A, Liu P, et al. Cardiac disease-free survival in patients with thalassemia major treated with subcutaneous deferoxamine. Ann NY Acad Sci 1990;612:585–586.
40. Ignarro LJ, Adams JB, Horwitz PM, et al. Activation of soluble guanylate cyclase by NO-hemoproteins involves NO-heme exchange: comparison of heme-containing and heme-deficient enzyme forms. J Biol Chem 1986;261:4997–5002.
41. Link G, Pinson A, Hershko C. Iron loading of cultured cardiac myocytes modifies sarcolemmal structure and increases lysosomal fragility. J Lab Clin Med 1993;121:127–134.
42. Figueiredo MS, Baffa O, Barbieri Neto J, et al. Liver injury and generation of hydroxyl free radicals in experimental secondary hemochromatosis. Res Exp Med 1993;193:27–37.
43. Hockenberg DM, Oltavai ZN, Yin XM, et al. Bcl-2 functions in an antioxidant pathway to prevent apoptosis. Cell 1993;75:241–251.

44. Luo XP, Yazdanpanah M, Bhooi N, et al. Determination of aldehydes and other lipid peroxidation products in biological samples by gas chromatography-mass spectrometry. Anal Biochem 1995;228:294–298.
45. Liu P, Henkelman RM, Joshi J, et al. Quantification of tissue iron by nuclear magnetic resonance relaxometry in a novel murine thalassemia-cardiac iron overload model. Can J Cardiol 1996;12:155–164.
46. Bartfay WJ, Dawood F, Wen WH, et al. Cardiac function and cytotoxic aldehyde production in a murine model of chronic iron overload. Cardiovasc Res 1999;43:892–900.
47. Bartfay WJ, Butany J, Lehotay DC, et al. A biochemical, histochemical and electron microscopic study on the effects of iron loading in hearts of mice. Cardiovasc Pathol 1999;8:305–314.
48. Bartfay WJ, Hou D, Brittenham GM, et al. The synergistic effect of vitamin E and selenium in iron overloaded mouse hearts. Can J Cardiol 1998;14:937–941.
49. Bartfay WJ, Hou D, Lehotay DC, et al. Cardioprotective effects of selenium and morin hydrate in a murine model of chronic iron overload. J Trace Elements Exp Med 2000;13:285–297.
50. Bartfay WJ, Lehotay DC, Sher GD, et al. Comparison of cytotoxic aldehydes in beta-thalassemia patients chelated with deferoxamine or deferiprone (L1) versus no chelation. Hematology 1999;4:67–76.
51. Bartfay WJ, Lehotay DC, Sher GD, et al. Effect of transfusion on lipid peroxidation products in plasma of thalassemia patients. Transfusion 1999;39:333–343.
52. Mak S, Lehotay DC, Yazdanpanah M, et al. Unsaturated aldehydes including 4-OH-nonenal are elevated in patients with congestive heart failure. J Cardiac Fail 2000;6:108–114.
53. Parola M, Robino G, Marra F, et al. HNE interacts directly with JNK isoforms in human hepatic stellate cells. J Clin Invest 1998;102:1942–1950.
54. Irwin M, Mak S, Mann D, et al. Tissue expression and immunolocalization of tumor necrosis factor-alpha in post-infarction dysfunctional myocardium. Circulation 1999;99:1492–1498.
55. Penninger JM, Pummerer C, Liu P, et al. Cellular and molecular mechanisms of murine autoimmune myocarditis. APMIS 1997;105:1–13.
56. Torre-Amione G, Kapadia S, Lee J, et al. Tumor necrosis factor-alpha and tumor necrosis factor receptors in the failing human heart. Circulation 1996;93:704–711.
57. Zhai Y, Ni J, Jiang GW, et al. VEGI, a novel cytokine of the tumor necrosis factor family, is an angiogenesis inhibitor that suppresses the growth of colon carcinomas in vivo. FASEB J 1999;13:181–189.
58. Levine B, Kalman J, Mayer L, et al. Elevated circulating levels of tumor necrosis factor in severe chronic heart failure. N Engl J Med 1990;323:236–241.
59. McMurray J, Abdullah I, Dargie HJ, et al. Increased concentrations of tumour necrosis factor in "cachectic" patients with severe chronic heart failure. Br Heart J 1991;66:356–358.
60. Wiedermann CJ, Beimpold H, Herold M, et al. Increased levels of serum neopterin and decreased production of neutrophil superoxide anions in chronic heart failure with elevated levels of tumor necrosis factor-alpha. J Am Coll Cardiol 1993;22:1897–1901.
61. Matsumori A, Yamada T, Suzuki H, et al. Increased circulating cytokines

in patients with myocarditis and cardiomyopathy. Br Heart J 1994;72:561–566.

62. Ferrari R, Bachetti T, Confortini R, et al. Tumor necrosis factor soluble receptors in patients with various degrees of advanced congestive heart failure. Circulation 1995;1995:1479–1486.

63. Testa M, Yeh M, Lee P, et al. Circulating levels of cytokines and their endogenous modulators in patients with mild to severe congestive heart failure due to coronary artery disease or hypertension. J Am Coll Cardiol 1996; 28: 964–971.

64. Anker SD, Swan JW, Volterrani M, et al. The influence of muscle mass, strength, fatigability and blood flow on exercise capacity in cachectic and non-cachectic patients with chronic heart failure. Eur Heart J 1997;18:259–269.

65. Torre-Amione G, Kapadia S, Lee J, et al. Expression and functional significance of tumor necrosis factor receptors in human myocardium. Circulation 1995;92:1487–1493.

66. Moe G, Qu R, Liu P. Cardiac production and expression of tumor necrosis factor alpha in canine model of pacing-induced heart failure. Circulation, submitted.

67. Liu P, Aitken K, Kong YY, et al. Essential role for the tyrosine kinase p56lck in coxsackievirus B3-mediated heart disease. Nature Med 2000;6:429–434.

68. Opavsky MA, Penninger J, Aitken K, et al. Susceptibility to myocarditis is dependent on the response of ab T lymphocytes to coxsackieviral infection. Circ Res 1999;85:551–558.

69. Bachmaier K, Neu N, Yeung RS, et al. Generation of humanized mice susceptible to peptide-induced inflammatory heart disease. Circulation 1999;99: 1885–1891.

70. Sawyer DB, Colucci WS. Mitochondrial oxidative stress in heart failure: "oxygen wastage" revisited. Circ Res 2000;86:119–120.

71. Darley-Usmar V, White R. Disruption of vascular signaling by the reaction of nitric oxide with superoxide: implications for cardiovascular disease. Exp Physiol 1994;82:305–316.

72. Bryant D, Becker L, Richardson J, et al. Cardiac failure in transgenic mice with myocardial expression of tumor necrosis factor-alpha. Circulation 1998; 97:1375–1381.

73. Kubota T, McTiernan CF, Frye CS, et al. Dilated cardiomyopathy in transgenic mice with cardiac-specific overexpression of tumor necrosis factor-alpha. Circ Res 1997;81:627–635.

74. Kapadia S, Torre-Amione G, Yokoyama T, et al. Soluble TNF binding proteins modulate the negative inotropic properties of TNF-alpha in vitro. Am J Physiol 1995;268:H517–525.

75. Krown KA, Page MT, Nguyen C, et al. Tumor necrosis factor alpha-induced apoptosis in cardiac myocytes: involvement of the sphingolipid signaling cascade in cardiac cell death. J Clin Invest 1996;98:2854–2865.

76. de Moissac D, Zheng H, Kirshenbaum LA. Linkage of the BH4 domain of Bcl-2 and the nuclear factor κB signaling pathway for suppression of apoptosis. J Biol Chem 1999;274:29505–29509.

77. Liu ZG, Hsu H, Goeddel DV. Dissection of TNF receptor 1 effector function: JNK activation is not linked to apoptosis while NF-κB activation prevents cell death. Cell 1996;87:565–576.

78. Li P-F, Dietz R, von Harsdorf R. Superoxide induces apoptosis in cardiomyocytes, but proliferation and expression of transforming growth factor-beta1 in cardiac fibroblasts. FEBS Lett 1999;448:206–210.

79. von Harsdorf R, Li P-F, Dietz R. Signaling pathways in reactive oxygen species-induced cardiomyocyte apoptosis. Circulation 1999;99:2934–2941.
80. Tsutsui H, Ide T, Hayashidani S, et al. Greater susceptibility of failing cardiac myocytes to oxygen free radical-mediated injury. Cardiovasc Res 2001; 49:103–109.
81. Wang G-W, Zhou Z, Klein JB, et al. Inhibition of hypoxia/reoxygenation-induced apoptosis in metallothionein-overexpressing cardiomyocytes. Am J Physiol 2001;280:H2292–H2299.
82. Brenner DA, O'Hara M, Angel P, et al. Prolonged activation of jun and collagenase genes by tumor necrosis factor-alpha. Nature 1989;337:661–663.
83. Nakamura H, Yamamoto T, Yamamura T, et al. Repetitive coxsackievirus infection induces cardiac dilatation in post-myocarditic mice. Japan Circ J 1999; 7:802–804.
84. Okamoto T, Akaike T, Sawa T, et al. Activation of matrix metalloproteinase by peroxynitrite-induced protein S-glutathiolation via disulfide S-oxide formation. J Biol Chem 2001;276:29596–29602.
85. Fyfe A, Dawood F, Wen WH, et al. Tumour necrosis factor alpha depresses myocardial function through impaired calcium recycling. Can J Cardiol 1991; 7:121.
86. Yokoyama T, Vaca L, Rossen RD, et al. Cellular basis for the negative inotropic effects of tumor necrosis factor-alpha in the adult mammalian heart. J Clin Invest 1993;92:2303–2312.
87. Panas D, Khadour FH, Szabo C, et al. Proinflammatory cytokines depress cardiac efficiency by a nitric oxide-dependent mechanism. Am J Physiol 1998;275: H1016–1023.
88. Schulz R, Nava E, Moncada S. Induction and potential biological relevance of Ca^{2+}-independent nitric oxide synthase in the myocardium. Br J Pharmacol 1992;105:3629–3632.
89. Liu P. The role of inducible nitric oxide synthase (iNOS) in myocardial disease: a functional duality. In: Lewis MJ, Shah AJ, eds. Endothelial Modulation of Cardiac Function. Harwood Academic Publishers, London, 1997; 91–102.
90. Ungureanu-Langois D, Balligand JL, Kelly RA, et al. Myocardial contractile dysfunction in the systemic inflammatory response syndrome: role of a cytokine-inducible nitric oxide synthase in cardiac myocytes. J Mol Cell Cardiol 1995;27:155–167.
91. Ungureanu-Langois D, Balligand JL, Simmons WW, et al. Induction of nitric oxide synthase activity by cytokines in ventricular myocytes is necessary but not sufficient to decrease contractile responsiveness to beta-adrenergic agonists. Circ Res 1995;77:494–502.
92. Chung MK, Gulick TS, Rotondo RE, et al. Mechanism of cytokine inhibition of beta-adrenergic agonist stimulation of cyclic AMP in rat cardiac myocytes: impairment of signal transduction. Circ Res 1990;67:753–763.
93. Yasmin W, Strynadka KD, Schulz R. Generation of peroxynitrite contributes to ischemia-reperfusion injury in isolated rat hearts. Cardiovasc Res 1997; 33:422–432.
94. Ferdinandy P, Danial H, Ambrus I, et al. Peroxynitrite is a major contributor to cytokine-induced myocardial contractile failure. Circ Res 2000;87:241–247.
95. Keith ME, Jeejeebhoy KN, Langer A, et al. A controlled clinical trial of vitamin E supplementation in patients with congestive heart failure. Am J Clin Nutrition 2001;73:219–224.
96. Rajagopalan S, Kurz S, Munzel T, et al. Angiotensin induces vasoconstric-

tion via free radicals generated by NADPH oxidase. J Clin Invest 1996;97: 1916–1923.

97. Kukin M, Kalman J, Charney RH, et al. Prospective, randomized comparison of effect of long-term treatment with metoprolol or carvedilol on symptoms, exercise, ejection fraction, and oxidative stress in heart failure. Circulation 1999;99:2645–2651.

• 7 •

Adrenergic and Mechanical Regulation of Oxidative Stress in the Myocardium

Deborah A. Siwik, PhD, David R. Pimentel, MD, Lei Xiao, PhD, Krishna Singh, PhD, Douglas B. Sawyer, MD, PhD, and Wilson S. Colucci, MD

Introduction

Myocardial remodeling is a fundamental response to hemodynamic overload, which is characterized by cardiac enlargement, altered chamber geometry, and pump dysfunction.[1] Progressive remodeling often results in clinical heart failure, a syndrome associated with disabling symptoms, exercise limitation, and death. Mechanical overload is the primary or initiating stimulus for myocardial remodeling in most circumstances: The type, intensity, and duration of hemodynamic overload are important determinants of the form (e.g., eccentric versus concentric), extent, and functional impact of myocardial remodeling. In addition, secondary pathways that are activated in response to hemodynamic dysfunction (e.g., the renin-angiotensin and sympathetic nervous systems) play an important role in modifying the process and perhaps in determining whether the remodeling is adaptive or maladaptive.

Progress in understanding the mechanisms that mediate myocardial remodeling at the cellular level has led to the identification of a variety of intracellular signaling pathways that can regulate the phenotype of car-

From: Kukin ML, Fuster V (eds). *Oxidative Stress and Cardiac Failure.* Armonk, NY: Futura Publishing Co., Inc. ©2003.

diac myocytes and fibroblasts. Reactive oxygen species (ROS) in high levels, as may occur with ischemia followed by reperfusion, have long been recognized to exert toxic effects on cells, resulting in necrosis. Emerging observations suggest that ROS, albeit at much lower levels, can also serve as intracellular signaling molecules in many cell types.[2,3] For example, in fibroblasts, it was shown that several ligands, including epidermal growth factor, platelet-derived growth factor, tumor necrosis factor-α, and interleukin-1β, cause an increase in intracellular ROS levels.[4] Likewise, it was found that overexpression of the small GTP-binding proteins *ras* or *rac* increased intracellular ROS levels and that the increase in ROS caused by either extracellular ligands or *ras* expression was inhibited by a dominant negative to *rac*.[4] It was further shown that cell growth in *ras*-transformed fibroblasts was dependent on ROS.[5] Griendling and colleagues made the important observation that the growth-promoting effect of angiotensin in vascular smooth muscle cells is ROS-dependent and involves activation of an NAD(P)H oxidase.[6,7] In this chapter, several observations will be summarized that suggest that ROS can act as intracellular signaling molecules in cardiac myocytes and fibroblasts, and may thus play a central role in determining the myocardial response to important extracellular remodeling stimuli such as mechanical strain and neurohormones.

Cellular Mechanisms of Myocardial Remodeling

At the cellular level, myocardial remodeling is associated with characteristic changes in the phenotype of cardiac myocytes and the composition of the extracellular matrix (Figure 1), the latter primarily reflecting changes in the phenotype of cardiac fibroblasts.[8,9] Cardiac hypertrophy is due to myocyte growth and/or accumulation of extracellular matrix. Chamber dilation may reflect myocyte lengthening,[10] myocyte apoptosis,[11] and/or myocyte slippage,[12] the latter perhaps caused by depletion of fibrillar collagen struts due to activation of metalloproteinases (MMPs).[13,14] Pump dysfunction may reflect abnormal chamber geometry, loss of functional myocytes, and/or a shift in myocyte contractile phenotype with the reexpression of fetal isoforms involved in contraction (e.g., β-myosin heavy chain)[15] and/or calcium homeostasis (e.g., sarcoplasmic reticulum Ca^{++} ATPase).[16]

Stimuli for Myocardial Remodeling

The primary stimulus for myocardial remodeling is most often hemodynamic overload (Figure 1). The effects of hemodynamic overload are

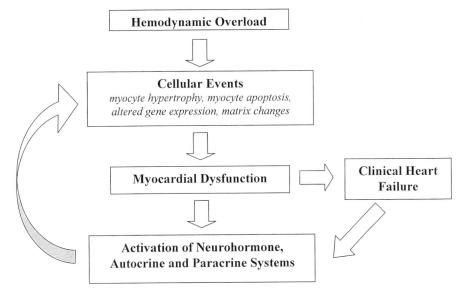

Figure 1. Overview of the regulation of myocardial remodeling. Hemodynamic overload leads to cellular responses including, but not limited to, myocyte hypertrophy, myocyte apoptosis, altered gene expression, and changes in the quantity and quality of the interstitial matrix. Hemodynamic dysfunction may result in overt clinical heart failure. Myocardial dysfunction and heart failure, in turn, activate a variety of neurohormone, autocrine, and paracrine pathways that may exert additional direct effects on the phenotype of cardiac myocytes and fibroblasts.

mediated by an increase in myocardial wall stress, which, depending on the nature of the insult, may occur primarily during systole (e.g., aortic stenosis) or diastole (e.g., mitral regurgitation or myocardial infarction). In addition, it is now clear that neurohormones (e.g., norepinephrine, angiotensin) that are activated systemically in response to hemodynamic dysfunction and peptides (e.g., tumor necrosis factor-α, endothelin) that are produced locally in the myocardium can exert important direct effects on cardiac myocytes and fibroblasts, thereby further promoting and modifying the remodeling process (Figure 1). The importance of these secondary systems has been suggested by the effectiveness of specific inhibitors (e.g., ACE inhibitors and beta-blockers) to slow or even reverse remodeling and to improve the clinical outcome of patients.[17]

Oxidative Stress in Failing Myocardium

There is indirect evidence that oxidative stress is elevated systemically[18–20] and in the myocardium[21] of patients with chronic systolic failure. More direct evidence of increased oxidative stress can be obtained in myocardium from animals with postmyocardial infarction (MI) remodeling,[22] pressure overload-induced failure,[23] or pacing-induced failure.[24] Singal and Dhalla were among the first to suggest that oxidative stress plays a role in myocardial remodeling.[25,26] Evidence that ROS were of pathophysiological significance was provided by the demonstration that the transition from compensated hypertrophy to failure in guinea pigs with pressure overload due to aortic constriction was prevented by administration of the antioxidant, vitamin E.[27] Likewise, they showed that probucol, a lipid-lowering agent with antioxidant properties, protected against Adriamycin-induced myocardial failure[28] and diabetic cardiomyopathy.[29] These observations, together with the evidence that oxidative stress is increased in failing myocardium, led them to propose that chronically elevated oxidative stress in the myocardium is of pathophysiological relevance in conditions associated with cardiac remodeling.

Regulation of Oxidative Stress in Normal and Failing Myocardium

Oxidative stress may result when there is an increase in ROS production, a decrease in the clearance of ROS, or both. Although the cause of increased myocardial oxidative stress during remodeling and failure is not known, there is indirect evidence for more than one mechanism. The myocardium performs a high level of oxidative metabolism, and therefore has the potential to generate ROS. There is evidence that mitochondrial production of ROS is increased in the myocardium of dogs with pacing-induced heart failure[24] in association with a decrease in the function of complex I of the electron transport chain.[30] This observation raises the possibility that there is a leakage of electrons from the mitochondria, and is consistent with the concept of "oxygen wastage," a term that in the past has been used to describe the decreased efficiency of oxygen usage in the failing myocardium.[31,32] It is possible that certain stimuli (e.g., catecholamines, mechanical strain) act directly or indirectly to cause electron "leakage" by increasing electron flux and/or depressing electron transport function. The latter might occur via phosphorylation of a component or components of complex I. It is also possible that cytochrome c released by apoptotic stimuli leads to increased ROS generation through its effects on electron transport.[33,34] Increased myocardial ROS levels might also reflect increased activation of cytosolic oxidases, including NAD(P)H oxidase,[35] xanthine oxidase,[36] and/or nitric oxide synthase 2.[37] NAD(P)H oxidase is a plasmalemmal enzyme

that has been shown to mediate the ROS-dependent effects of angiotensin in vascular smooth muscle cells.[6]

Multiple antioxidant enzymes in the myocardium protect cells by
maintaining O_2^- and H_2O_2 at low levels. Three isoforms of superoxide dismutase (SOD) are present in the myocardium. MnSOD makes up approximately 70% of the SOD activity in the heart and approximately 90%
of the activity in cardiac myocytes,[38] the remaining fraction consisting
primarily of CuZnSOD, which is the major isoform of SOD in the cytosol.
Extracellular SOD is the least prevalent isoform in the myocardium. An
inappropriate decrease in SOD activity has been observed in failing myocardium, raising the possibility that impaired antioxidant capacity may
contribute to increased oxidative stress.[19,22] As the only SOD located in
the mitochondria, MnSOD plays a critical role in the control of mitochondrial O_2^- generation during normal oxidative phosphorylation. The importance of MnSOD in the regulation of ambient O_2^- levels in the myocardium is highlighted by the demonstration that homozygous knockout
mice deficient in MnSOD develop normally but die soon after birth with
dilated cardiomyopathy.[39] H_2O_2, the product of SOD, is handled by glutathione peroxidase (GPx) and catalase. GPx is a selenium-containing enzyme that catalyzes the removal of H_2O_2 through oxidation of reduced
glutathione, which is recycled from oxidized glutathione by glutathione
reductase.

Reactive Oxygen Species Regulate Myocyte Phenotype In Vitro

If oxidative stress plays a role in myocardial remodeling, an increase
in ROS should mimic the cellular hallmarks of myocardial remodeling. To
test this basic premise, we performed experiments in neonatal rat cardiac
myocytes in vitro.[40] The copper chelator diethyldithiocarbamic acid (DDC)
was used to inhibit SOD activity; DDC caused a concentration-dependent
inhibition of SOD activity at concentration of 1–1000 μM. The addition of
DDC to cultured myocytes caused a graded increase in intracellular O_2^-
levels, as assessed by lucigenin chemiluminescence or NBT reduction, and
the increases in O_2^- levels were prevented by the antioxidant Tiron or the
SOD-mimetic Euk-8.

Exposure to the low concentration of DDC (1 μM) for 24 hours
caused a hypertrophic phenotype associated with increased protein synthesis, increased myocyte size, induction of *c-fos* expression, and reexpression of a fetal gene program with an increase in ANF mRNA (Figure 2A) and a decrease in SERCA2 mRNA. In contrast, exposure to high
concentrations of DDC (≥100 μM) caused myocyte apoptosis (Figure 2B)

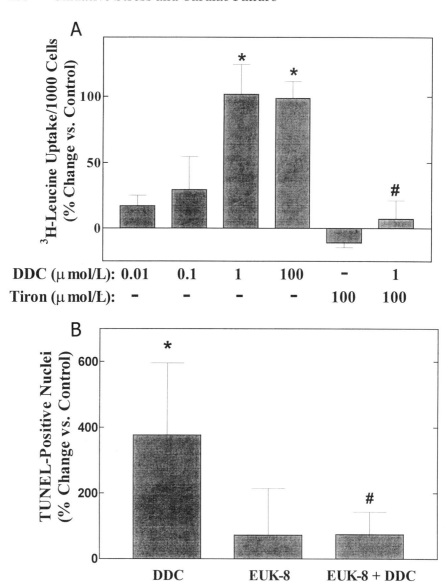

Figure 2. Graded effects of ROS on cardiac myocyte phenotype. To test the overall thesis that nontoxic levels of ROS can regulate the phenotype of cardiac myocytes, cultured myocytes obtained from neonatal rat hearts were treated with diethyldithio-carbamic acid (DDC), a copper chelator that inhibits superoxide dismutase and causes a modest increase in ROS levels. (A) At low concentrations of DDC ($\leq$1 μM), there was myocyte hypertrophy associated with the reexpression of fetal genes such as atrial natriuretic factor. (B) At higher DDC concentrations ($\geq$100 μM), apoptosis occurred. Both the hypertrophic and apoptotic effects of DDC were prevented by co-treatment with the superoxide dismutase mimetics, thus indicating that the observed effects of DDC were mediated by ROS. Adapted from reference 52.

as well as hypertrophy. The apoptotic phenotype was associated with increased expression of mRNA for the pro-apoptotic protein, bax. The effects of both the low and high concentrations of DDC on cell growth, gene expression, and apoptosis were inhibited by the antioxidants Tiron or Euk-8, and were mimicked by exogenous O_2^- generation by the addition of xanthine/xanthine oxidase. Similar observations were made by von Harsdorf et al.,[41] who demonstrated that exposing neonatal rat cardiac myocytes to either an exogenous source of superoxide or H_2O_2 for 24 hours resulted in apoptosis. Thus, ROS can modify the phenotype of cardiac myocytes. These experiments further demonstrate that ROS can exert a graded effect on myocyte phenotype, with hypertrophy at lower concentrations and apoptosis at higher concentrations. Since these effects were caused by inhibition of SOD, it appears that endogenous production of ROS is sufficient to cause important changes in myocyte phenotype.

Reactive Oxygen Species Regulate Collagen Metabolism by Cardiac Fibroblasts

Cardiac fibroblasts play an important role in regulating the composition and quantity of interstitial matrix proteins. A particularly important component of the interstitium is collagen, which contributes to the structural integrity of the myocardium. The quantity of collagen in the interstitium is regulated by the balance between synthesis and degradation, the latter primarily due to the action of matrix metalloproteinases (MMPs). To determine the role of ROS in the regulation of cardiac fibroblast function, fibroblasts from adult and neonatal rats were cultured and exposed to an increase in ROS caused by exposure for 24 hours to the superoxide-generating system of xanthine plus xanthine oxidase (XXO), the SOD inhibitor DDC, or H_2O_2.[42] MMP activity, measured by in-gel zymography, was increased by approximately 40–50% by each of the ROS sources (XXO, DDC, and H_2O_2), due primarily to increases in the activities of MMP1, MMP2, and MMP9 (Figure 3A). In parallel, collagen synthesis, measured as collagenase-sensitive [³H]-proline incorporation, was decreased by each of the ROS sources (Figure 3B). The decreases in collagen synthesis were associated with reduced expression of mRNA for the procollagens $\alpha 1$(I), $\alpha 2$(I), and $\alpha 1$(III). These experiments demonstrate that ROS can both activate MMPs and decrease collagen synthesis in cardiac fibroblasts, and thus raise the possibility that ROS contribute to myocardial remodeling, in part through their effects on intercellular matrix turnover.

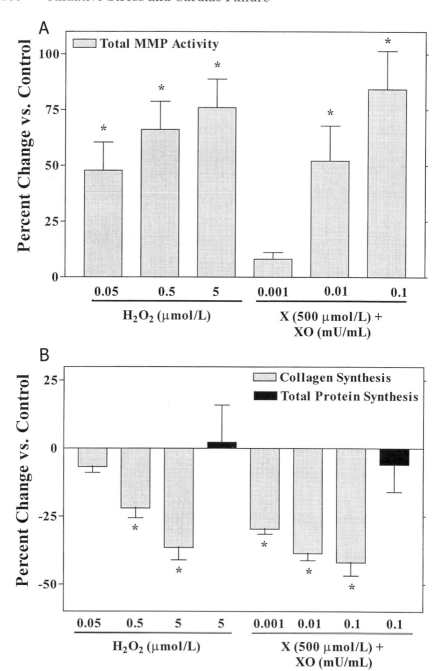

Figure 3. ROS regulation of collagen synthesis and degradation by cardiac fibroblasts. Cardiac fibroblasts cultured from neonatal rat hearts were exposed to either H_2O_2 or the superoxide-generating system of xanthine 1 and xanthine oxidase (XXO) for 24 hours. H_2O_2 and XXO each caused increases in the activity of metalloproteinases (**A**) and decreases in collagen synthesis (**B**). Adapted from reference 51.

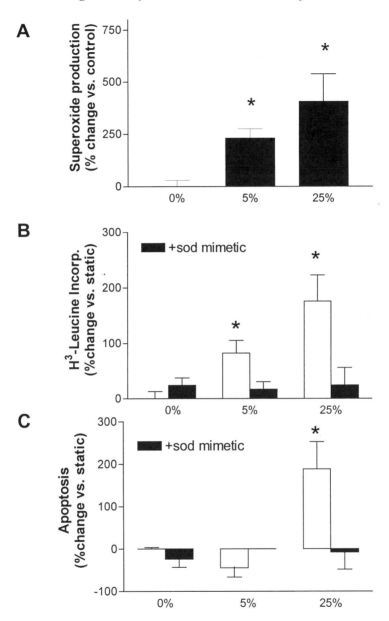

Figure 4. Role of ROS in mediating the effects of mechanical strain on cardiac myocytes. Cardiac myocytes cultured from neonatal rat hearts were subjected to cyclic stretching at 60 Hz for 24 hours. At a low level of strain (5% stretch), there was a modest increase in ROS (**A**) that was associated with increased protein synthesis (**B**). At a higher level of strain (25% stretch), there was a greater increase in ROS levels (**A**), which was also associated with myocyte hypertrophy (**B**). In addition, high strain caused myocyte apoptosis (**C**). The effects of both low and high strain were prevented by co-treatment with superoxide dismutase mimetics, thus implicating ROS in the observed responses to mechanical strain.

Mechanical Strain Regulates Myocyte Phenotype via an ROS-Dependent Mechanism In Vitro

There is evidence that mechanical strain can increase ROS levels. Ansersa and colleagues showed that mechanical strain increases ROS levels in rat papillary muscle.[43] Likewise, it has been shown that mechanical strain can increase ROS in cardiac fibroblasts.[44] To determine the relationship between mechanical strain, ROS, and cardiac myocyte phenotype, we subjected neonatal rat ventricular myocytes to cyclic mechanical strain at a frequency of 1 Hz for 24 hours, and ROS levels were assessed with lucigenin. Low-amplitude strain (5% nominal stretch) caused a small increase in ROS associated with small increases in protein synthesis and ANF expression, but had no effect on the frequency of apoptosis as measured by TUNEL or DNA laddering (Figure 4A, B). In contrast, myocytes stretched at high-amplitude strain (25% nominal stretch) had larger increases in ROS, associated with larger increases in protein synthesis and ANF expression (versus cells with low-amplitude strain) (Figure 4A, C). Of note, at high-amplitude strain there was an increase in the number of apoptotic myocytes, which did not occur with low-level stretch. Treatment of myocytes with the SOD-mimetic MnTMPyP prevented stretch-induced hypertrophy and apoptosis.

These observations suggest that mechanical strain causes a graded increase in ROS that mediates myocyte hypertrophy, fetal gene expression, and apoptosis. As with the effects of SOD inhibition, the smaller increase in ROS caused by low-amplitude strain resulted in hypertrophy and fetal gene expression, whereas the larger increase in ROS caused by high-amplitude strain also resulted in apoptosis. These observations support the thesis that ROS play a critical role in mediating the phenotypic response of cardiac myocytes to a primary remodeling stimulus (mechanical strain), and further suggest that the amount of ROS may be a determinant of the resulting phenotype.

Alpha$_1$-Adrenergic Receptor-Stimulated Hypertrophy Is ROS-Dependent

Alpha$_1$-adrenergic stimulation causes hypertrophy in cardiac myocytes in culture.[45,46] In primary cultures of adult rat cardiac myocytes, we found that stimulation with norepinephrine (NE) (1 μM) for 48 hours caused hypertrophy as evidenced by an increase in total protein per cell and ^{3}H-leucine incorporation, associated with reexpression of a fetal gene program as reflected by an increase in atrial natriuretic peptide mRNA and a decrease in SERCA2 mRNA.[47] The increase in protein synthesis is inhibited completely by prazosin, but not by propranolol, indicating that it was mediated by α_1-AR. Stimulation with NE caused an increase in ROS levels as assessed by lucigenin chemiluminescence, and addition of the SOD-mimetic MnTMPyP (50 μM) inhibited α_1-AR-stimulated myocyte hypertrophy, suggesting that α_1-AR-stimulated myocyte hypertrophy is ROS-dependent (Figure 5). To further clarify the cellular site at which α_1-AR-stimulated myocyte hypertrophy is ROS-dependent, myocytes were infected with an adenoviral vector expressing CuZnSOD, which localizes to the cytosol (Figure 6). In cells overexpressing CuZn-SOD, α_1-AR-stimulated myocyte hypertrophy was prevented, suggesting that the ROS-dependent step is located in the cytosol. Recently, Tanaka et al. reported very similar findings.[48] They found that in adult rat cardiac myocytes, the hypertrophic responses to both α_1-AR stimulation and endothelin were associated with an increase in ROS and were inhibited by the addition of antioxidants. Other putative remodeling stimuli for cardiac myocytes, including angiotensin and tumor necrosis factor-α, have also been shown to increase oxidative stress in cardiac cells or tissue and to cause ROS-dependent myocyte hypertrophy.[49]

The NAD(P)H oxidase is a cytosolic system that has been implicated in mediating ROS production and the ROS-dependent growth effects of angiotensin in vascular smooth muscle cells.[35] We therefore examined

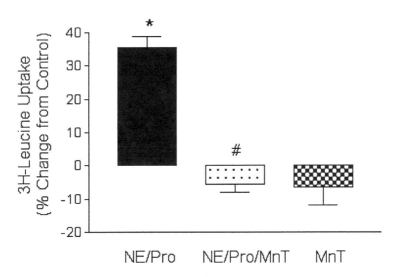

Figure 5. Role of ROS in mediating myocyte hypertrophy in response to α_1-adrenergic receptor (α_1-AR) stimulation. Adult rat cardiac myocytes were exposed to α_1-AR stimulation with norepinephrine (NE) in the presence of propranolol (Pro) for 24 hours. α_1-AR stimulation increased protein synthesis. This effect was prevented by addition of the SOD-mimetic MnTMPyP (MnT). Adapted from reference 62.

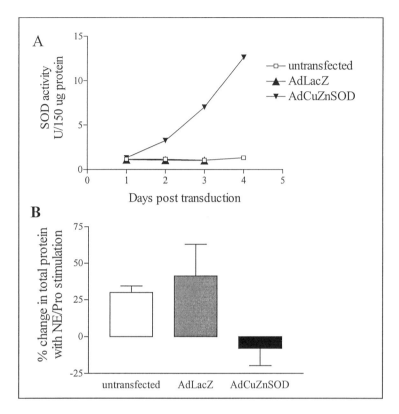

Figure 6. Inhibition of α_1-AR-stimulated protein synthesis by CuZnSOD. (A) CuZn-SOD was overexpressed in adult rat cardiac myocytes using an adenoviral vector, resulting in a time-dependent increase in SOD activity. (B) In myocytes overexpressing CuZnSOD, α_1-AR-stimulated protein synthesis was abolished (n=4). α_1-AR-stimulated protein synthesis was not affected in cells infected only with a control vector expressing LacZ (AdLacZ).

whether activation of NAD(P)H oxidase might be involved in α_1-AR-stimulated hypertrophy of cardiac myocytes. In adult rat cardiac myocytes, the NAD(P)H oxidase inhibitor diphenylene iodonium (DPI) completely prevented the α_1-AR-stimulated activation of Erk1/2. In contrast, inhibition of the mitochondrial respiratory chain complex I, another likely source of ROS in myocytes, with rotenone had no effect on the α_1-AR-stimulated activation of Erk1/2. These observations suggest that NAD(P)H oxidase is a source of ROS in response to α_1-AR-stimulation.[50] Although the presence of an active NAD(P)H oxidase system in cardiac myocytes has not been established, we have identified several subunits of NAD(P)H oxidase by rtPCR in adult rat cardiac myocytes. Likewise,

Tanaka et al.[48] have recently reported that α_1-AR stimulation and endothelin caused activation of Erk1/2 and that both hypertrophy and Erk1/2 activation were inhibited by DPI. Thus, taken together, these observations suggest that cardiac myocytes possess an NAD(P)H oxidase system that plays a role in mediating the hypertrophic response to α_1-AR stimulation. The role of this system in mediating the responses to other growth stimuli that have been shown to be ROS-dependent remains to be determined.

α_1-Adrenergic stimulation is known to activate stress-activated kinases in cardiac myocytes.[51] In adult rat cardiac myocytes, we found that α_1-AR stimulation caused marked activation of the Ras-MEK1/2-Erk1/2 pathway, but did not activate p38kinases or JNKs.[50] The MEK1/2 inhibitor PD98059 abolished α_1-AR-stimulated hypertrophy. Likewise, Western blotting for activated Erk1/2 in lysates from the myocytes after α_1-AR stimulation showed a robust increase in phospho-Erk1/2 at 15 minutes that was completely prevented by the SOD-mimetic MnTMPyP, suggesting that in adult cardiac myocytes, α_1-AR-stimulated hypertrophy involves an ROS-dependent activation of Erk1/2.

β_1-Adrenergic Receptor (-AR)-Stimulated Apoptosis Is ROS-Dependent

We[52] and others[53] have found that β-AR stimulation for 24 hours causes apoptosis in adult rat cardiac myocytes as evidenced by increased DNA laddering and an increase in the percentage of cells stained by terminal deoxynucleotidyl transferase-mediated nick end-labeling (TUNEL). β-AR-stimulated apoptosis was mimicked by isoproterenol and forskolin, abolished by propranolol (but not by prazosin), and inhibited by the adenylyl cyclase inhibitor H89 and the voltage-dependent calcium channel blocker diltiazem. The apoptotic effect of β-AR stimulation was inhibited by the β_1-AR-selective antagonist CGP-20712A, whereas the β_2-AR-selective antagonist ICI-118,551 increased the amount of apoptosis. The anti-apoptotic action of β_2-AR stimulation was abolished by pertussis toxin and mimicked by the Gi activator carbachol, implicating Gi in an anti-apoptotic pathway. These observations suggest that NE can stimulate apoptosis via β_1-ARs that are coupled to Gs-adenylyl cyclase-calcium influx, whereas β_2-ARs exert an anti-apoptotic action via coupling to Gi.

To test the role of ROS in β_1-AR-stimulated apoptosis, myocytes were exposed to β-AR stimulation in the presence or absence of the SOD-mimetics MnTmPyP or Euk-134. β-AR-stimulated apoptosis was abolished by either MnTmPyP or Euk 134, suggesting that ROS are involved in β_1-AR-stimulated apoptosis.[54] The source of ROS that mediates the apoptotic effect of β-AR stimulation is not known. However, there is indirect evidence that the mechanism may involve mitochondria. For example, we found that β-AR-stimulated apoptosis was associated with increased expression of bax and decreased expression of Bcl-x$_L$ at 6 hours. Likewise, Zaugg et al.[53] found that β-AR stimulation in adult rat cardiac myocytes increased the ratio of bax to Bcl-2, and this effect was prevented by the β$_1$-AR-selective antagonist atenolol. Bax and bak, pro-apoptotic members of the Bcl-2 family of proteins, interact with the mitochondrial permeability transition pore, thereby promoting cytochrome *c* release and dissipation of the membrane potential.[55-57] The mitochondrial transition pore regulates the release of cytochrome *c* from the intermembrane space, leading to the activation of caspase 3, an early step in the regulation of myocyte apoptosis.[58] We found that β$_1$-AR stimulation increased the translocation of cytochrome *c*, as assessed by Western blotting, from the mitochondria to the cytosol, and increased caspase-3 activity.[54] Zaugg et al.[53] found that β$_1$-AR stimulation increased the activity of caspase 9, but not caspase 8. Taken together, these observations provide circumstantial evidence for the involvement of mitochondria in β-AR-stimulated apoptosis.

Stress-activated protein kinases (SAPKs) are well known to be activated by ROS[59] and have been implicated in the regulation of cardiac myocyte apoptosis.[60] To examine whether SAPKs play a role in β-AR-stimulated apoptosis, we examined the JNK and p38 kinase activity in adult rat cardiac myocytes. β-AR stimulation caused rapid (15 min) activation of both JNK and p38, and to a lesser extent, Erk1/2, which was not evident until 90 minutes.[61] Inhibition of Erk1/2 with PD98059 had no effect on the amount of β-AR-stimulated apoptosis, suggesting that Erk1/2 neither promoted nor inhibited apoptosis under these circumstances. In contrast, inhibition of p38 with SB202190 (10 μM) increased the amount of apoptosis. This observation raised the possibility that one or more p38 isoforms exert an anti-apoptotic effect. However, subsequent work in mouse cardiac myocytes has suggested that the protective effect of β$_2$-AR stimulation is mediated by activation of PI3kinase, rather than p38, and that the effect of SB202190 that was observed may thus have been due to nonspecific inhibition of PI3kinase by the drug.[62] Further experiments using molecular probes will be required to clarify this issue. The role of JNK in β-AR-stimulated apoptosis is not known, due in large part to the current lack of selective pharmacological inhibitors of JNK. Given the involvement of JNK in the regulation of myocyte growth and apoptosis and their well-recognized stimulation by oxidative stress,[63] it is possible that they are involved in mediating the ROS-dependent effects of β-AR stimulation.

Conclusion

We have formulated a working model to describe the role of ROS in mediating myocardial remodeling in response to mechanical overload and excessive adrenergic stimulation (Figure 7). α$_1$-AR stimulation appears to

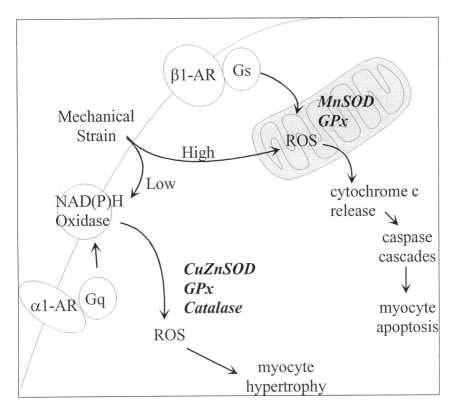

Figure 7. Illustration of a working model for the relationship between remodeling stimuli and ROS in cardiac myocytes. According to this model, low-level mechanical strain and α_1-AR stimulation result in a hypertrophic phenotype that is mediated primarily by NAD(P)H oxidase, whereas high-level mechanical strain and β_1-AR stimulation lead to an apoptotic phenotype by activation via a mitochondrial pathway.

mediate myocyte hypertrophy via activation of a plasmalemmal NAD(P)H oxidase that would be expected to increase both O_2^- and H_2O_2 in the cytosol. CuZnSOD dismutates O_2^- to H_2O_2, which is then converted to H_2O by catalase and GPx. It remains to be determined whether O_2^-, H_2O_2, or both, is responsible for the hypertrophic phenotype. Low-level mechanical strain causes a hypertrophic phenotype similar to α_1-AR stimulation, which may also be mediated by NAD(P)H oxidase. In contrast, α_1-AR stimulation causes an apoptotic phenotype, which appears to involve mitochondrial pathways and ROS. It remains to be determined whether ROS act upstream and/or downstream of mitochondria in signaling the response to β_1-AR. Increased O_2^- production in the mitochondria may also result in the generation of $OH^{\cdot}$ via the Fenton reaction and increased levels of H_2O_2 due to dismutation by MnSOD. The precise relationship between extracellular stimuli for remodeling, ROS, and various intracellular signaling pathways remains to be determined, and likely will hold important complexities that dictate the ensuing phenotype. Understanding the role of ROS in myocardial remodeling may allow for the therapeutic manipulation of this important process in patients at risk for myocardial failure.[64,32]

References

1. Cohn JN. Structural basis for heart failure: ventricular remodeling and its pharmacological inhibition. Circulation 1995;91:2504–2507.
2. Griendling KK, Ushio-Fukai M. Redox control of vascular smooth muscle proliferation. J Lab Clin Med 1998;132:9–15.
3. Sundaresan M, Yu ZX, Ferrans VJ, et al. Requirement for generation of H_2O_2 for platelet-derived growth factor signal transduction. Science 1995;270:296–299.
4. Sundaresan M, Yu ZX, Ferrans VJ, et al. Regulation of reactive-oxygen-species generation in fibroblasts by Rac1. Biochem J 1996;318:379–382.
5. Irani K, Xia Y, Zweier JL, et al. Mitogenic signaling mediated by oxidants in Ras-transformed fibroblasts. Science 1997;l275:1649–1652.
6. Griendling KK, Minieri CA, Ollerenshaw JD, et al. Angiotensin II stimulates NADH and NADPH oxidase activity in cultured vascular smooth muscle cells. Circ Res 1994;74:1141–1148.
7. Ushio-Fukai M, Zafari AM, Fukui T, et al. p22phox is a critical component of the superoxide-generating NADH/NADPH oxidase system and regulates angiotensin II-induced hypertrophy in vascular smooth muscle cells. J Biol Chem 1996;271:23317–23321.
8. Colucci WS. Molecular and cellular mechanisms of myocardial failure. Am J Cardiol 1997;80:15L–25L.
9. Katz AM. The cardiomyopathy of overload: an unnatural growth response in the hypertrophied heart. Ann Intern Med 1994;121:363–371.
10. Gerdes AM, Liu Z, Zimmer HG. Changes in nuclear size of cardiac myocytes during the development and progression of hypertrophy in rats. Cardioscience 1994;5:203–208.
11. MacLellan WR, Schneider MD. Death by design: programmed cell death in cardiovascular biology and disease. Circ Res 1997;81:137–144.
12. Olivetti G, Capasso JM, Sonnenblick EH, et al. Side-to-side slippage of myocytes participates in ventricular wall remodeling acutely after myocardial infarction in rats. Circ Res 1990;67:23–34.
13. Mann DL, Spinale FG. Activation of matrix metalloproteinases in the failing human heart: breaking the tie that binds [editorial]. Circulation 1998;98:1699–1702.
14. Weber KT, Anversa P, Armstrong PW, et al. Remodeling and reparation of the cardiovascular system. J Am Coll Cardiol 1992;20:3–16.
15. Litwin SE, Bridge JH. Enhanced Na(+)-Ca^{2+} exchange in the infarcted heart: implications for excitation-contraction coupling. Circ Res 1997;81:1083–1093.
16. Morgan JP, Erny RE, Allen PD, et al. Abnormal intracellular calcium handling, a major cause of systolic and diastolic dysfunction in ventricular myocardium from patients with heart failure. Circulation 1990;81(Suppl):III21–32.

17. The SOLVD Investigators. Effect of enalapril on survival in patients with re-
    duced left ventricular ejection fractions and congestive heart failure. N Engl
    J Med 1991;325:293–302.
18. Diaz-Velez CR, Garcia-Castineiras S, Mendoza-Ramos E, et al. Increased
    malondialdehyde in peripheral blood of patients with congestive heart fail-
    ure. Am Heart J 1996;131:146–152.
19. Ghatak A, Brar MJ, Agarwal A, et al. Oxy free radical system in heart fail-
    ure and therapeutic role of oral vitamin E. Int J Cardiol 1996;57:119–127.
20. Keith M, Geranmayegan AJ, Sole MJ, et al. Increased oxidative stress in pa-
    tients with congestive heart failure. J Am Coll Cardiol 1998;31:1352–1356.
21. Mallat Z, Philip I, Lebret M, et al. Elevated levels of 8-iso-prostaglandin F2al-
    pha in pericardial fluid of patients with heart failure: a potential role for in
    vivo oxidant stress in ventricular dilatation and progression to heart failure.
    Circulation 1998;97:1536–1539.
22. Hill MF, Singal PK. Antioxidant and oxidative stress changes during heart fail-
    ure subsequent to myocardial infarction in rats. Am J Pathol 1996;148:291–300.
23. Dhalla AK, Singal PK. Antioxidant changes in hypertrophied and failing
    guinea pig hearts. Am J Physiol 1994;266:H1280–H1285.
24. Ide T, Tsutsui H, Kinugawa S, et al. Direct evidence for increased hydroxyl
    radicals originating from superoxide in the failing myocardium. Circ Res
    2000;86:152–157.
25. Singal PK, Dhalla AK, Hill M, et al. Endogenous antioxidant changes in the
    myocardium in response to acute and chronic stress conditions. Mol Cell
    Biochem 1993;129:179–186.
26. Singal PK, Kapur N, Dhillon KS, et al. Role of free radicals in catecholamine-
    induced cardiomyopathy. Can J Physiol Pharmacol 1982;60:1390–1397.
27. Dhalla AK, Hill MF, Singal PK. Role of oxidative stress in transition of hy-
    pertrophy to heart failure. J Am Coll Cardiol 1996;28:506–514.
28. Singal PK, Siveski-Iliskovic N, Hill M, et al. Combination therapy with probu-
    col prevents Adriamycin-induced cardiomyopathy. J Mol Cell Cardiol 1995;27:
    1055–1063.
29. Kaul N, Siveski-Iliskovic N, Thomas TP, et al. Probucol improves antioxidant
    activity and modulates development of diabetic cardiomyopathy. Nutrition
    1995;11:551–554.
30. Ide T, Tsutsui H, Kinugawa S, et al. Mitochondrial electron transport com-
    plex I is a potential source of oxygen free radicals in the failing myocardium.
    Circ Res 1999;85:357–363.
31. Opie LH, Thandroyen FT, Muller C, et al. Adrenaline-induced "oxygen-
    wastage" and enzyme release from working rat heart: effects of calcium an-
    tagonism, beta-blockade, nicotinic acid and coronary artery ligation. J Mol
    Cell Cardiol 1979;11:1073–1094.
32. Sawyer DB, Colucci WS. Mitochondrial oxidative stress in heart failure: "oxy-
    gen wastage" revisited. Circ Res 2000;86:119–120.
33. Kojima H, Endo K, Moriyama H, et al. Abrogation of mitochondrial cyto-
    chrome c release and caspase-3 activation in acquired multidrug resistance.
    J Biol Chem 1998;273:16647–16650.
34. Reed JC. Cytochrome *c:* can't live with it—can't live without it [comment].
    Cell 1997;91(5):559–562.
35. Griendling KK, Sorescu D, Ushio-Fukai M. NAD(P)H oxidase: role in cardio-
    vascular biology and disease. Circ Res 2000;86:494–501.
36. Ekelund UE, Harrison RW, Shokek O, et al. Intravenous allopurinol de-
    creases myocardial oxygen consumption and increases mechanical efficiency
    in dogs with pacing-induced heart failure. Circ Res 1999;85:437–445.

37. Xia Y, Dawson VL, Dawson TM, et al. Nitric oxide synthase generates super-oxide and nitric oxide in arginine-depleted cells leading to peroxynitrite-mediated cellular injury. Proc Natl Acad Sci USA 1996;93:6770–6774.
38. Assem M, Teyssier JR, Benderitter M, et al. Pattern of superoxide dismutase enzymatic activity and RNA changes in rat heart ventricles after myocardial infarction. Am J Pathol 1997;151:549–555.
39. Li Y, Huang TT, Carlson EJ, et al. Dilated cardiomyopathy and neonatal lethality in mutant mice lacking manganese superoxide dismutase. Nature Genetics 1995;11:376–381.
40. Siwik DA, Tzortzis JD, Pimentel DR, et al. Inhibition of copper-zinc super-oxide dismutase induces cell growth, hypertrophic phenotype, and apoptosis in neonatal rat cardiac myocytes in vitro. Circ Res 1999;85:147–153.
41. von Harsdorf R, Li PF, Dietz R. Signaling pathways in reactive oxygen species-induced cardiomyocyte apoptosis. Circulation 1999;99:2934–2941.
42. Siwik DA, Pagano PJ, Colucci WS. Oxidative stress regulates collagen syn-thesis and matrix metalloproteinase activity in cardiac fibroblasts. Am J Phys-iol Cell Physiol 2001;280:C53–C60.
43. Cheng W, Li B, Kajstura J, et al. Stretch-induced programmed myocyte cell death. J Clin Invest 1995;96:2247–2259.
44. Tyagi SC, Lewis K, Pikes D, et al. Stretch-induced membrane type matrix metalloproteinase and tissue plasminogen activator in cardiac fibroblast cells. J Cell Physiol 1998;176:374–382.
45. Schluter KD, Piper HM. Regulation of growth in the adult cardiomyocytes. FASEB J 1999;13(Suppl):S17–22.
46. Simpson P. Stimulation of hypertrophy of cultured neonatal rat heart cells through an alpha 1-adrenergic receptor and induction of beating through an alpha 1- and beta 1-adrenergic receptor interaction. Evidence for independ-ent regulation of growth and beating. Circ Res 1985;56:884–894.
47. Amin JK, Xiao L, Pimentel DR, et al. Reactive oxygen species mediate alpha-adrenergic receptor-stimulated hypertrophy in adult rat ventricular myo-cytes. J Mol Cell Cardiol 2001;33:131–139.
48. Tanaka K, Honda M, Takabatake T. Redox regulation of MAPK pathways and cardiac hypertrophy in adult rat cardiac myocyte. J Am Coll Cardiol 2001;37:676–685.
49. Nakamura K, Fushimi K, Kouchi H, et al. Inhibitory effects of antioxidants on neonatal rat cardiac myocyte hypertrophy induced by tumor necrosis factor-alpha and angiotensin II. Circulation 1998;98:794–799.
50. Xiao L, Pimentel DR, Amin JK, et al. MEK1/2-ERK1/2 mediates alpha1-adrenergic receptor-stimulated hypertrophy in adult rat ventricular myo-cytes. J Mol Cell Cardiol 2001;33:779–787.
51. Bogoyevitch MA, Andersson MB, Gillespie-Brown J, et al. Adrenergic recep-tor stimulation of the mitogen-activated protein kinase cascade and cardiac hypertrophy. Biochem J 1996;314:115–121.
52. Communal C, Singh K, Pimentel DR, et al. Norepinephrine stimulates apop-tosis in adult rat ventricular myocytes by activation of the β-adrenergic path-way. Circulation 1998;98:1329–1334.
53. Zaugg M, Xu W, Lucchinetti E, et al. Beta-adrenergic receptor subtypes dif-ferentially affect apoptosis in adult rat ventricular myocytes. Circulation 2000; 102:344–350.
54. Communal C, Xie Z, Sawyer DB, et al. Beta-adrenergic receptor-stimulated apoptosis involves mitochondrial pathways and reactive oxygen species. Cir-culation 2000;102(Suppl 2):II-9.

55. Jurgensmeier JM, Xie Z, Deveraux Q, et al. Bax directly induces release of cytochrome c from isolated mitochondria. Proc Natl Acad Sci USA 1998;95: 4997–5002.
56. Narita M, Shimizu S, Ito T, et al. Bax interacts with the permeability transition pore to induce permeability transition and cytochrome *c* release in isolated mitochondria. Proc Natl Acad Sci USA 1998;95:14681–14686.
57. Rosse T, Olivier R, Monney L, et al. Bcl-2 prolongs cell survival after Bax-induced release of cytochrome *c* [see comments]. Nature 1998;391:496–499.
58. Cai J, Jones DP. Superoxide in apoptosisL nitochondrial generation triggered by cytochrome c loss. J Biol Chem 1998;273:11401–11404.
59. Clerk A, Michael A, Sugden PH. Stimulation of multiple mitogen-activated protein kinase sub-families by oxidative stress and phosphorylation of the small heat shock protein, HSP25/27, in neonatal ventricular myocytes. Biochem J 1998;333:581–589.
60. Sugden PH, Clerk A. Cellular mechanisms of cardiac hypertrophy. J Mol Med 1998;76:725–746.
61. Communal C, Colucci WS, Singh K. p38 Mitogen-activated protein kinase pathway protects adult rat ventricular myocytes against beta-adrenergic receptor-stimulated apoptosis: evidence for Gi-dependent activation. J Biol Chem 2000;275:19395–19400.
62. Zhu WZ, Zheng M, Koch WJ, et al. Dual modulation of cell survival and cell death by beta(2)-adrenergic signaling in adult mouse cardiac myocytes. Proc Natl Acad Sci USA 2001;98:1607–1612.
63. Clerk A, Fuller SJ, Michael A, et al. Stimulation of "stress-regulated" mitogen-activated protein kinases (stress-activated protein kinases/c-Jun N-terminal kinases and p38-mitogen-activated protein kinases) in perfused rat hearts by oxidative and other stresses. J Biol Chem 1998;273:7228–7234.
64. Givertz MM, Colucci WS. New targets for heart-failure therapy: endothelin, inflammatory cytokines, and oxidative stress. Lancet 1998;352(Suppl 1):SI34–38.

III

Therapeutic Pathways and
Modulation of Oxidative Stress

• 8 •

Beta-Blockers and Oxidative Stress

Marrick L. Kukin, MD

Introduction

The chemistry and biology of oxidative stress have been superbly described in the previous chapters with convincing data that oxidative stress contributes to the pathogenesis and progression of heart failure.

Many pharmaceutical approaches for heart failure have been developed and some have proven to be efficacious. In the next six chapters, the specific antioxidant effects of different classes of heart failure drugs will be explored. In this chapter, the mortality benefits of beta-blockers will be reviewed before exploring evidence for the specific antioxidant effects of beta-blockers.

Mortality Trials

Data from placebo-controlled mortality trials that each enrolled more than 1000 patients definitively shows that beta-blockers reduce mortality in chronic heart failure.

CIBIS II[1] randomized 2647 patients with moderate-to-severe heart failure secondary to nonischemic or ischemic cardiomyopathy on background therapy (digoxin, diuretic, and ACE inhibitor) to receive the β-1 selective agent bisoprolol or placebo. The trial was prematurely terminated by the Data Safety Monitoring Board (DSMB) due to a highly significant 34% reduction in all-cause mortality in the bisoprolol group ($P<0.0001$),

From: Kukin ML, Fuster V (eds). *Oxidative Stress and Cardiac Failure*. Armonk, NY: Futura Publishing Co., Inc. ©2003.

with a significant 42% reduction of sudden death among patients on biso-prolol.

The Metoprolol CR/XL Randomized Intervention Trial in Congestive Heart Failure (MERIT-HF)[2] enrolled 3991 patients with mild-to-moderate or moderate-to-severe heart failure due to either ischemic or nonischemic causes. Patients were randomized to receive either placebo or metoprolol succinate controlled release/extended release (CR/XL), which is also β-1 selective, in addition to background therapy. This preparation of meto-prolol provides more pronounced steady-state beta-blockade over the course of 24 hours[3] than the twice daily metoprolol tartrate, which may be im-portant in protecting the heart from surges of sympathetic activity that may trigger lethal arrhythmias.[4] Showing a nearly identical result as in CIBIS-II, there was a 34% reduction in mortality (P=0.00009) with meto-prolol succinate.

Although a substantial body of evidence in the medical literature supports the use of beta-blockers in patients with mild-to-moderate heart failure, data regarding the long-term safety and efficacy of beta-blockers in patients with severe heart failure are limited.[5] The COPERNICUS trial evaluated the beta nonselective agent carvedilol in 2289 patients with severe heart failure and an LVEF ≤25%.[6] Patients randomized to carvedilol treatment received an initial dose of 3.125 mg twice daily for 2 weeks, which was doubled at 2-week intervals to a maximum target dose of 25 mg twice daily as tolerated. The trial was discontinued early by the DSMB due to the mortality benefits observed with carvedilol. Final analysis of the data showed that patients in the carvedilol group had a 35% risk reduction in total mortality (P=.0014), with cumulative risk of death at 1 year of 18.5% in the placebo group and 11.4% in the carvedilol group. These data are consistent with the results of MERIT-HF and CIBIS-II and extend the results of beta-blocker trials to the sickest group of patients.

However, all of the recent data on beta-blockers in chronic heart fail-ure have not been positive. The Beta-Blocker Evaluation Survival Trial (BEST)[7] was a randomized, placebo-controlled, double-blind trial assess-ing the efficacy of the vasodilating beta-blocker bucindolol compared with placebo in reducing mortality in patients with chronic heart failure with predominantly class III chronic heart failure and a mean ejection fraction of 23%. The study was terminated by the DSMB due to the absence of a significant survival advantage with bucindolol. Whether the nonsignifi-cant survival result is an effect specific to bucindolol or reflects specific characteristics of the BEST population remains to be determined.

The cumulative effect of these data has helped make beta-blockers part of the accepted new standard of "quadruple" therapy for NYHA II-III heart failure[8] 25 years after Waagstein's pioneering work with beta-blockers in chronic heart failure.[9]

Antioxidant Effects of Carvedilol

Carvedilol is a unique pharmacological compound that has multiple pharmacological properties. It blocks β1 and β2 receptors as well as alpha receptors. Additionally, it has a specific antioxidant moiety as part of its chemical structure.

Initial studies with carvedilol using rat brain homogenates demonstrated inhibition of lipid peroxidation[10] through the formation of TBARS (thiobarbituric acid reactive substances) using a malondialdehyde (MDA) standard curve. Compared to five other beta-blockers (celiprolol, labetalol, propranolol, atenolol, and pindolol), carvedilol had the most potent effect of inhibiting iron-induced and vitamin C-induced lipid peroxidation. Using spin trapping (DMPO – dimethyl pyrrolidine oxide) techniques, carvedilol was shown to be a free radical scavenger as well.

Carvedilol is highly lipophilic and extensively distributed in tissue.[11] Continued dosing of carvedilol may allow for cell membranes to accumulate drug levels and potentiate antioxidant activity. Whether the in vitro effects can be demonstrated in vivo specifically for carvedilol and not other beta-blockers remains an unanswered question.

In a direct comparison of carvedilol and metoprolol in heart failure patients,[12] we specifically measured oxidative stress and changes in these levels with beta-blocker therapy. TBARS were chosen as the indirect measure for oxidative stress following the previous work of Belch and colleagues (see Chapter 4). TBARS were measured twice at baseline (weeks –2 and 0) and then again at months 4 and 6 of beta-blocker therapy.

Sixty-seven patients were enrolled in this randomized trial. Thirty received metoprolol tartrate (target dose 25 mg bid), and 37 received carvedilol (target dose 25 mg bid). The groups were similar at baseline. In terms of clinical outcome, there were parallel improvements in symptom score, Minnesota Living With Heart Failure Questionnaires, 6-minute walk, peak VO_2, and ejection fraction for both metoprolol and carvedilol with no between group differences.

Surprisingly, there was no difference in antioxidant activity. Elevated TBAR levels declined with metoprolol from 4.7 ± 0.9 nmol/mL at baseline to 4.2 ±1.5 at month four to 3.9 ± 1 at month 6 ($P<0.0001$). With carvedilol, there was a parallel decline from 4.7 ± 1.4 nmol/mL to 4.2 ± 1.3 to 4.1 ± 1.2 over the same time frame ($P<0.025$), with no between group differences in these changes (Figure 1). Thus, as patients improved clinically over 6 months, this measure of oxidative stress declined in parallel for both metoprolol- and carvedilol-treated patients.

Two other small trials[13,14] directly compared metoprolol and carvedilol, finding similar chronic improvements for both beta-blockers with ejection fraction and clinical parameters. Neither of these studies measured oxidative stress.

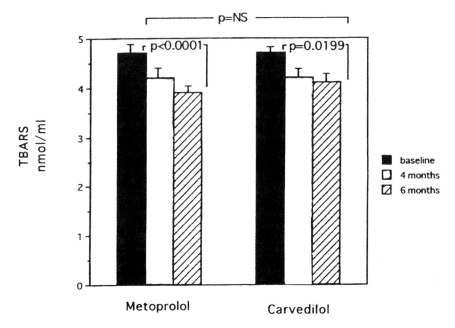

Figure 1. TBARS values for those who completed the protocol at baseline, month 4, and month 6 for metoprolol and carvedilol, respectively. Values are mean ±SEM; *P* values inside box are within group by paired *t* tests between baseline and month 6; *P* value above box is between groups by ANOVA for all time points.

In a substudy of their beta-blocker trial, Sanderson and colleagues[15] compared antioxidant properties of carvedilol and metoprolol. They did not measure TBARS, but rather compared assays of total antioxidant status (TAS), glutathione peroxidation (GPx), and sodium dismutase (SOD). Thirteen patients received metoprolol and 11 received carvedilol. There was no significant change over 12 weeks in TAS. Over this period, SOD and GPx slightly decreased with carvedilol (within group), but the changes were not significant when compared between groups.

In a recent study, Lysko[16] and colleagues of GlaxoSmith Kline examined antioxidant activity of metoprolol and carvedilol directly in cells and tissues of rats exposed to oxidative stress. Carvedilol and not metoprolol prevented an increase in TBARS when exposed to oxidative stress (FeCl2/ascorbate). Similar results were seen with cultured cerebellar granular cells with measurement of superoxide anion. The authors speculate whether these results differ from the decrease in TBARS with both carvedilol and metoprolol seen in the Kukin clinical studies may be due to further metabolism of metoprolol in vivo.

The demonstration of antioxidant effects of beta-blockers in vivo clearly varies with the antioxidant assay chosen and the beta-blocker studied. Berdeaux and colleagues[17] randomized 50 patients to carvedilol or placebo. They measured antioxidant status at baseline and at 6 months with the addition of an oxygen radical donor (2,2-azobis [2-amidino propane] dihydrochloride, AAPH) to a red blood cell suspension and measured LDH activity as percentage of hemolysed erythrocytes (PHE) opposing AAPH-induced oxidative stress as well as the effects of plasma opposing the AAPH reaction (IVP50). Despite the improved ejection fraction with carvedilol, there was no effect on IVP50 or PHE antioxidant test parameters.

In a study of non-heart failure human specimens testing force of contraction in the presence of OH· radicals, no significant differences were seen between metoprolol and carvedilol.[18] Serum from chronic heart failure patients was shown to induce apoptosis in human umbilical vein endothelial cells, but in serum from chronic heart failure patients on carvedilol, there was suppression of the apoptotic induction.[19] No serum from metoprolol-treated patients was tested, so a beta-blocking effect cannot be discounted.

In a study of eight normal volunteers, generation of reactive oxygen species (ROS) by polymorphonuclear leukocytes and monocytes was reduced after carvedilol administration.[20]

Using PET scanning to measure oxidative metabolism in a double-blind placebo controlled study, Beanlands et al.[21] studied 40 patients with chronic heart failure on metoprolol 50 tid or placebo. The metoprolol group had a significant decrease in oxidative metabolism as measured by C-11 acetate PET acquisition compared to placebo. There was no carvedilol patient comparative group.

Conclusion

There is evidence for beneficial reductions of oxidative stress in heart failure patients with beta-blocker therapy. Whether this benefit is found solely with carvedilol is controversial. Part of the difficulty is comparing studies with cultured cells or tissue homogenates with clinical in vivo studies. Another difficulty is in the multitude of assays used to indirectly demonstrate oxidative stress reductions. Finally, most of the clinical studies compared beta-blockers with placebo as opposed to comparisons of different beta-blockers within the same study.

While beta-blockers are clearly of benefit in heart failure patients, the contribution of reducing oxidative stress and the relative merits of each beta-blocker in this regard requires further study.

References

1. CIBIS-II Investigators and Committees. The Cardiac Insufficiency Bisoprolol Study II (CIBIS-II): a randomised trial. Lancet 1999;353:9–13.
2. The MERIT-HF Study Group. Effect of metoprolol CR/XL in chronic heart failure: Metoprolol CR/XL Randomised Intervention Trial in Congestive Heart Failure (MERIT-HF). Lancet 1999;353:2001–2007.
3. Sandberg A, Ragnarsson G, Jonsson UE, et al. Design of a new multiple-unit controlled-release formulation of metoprolol: metoprolol CR/XL. Eur J Clin Pharmacol 1988;33(Suppl):S3–7.
4. Wikstrand J, Kendall M. The role of beta receptor blockade in preventing sudden death. Eur Heart J 1992;13(Suppl D):111–120.
5. Heart Failure Society of America. HFSA guidelines for management of patients with heart failure caused by left ventricular systolic dysfunction: pharmacological approaches. Pharmacotherapy 2000;20:495–521.
6. Packer M, Coats AJS, Fowler MB, et al. Effect of carvedilol on survival in severe chronic heart failure. N Engl J Med 2001;344:1651–1658.
7. The Beta-Blocker Evaluation of Survival Trial Investigators. A trial of the beta-blocker bucindolol in patients with advanced chronic heart failure. N Engl J Med 2001;344:1659–1667.
8. Packer M, Cohn JN, on behalf of the Steering Committee and membership of the Advisory Council to Improve Outcomes Nationwide in Heart Failure. Consensus recommendations for the management of heart failure. Am J Cardiol 1999;83(Suppl 2A):17A–22A.
9. Waagstein F, Hjalmarson A, Varnauskas E, et al. Effect of chronic beta-adrenergic receptor blockade in congestive cardiomyopathy. Br Heart J 1975;37:1022–1036.
10. Yue TL, Cheng HY, Lysko PG, et al. Carvedilol, a new vasodilator and beta adrenoceptor antagonist, is an antioxidant and free radical scavenger. J Pharmacol Exp Therap 1992;263:92–98.
11. Fuerstein G, Yue TL, Ma XL, et al. A novel multiple-action antihypertensive drug that provides major organ protection. Cardiovasc Drug Rev 1994;12:85–104.
12. Kukin ML, Kalman J, Charney RH, et al. Prospective, randomized comparison of effect of long-term treatment with metoprolol or carvedilol on symptoms, exercise, ejection fraction, and oxidative stress in heart failure. Circulation 1999;99:2645–2651.
13. Metra M, Giubbini R, Nodari S, et al. Differential effects of β-blockers in patients with heart failure: a prospective, randomized, double-blind comparison of the long-term effects of metoprolol versus carvedilol. Circulation 2000;102:546–551.
14. Sanderson JE, Chan SKW, Yip G, et al. Beta-blockade in heart failure: a comparison of carvedilol with metoprolol. J Am Coll Cardiol 1999;34:1522–1528.
15. Arumanayagam M, Chan S, Tong S, et al. Antioxidant properties of carvedilol and metoprolol in heart failure: a double-blind randomized controlled trial. J Cardiovasc Pharmacol 2001;37:48–54.
16. Lysko PG, Webb CL, Gu JL, et al. A comparison of carvedilol and metoprolol antioxidant activities in vitro. J Cardiovasc Pharmacol 2000;36:277–281.
17. Berdeaux A, Abella A, Lindenbaum A, et al. Lack of antioxidant effect of six months carvedilol treatment in patients with chronic heart failure. Circulation 2000; supplement.

18. Flesch M, Maack C, Cremers B, et al. Effect of beta-blockers on free radical-induced contractile dysfunction. Circulation 1999;100:346–353.
19. Rossig L, Haendeler J, Malat Z, et al. Congestive heart failure induces endothelial cell apoptosis: protective role of carvedilol. J Am Coll Cardiol 2000; 36:2081–2089.
20. Dandona P, Karne R, Ghanim H, et al. Carvedilol inhibits reactive oxygen species generation by leukocytes and oxidative damage to amino acids. Circulation 2000;101:122–124.
21. Beanlands RSB, Nahmias C, Gordon E, et al. The effects of beta1-blockade on oxidative metabolism and the metabolic cost of ventricular work in patients with left ventricular dysfunction: a double-blind, placebo-controlled, positron-emisssion tomography study. Circulation 2000;102:2070–2075.

• 9 •

Angiotensin-Converting Enzyme Inhibitors and Oxidative Stress

Balkrishna Singh, MD,
and William T. Abraham, MD

Introduction

Myocardial dysfunction leading to congestive heart failure (CHF) is a progressive condition. It is now well understood that the initial insult (e.g., myocardial infarction) may be mild, and may not produce immediate reduction in overall pump function. However, with time, there is a relentless deterioration in both the structure and function of the ventricle. Pathological remodeling is thus central to the progression of myocardial failure. Although the process is not fully understood, several factors such as mechanical stress, neurohormonal activation (e.g., increased angiotensin II and norepinephrine), and a variety of molecular and cellular events are involved. Several additional mechanisms such as activation of proinflammatory cytokines, nitric oxide (NO), endothelin, and peptide growth factors are also implicated in this process. Angiotensin-converting enzyme (ACE) inhibition, in addition to beta-blockade and aldosterone antagonism, is known to counteract some of these factors and to slow the progression of heart failure.

In this context, the role of free radicals and oxidative stress in heart failure is being increasingly recognized. A relative deficit in the myocardial antioxidant reserve is associated with an increase in myocardial oxidative stress. Increased oxidative stress is capable of causing subcellular abnormalities that can lead to depressed contractile function, myocyte loss, and heart failure. Animal and human studies suggest that treat-

From: Kukin ML, Fuster V (eds). *Oxidative Stress and Cardiac Failure.* Armonk, NY: Futura Publishing Co., Inc. ©2003.

ment with antioxidants can protect against oxidative stress-induced myocardial damage and thus potentially attenuate the onset and progression of CHF.

As mentioned, ACE inhibition has been proven to be beneficial in the treatment of heart failure and causes a favorable alteration in the adverse remodeling process.[1-3] Moreover, treatment with ACE inhibitors reduces both morbidity and mortality in chronic CHF.[1,2] The exact mechanism of benefit of ACE inhibitor treatment remains unclear. ACE inhibition undoubtedly improves hemodynamics and exerts a variety of beneficial effects on the heart, vasculature, and kidneys in the setting of heart failure. However, a growing number of cellular, animal, and human studies suggest that ACE inhibitors have important antioxidant effects. This chapter summarizes what is known about the role of angiotensin II and, in particular, ACE inhibition on oxidative stress in CHF.

Oxidative Stress and Heart Failure

The discovery of superoxide dismutase, an antioxidant enzyme, in 1969[4] led to a plethora of free radical research in various fields of medicine. Most of this research has focused on the measurement of products of oxidative stress, such as lipid peroxidation. Products such as malondialdehyde (MDA), thiobarbituric acid reactive substances (TBARS), and the ratio of reduced to oxidized glutathione are considered indicative of changes in oxidative stress. Similarly, the measurement of different antioxidant enzymes such as superoxide dismutase (SOD), glutathione peroxidase, and catalase has furthered our understanding of the role of oxidative stress in human illness. These antioxidant substances are viewed as protective and may reduce the damage caused by increased oxidative stress. It is increasingly being recognized that an optimal balance between various antioxidant enzymes and oxidative stress may play a crucial role in maintaining the structural and functional integrity of cells, including myocytes. Although incomplete, a growing body of evidence suggests that changes in oxidative stress are involved as either a primary and/or a secondary event that alters myocyte structure and function in CHF. Moreover, emerging data suggest that treatment with antioxidants may have a favorable effect on the disease process.

Free radicals have been implicated in the pathogenesis of certain types of acute myocardial dysfunction such as reperfusion injury and stunning.[5,6] Moreover, evidence for increased lipid peroxidation has been reported in experimental models of CHF, such as in the cardiomyopathic hamster.[7] Increases in oxidative stress have been shown to cause myocardial cell damage and loss of contractile function in ex vivo studies.[8,9] In an experiment by Singal and colleagues,[10] a role for oxygen radical metabolism in the transition from hypertrophy to heart failure was suggested. According to this hypothesis, activated oxygen radical formation during hypertrophy is compensated by an adaptive increase in enzymatic antioxidative defenses (e.g., glutathione peroxidase and SOD). Thus, an imbalance between oxygen radical formation and detoxification, that results in increased oxidative stress, may be prevented and the heart function stabilized during the compensated, hypertrophic stage. However, because of the limited adaptive capacity of the heart, a rise in oxidative stress may ultimately lead to a deficit in antioxidative defenses favoring damaging reactions such as lipid peroxidation. These mechanisms may contribute to the transition from hypertrophy to heart failure, as characterized by progressive dilation and depressed cardiac function. Observations from Belch et al.[11] also support such a role for oxygen free radicals in CHF.

Mounting evidence from human studies also supports a role for oxidative stress in heart failure. An increase in lipid peroxidation, measured by expired pentane content, has been shown to occur in patients with CHF[12] and also during acute myocardial infarction.[13] In a study of 29 patients, McMurray and associates[14] demonstrated that, in patients with CHF, the levels of MDA were significantly increased compared to controls. Similarly, the concentration of thiol (thought to act as a free radical scavenger) was reduced in these patients. Another study has shown that there is a progressive increase in TBARS with worsening NYHA functional class.[15] Moreover, antiadrenergic therapy of heart failure with either metoprolol or carvedilol, a treatment strategy shown to reduce CHF morbidity and mortality, improves TBARS levels in patients with chronic heart failure.[16]

A variety of sources or stimuli of oxidative stress have been described. Many of these relate directly or indirectly to various neurohormonal systems and proinflammatory cytokines that are activated in CHF. As summarized in Table 1, these include NO, prostaglandins, norepi-

Table 1
Potential Mediators of Increased Oxidative Stress
in Congestive Heart Failure

Nitric oxide
Proinflammatory cytokines
Prostaglandins
Auto-oxidation of catecholamines
Activation of polymorphonuclear leukocytes and ischemia-induced xanthine-
 xanthine oxidase
Myocardial stretch
Angiotensin II

nephrine, polymorphonuclear leucocytes, ischemia, increased myocardial stretch, angiotensin II, and others.[17,18]

Angiotensin II and Oxidative Stress

Angiotensin II may contribute to increased oxidative stress via numerous mechanisms (Figure 1). For example, angiotensin II activates membrane-associated nicotinamide adenine dinucleotide phosphate (NADPH)-dependent oxidase, an important vascular source of oxygen radicals.[19,20] Rajagopalan and associates[21] have implicated the angiotensin II AT-1 receptor pathway in this vascular-mediated oxidative stress. They demonstrated that the hypertension caused by angiotensin II, in contrast to norepinephrine, was associated with increased vascular superoxide production and the mechanism of this superoxide production was related to activation of the NADH/NADPH oxidase. Impaired relaxation to acetylcholine, calcium ionophore A23187, and nitroglycerin was variably corrected by treatment of vessels with liposome-encapsulated SOD. Concomitant use of losartan normalized superoxide production and vascular

Role of Angiotensin II in Oxidative Stress

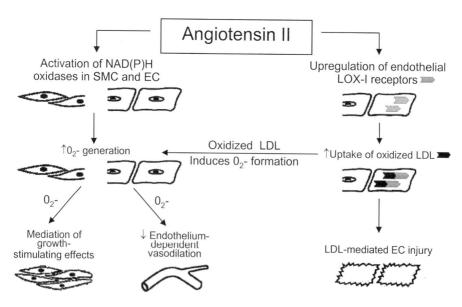

Figure 1. Angiotensin II and oxidative stress. Angiotensin II may contribute to increased oxidative stress via numerous mechanisms. See text for details.

relaxation, suggesting that the AT-1 receptor plays a role in these effects. The participation of AT-1 receptors in the generation of oxygen free radicals has been suggested by other studies as well.[22,23]

Angiotensin II also causes an augmentation of oxygen radical generation in human leucocytes.[24,25] Interestingly, the activity of ACE is increased in some tissues after the addition of oxidizing agents.[26] Thus, a vicious cycle including elevated angiotensin II levels and increased ACE activity may contribute to increased oxygen radical formation in heart failure. Given these observations, one may speculate that ACE inhibition should decrease oxygen radical formation. Contemporary evidence supports this notion.

Evidence for the Antioxidant Effect of ACE Inhibitors

Evidence for the antioxidant effect of ACE inhibition comes from several in vitro and in vivo animal and human studies.

In Vitro Studies

Ruiz-Munoz et al.[27] demonstrated the antioxidant effects of enalaprilat in cultured mesangial cells. In this study, the effect of ACE inhibition on hydrogen peroxide (H_2O_2) production by cultured murine mesangial cells exposed to 5.5 (basal condition), 30, or 50 mM glucose was evaluated over 8 hours. H_2O_2 production by mesangial cells exposed to 50 mM glucose was significantly increased after 1 hour compared to cells exposed to 5.5 and 30 mM glucose. Addition of enalaprilat 100 ng/mL to cells with 50 mM glucose significantly inhibited H_2O_2 production during the 8 hours of study. This response was similar to that obtained with catalase 100 ng/mL, a known antioxidant. Increasing enalaprilat concentrations (10, 50, and 100 ng/mL) also significantly decreased the constitutive H_2O_2 generation in the presence of 5.5 mM glucose. Angiotensin II and saralasin, both at 1 μM, did not modify H_2O_2 production by cells exposed to 5.5 mM glucose. In contrast, 1 μM staurosporine, a protein kinase C (PKC) antagonist, significantly decreased H_2O_2 generation in the presence of 50 mM glucose. These findings suggest that enalaprilat has an antioxidant effect in cultured mesangial cells and that this action is not linked to ACE inhibition per se, but may be related to an inhibition of the PKC system.

Similarly, Zahler and colleagues[28] demonstrated the antioxidant effect of the ACE inhibitor cilazaprilat in human umbilical vein endothelial cells (HUVECs) exposed to H_2O_2. Specifically, they studied the effect of cilazaprilat on redox status, expression of the adhesion molecule P-selectin, and neutrophil adhesion under conditions of oxidative stress in cultured

HUVECs. Incubation of cells with H_2O_2 (0.1 mM and 1 mM) for 15 minutes served as an oxidative stimulus. The intracellular and extracellular concentrations of reduced and oxidized glutathione were measured as indicators of endothelial redox status. Exposure of HUVECs to H_2O_2 caused a reduction in the ratio of reduced to oxidized glutathione. However, ACE inhibition could mitigate mild (0.1 mM H_2O_2) but not more severe redox stress in this model system. Finally, cilazaprilat reduced the upregulation of P-selectin at the higher H_2O_2 concentration, suggesting that this process is regulated independent of the cellular redox status.

Animal Studies

Ha et al.[29] studied the effect of captopril on diabetic proteinuria as a measure of oxidative stress in streptozotocin-induced diabetic rats. Chronic administration of captopril significantly reduced the urinary albumin excretion rate and decreased lipid peroxide excretion. Moreover, the urinary albumin excretion rate was significantly correlated with the lipid peroxide excretion rate. These results suggest that oxidative stress may be responsible, in part, for diabetic microalbuminuria, and that captopril can diminish the lipid peroxidation and ameliorate the microalbuminuria in diabetic rats.

Hayek et al.[30] demonstrated the antioxidative effect of captopril in atherosclerotic mice. The effect of captopril on the development of atherosclerosis in the apolipoprotein (apo) E-deficient mouse was studied. These mice develop severe hypercholesterolemia and extensive atherosclerotic lesions, similar to those found in humans, on chow diet. Furthermore, in these mice, accelerated atherosclerosis is associated with increased plasma lipid peroxidation. In this study, captopril reduced the aortic lesion area by 70% compared to a placebo control group. Captopril also increased the resistance of low-density lipoprotein (LDL) to $CuSO_4$-induced oxidative stress, as shown by a significant reduction in the LDL content of MDA by 30%, as well as by the prolongation of the lag time required for LDL oxidation from 55 minutes in the placebo-treated mice to 70 minutes in the captopril-treated animals, and reduction of maximum LDL oxidation at 150 minutes by 35%. These observations support the conclusion that captopril attenuates atherosclerosis in the apo E-deficient mouse and that this phenomenon may be related to its inhibitory effect on plasma LDL oxidation.

Similarly, Verbeelen et al.[31] demonstrated the antioxidant effect of enalapril and its benefit on renal function in 5/6 nephrectomized rats. Specifically, they investigated the influence of enalapril on the oxidative state of renal tissue and on renal function in these partially nephrectomized animals. Antioxidant enzyme activities were increased in the remnant renal cortex of enalapril-treated animals. Such increased antioxidant enzyme activities may thus contribute to the renal protective effects of this agent. In a similar experiment, Sugimoto and colleagues[32] demonstrated a rise in antioxidant levels with enalapril. However, this rise in antioxidant concentrations did not cause a fall in lipid peroxides. They attributed the beneficial effect of enalapril to other potential mechanisms. Three groups of rats were studied. One was a control group and the other two groups were nephrectomized (one treated with only the vehicle and the other with enalapril 5 mg/kg per day for 16 weeks). In these animals, lipid peroxides assessed by MDA content in the homogenate from the renal cortex significantly increased in the nephrectomized rats. This elevation of lipid peroxides was unaffected by enalapril. Antioxidant enzymes as measured by catalase and glutathione peroxidase activities in the vehicle-treated nephrectomized rats were significantly decreased compared to the control animals. Enalapril restored these enzyme activities to comparable levels seen in the control animals. Superoxide dismutase activity was not affected by nephrectomy or by drug treatment.

Thus, oxidative stress may contribute to the progression of renal injury in the nephrectomized rat. However, in the later study from Sugimoto, enalapril did not reduce the level of lipid peroxides despite the increase in some antioxidant enzymes. Although enalapril improved the balance between reactive oxygen intermediates and antioxidant enzymes in the remnant renal cortex, the protective effect of enalapril may have been mediated through mechanisms other than alterations in oxidative stress. On the other hand, others have shown that antioxidants reduce lipid peroxides and prevent renal dysfunction in various models of renal injury.

For example, the antioxidant and renal protective effects of enalapril and losartan have also been shown by Kedziora-Kornatowska et al.[33] in the animal model of streptozotocin-induced diabetes in rats. In this study, the effects of enalapril and losartan on lipid peroxidation and activities of Cu, Zn-SOD, catalase, and glutathione peroxidase in the kidneys of these rats following 6 and 12 weeks of treatment were examined. Streptozotocin-induced body weight changes and blood glucose concentrations were not affected by either drug, but both drugs decreased cholesterol and triglycerides, inhibited kidney weight gain, and decreased albuminuria. Both enalapril and losartan decreased the lipid peroxidation (MDA) and augmented the activities of antioxidant enzymes in the kidneys of these animals. These results seem to confirm the role of oxidative stress in the development of diabetic nephropathy during the early stages of development of diabetes and point to the possible antioxidative mechanism of the nephroprotective action of enalapril and losartan.

Using the animal model of adriamycin-induced nephritic syndrome in rats, Tesar et al.[34] studied the renoprotective effects of enalapril versus losartan by measuring the oxidative stress using MDA in blood, as well as urinary excretion of some eicosanoids and their metabolites. Proteinuria caused by adriamycin was not prevented by losartan but was blunted by enalapril. Both losartan and enalapril prevented adriamycin-induced increase of total MDA in serum, but urinary excretion of 8-isoprostane was increased in nephrotic rats treated by losartan compared to controls. There was no significant difference in the urinary excretion of other eicosanoids among different groups, but proteinuria correlated positively with urinary excretion of 8-isoprostane.

The authors concluded that adriamycin-induced nephropathy and proteinuria may be dependent on free radical generation and the formation of 8-isoprostane. The mild antiproteinuric effect of enalapril versus losartan may suggest a contributory role of the inhibition of kinin degradation in this model of nephritic syndrome.

In the rat model of high cholesterol diet-induced increases in blood pressure and renal injury, Atarashi et al.[22] studied the effects of the calcium channel antagonist amlodipine versus alacepril, an angiotensin-converting enzyme (ACE) inhibitor, on blood pressure, urinary protein, renal injury, and oxidative stress. In this study of male Sprague-Dawley rats, the ACE inhibitor, but not amlodipine, completely attenuated the MDA elevation induced by the high cholesterol diet. Although both amlodipine and alacepril decreased blood pressure and urinary protein and ameliorated renal injury, the renal effect of alacepril seems to be mediated by a decrease in oxidative stress as well as by reduction of blood pressure, since alacepril lowered the sclerosing score more than amlodipine and completely attenuated MDA, although the blood pressure reduction by alacepril was less than that seen with amlodipine.

In a recent study by de Cavanagh and associates,[35] the effect of enalapril and captopril on the enhancement of antioxidant defense mechanisms in mouse tissue was studied. The total glutathione content, selenium-dependent glutathione peroxidase, and glutathione reductase activities were investigated in mouse tissues, including liver, brain, kidneys, lung, and erythrocytes. Both enalapril and captopril caused an elevation of the antioxidant defenses as measured in these various tissues. In vitro erythrocyte oxidant stress was evaluated by TBARS production and phenylhydrazine-induced methemoglobin formation. Again, both ACE inhibitors caused a reduction in these measures of oxidant stress. Both of these ACE inhibitors also increased NO production. These findings support previous reports on the enalapril- and captopril-induced enhancement of endogenous antioxidant defenses and include new data on glutathione-dependent defenses, thus furthering current knowledge on the association of ACE inhibition and antioxidants.

Finally, other ACE inhibitors, such as ramipril, have been shown to inhibit the formation and the effects of oxygen radicals in in vitro experiments.[36]

Human Studies

Schneider et al.[37] demonstrated the antioxidative action of captopril in human hypertensive subjects. In this study of hypertensive volunteers, administration of sublingual captopril significantly raised the level of glutathione and glutathione peroxidase activity. The level of SOD and glutathione reductase activity remained high. The authors concluded that captopril may have concomitant scavenging action together with its antihypertensive action. Similarly, de Cavanagh et al.[38] studied the effect of enalapril on various antioxidant defenses in chronic hemodialysis patients. They demonstrated that there was a profound alteration in the circulating antioxidant systems of chronic hemodialysis patients and that additional oxidative stress occurs during the hemodialysis procedure. In patients treated chronically with ACE inhibition, the levels of several antioxidant defenses were greater than in those in untreated patients.

Mechanism of Antioxidant Effect of ACE Inhibitors

Because of the numerous circulatory and tissue effects of ACE inhibition and angiotensin II, the exact mechanism by which these agents improve left ventricular function and heart failure and lower oxidative stress is not yet fully defined. Moreover, the mechanism(s) may differ among some ACE inhibitors. In this regard, sulfhydryl groups in some agents (e.g., captopril) may act as free radical scavengers.[12,39] However captopril, like other ACE inhibitors, may also have a direct antioxidant effect.

Impairment of endothelium-dependent, flow-mediated vasodilatation of small arteries in CHF is altered by ACE inhibition. Varin et al.,[40] in a recent study, demonstrated that the ACE inhibitor-induced improvement in endothelial function and flow-mediated vasodilatation may be partly related to its antioxidant effect. Using perfused gracilis muscle arteries and treatment with perindopril, the role of NO, prostaglandin, and free radicals was assessed by pretreating the vessels with the NO synthase inhibitor Nw-nitro-L-arginine, the cyclooxygenase inhibitor diclofenac, or the free radical scavenger N-2-mercaptopropionyl-glycine (MPG). In animals with CHF, flow-mediated vasodilation was converted into vasoconstriction and was prevented by ACE inhibition. Flow-mediated dilation was abolished by Nw-nitro-L-arginine. In untreated CHF rats, flow-mediated dilation was increased by diclofenac and MPG. In contrast, in arteries from ACE inhibitor-treated rats, neither diclofenac nor MPG affected flow-mediated dilation. In parallel, ACE inhibition prevented the reduction of endothelial NO synthase (eNOS) mRNA by CHF. ACE inhibition normalized NO-dependent dilatation and suppressed the production of vasoconstrictor prostanoids, resulting in improved flow-mediated dilation. Notably, impaired flow-mediated dilation may be related to an increased production of vasoconstrictors such as prostanoids or to an increased production of oxygen-derived radicals. It may also be caused by a decrease in eNOS mRNA expression.

This latter notion has been examined. In a rat model of CHF, the effect of ACE inhibition to improve flow-mediated dilation was, in part, due to the normalization of NO bioavailabilty as well as an abolition of the release and/or the effect of vasoconstrictor prostanoids. This restoration of NO bioavalabilty may be partly related to a normalization of eNOS expression, together with a reduced degradation of NO by oxidative stress. Endothelial NOS expression is increased directly by increased flow. Thus, ACE inhibition augments eNOS expression and probably also decreases the degradation of NO. On the other hand, reactive oxygen species are potent inactivators of NO. Thus, ACE inhibition may exert a favorable effect on oxidative stress through a variety of mechanisms. Since NO inactivates oxygen-derived free radicals,[41] normalized production of NO by ACE inhibition may by itself reduce oxidative stress. Changes in oxidant stress may be related to flow. Indeed, in cultured endothelial cells, exposure to shear stress increases SOD.[42] Thus, the vasodilating effect of ACE inhibition may improve the oxidant/antioxidant milieu. Finally, since angiotensin II may trigger oxidant stress, the direct effect of ACE inhibition to lower angiotensin II production may have a favorable effect on the redox state.

Ruschitzka et al.[43] have described a bradykinin-dependent mechanism for the antioxidative effect of ACE inhibitors. Thus, the mechanism of benefit of ACE inhibition may be even more complex than that described above. Beyond inhibiting the renin-angiotensin system, ACE inhibition also diminishes the inactivation of bradykinin by ACE, thus leading to an augmentation of NO release. Massoudy and colleagues[44] have shown, in a guinea pig ischemia-reperfusion model, a bradykinin-mediated role of NO in the antioxidative effects of ramiprilat. In this study, the NO-synthase inhibitor Ng-nitro-L-arginine (NOLAG 10 μM) inhibited the effects of both ramiprilat and bradykinin. On the other hand, sodium nitroprusside used as a donor of NO improved the cardioprotective effects of the ACE inhibitor. Release of glutathione was decreased by all of the compounds known to cause increased NO concentration in the heart. It was concluded that NO was responsible for the bradykinin-mediated cardioprotective action of ramiprilat in this model, presumably by acting directly as an oxygen radical scavenger during reperfusion.

Barbagallo and associates[45] have demonstrated a role for intracellular magnesium in the antioxidant effect of sulfhydryl-containing ACE inhibitors, such as captopril. In contrast, nonsulfhydryl ACE inhibitors such as enalapril were not shown to increase intracellular magnesium. Magnesium (Mg) deficiency state enhances tissue sensitivity to ischemic damage, an effect reversed not only by Mg, but also by sulfhydryl-containing compounds. In this in vitro study of the model of RBC ischemia, oxygen depletion in the presence or absence of sulfhydryl compounds, including captopril, N-acetyl-L-cysteine (NAC), penicillamine, and N-(2-mercaptopropionyl)-glycine (MPG), was studied. The sulfhydryl compounds, but not the nonsulfhydryl compounds such as enalapril, significantly raised Mg concentrations in erythrocytes. Furthermore, the higher the initial Mg concentration and the greater the captopril-induced rise in intracellular Mg, the greater the metabolite-protective effect. Altogether, these data suggest that Mg influences the cellular response to ischemia, and the ability of sulfhydryl compounds such as captopril to ameliorate ischemic injury may, at least in part, be attributable to the ability of such compounds to increase cytosolic free Mg levels.

ACE inhibitors with thiol groups (e.g., captopril) as well as those without thiol groups (e.g., enalapril, lisinopril, ramipril) are known to act directly as oxygen radical scavengers. Engelman et al.,[46] using xanthine oxidase-hypoxanthine and xanthine oxidase-hypoxanthine-Fe for superoxide radical and hydroxyl radical generation, respectively, demonstrated that captopril is a weak scavenger of superoxide but a potent scavenger of hydroxyl radicals. The direct hydroxyl radical scavenging of captopril was confirmed by electron paramagnetic resonance (EPR) spectroscopy, as shown by Misik et al.[47] and Suzuki et al.[48] However, Suzuki also demonstrated that the nonthiol ACE inhibitors such as enalapril and delapril also had hydroxyl radical scavenging effects. Mira and associates[49] also demonstrated the scavenging activity of the nonthiol ACE inhibitors, including lisinopril and enalapril, using a chemiluminescence assay of oxidation of hypoxanthine by xanthine oxidase.

Finally, some have proposed hemodynamic improvement alone as a sufficient mediator of the antioxidant effect of ACE inhibitors. In a rat model of heart failure (LAD ligation), Khaper et al.[50] have demonstrated a reduction in lipid peroxidation both by ACE inhibitors and by the α_1-receptor antagonist, prazosin. Sham and experimental (postmyocardial infarction) animals were assessed for hemodynamic function as well as lung and liver weights at 1, 4, and 16 weeks after operation. At 4 weeks, some rats were treated with captopril (2 gm/L in drinking water) or prazosin (0.2 mg/kg body weight subcutaneously) daily and assessed at 16 weeks. Hearts were isolated to study the activity of SOD, glutathione peroxidase (GSHPx), and catalase as well as for TBARS.

SOD, GSHPx, and catalase activity in the untreated groups were decreased at 4 and 16 weeks. However, treatment with captopril resulted in a significant improvement in SOD, GSHPx, and catalase activity. Prazosin improved only the SOD activity. Lipid peroxidation as indicated by TBARS was significantly increased in the 16-week group, and both captopril and prazosin modulated this increase. The improvement in hemo-

194 · Oxidative Stress and Cardiac Failure

dynamics with such vasodilating agents may therefore alter vascular wall stress, causing a decrease in lipid peroxidation.

Despite the many observations supporting the antioxidant effects of ACE inhibitors, some studies have been negative.[51,52] However, when taken as a whole, the preponderance of evidence strongly supports such a role for ACE inhibition. These antioxidant effects may contribute to the improvement of heart failure associated with chronic ACE inhibitor therapy.

References

1. CONSENSUS Trial Study Group. Effects of enalapril on mortality in severe congestive heart failure. N Engl J Med 1987;316:1429–1435.
2. SOLVD Investigators. Effect of enalapril on survival in patients with reduced left ventricular ejection fractions and congestive heart failure. N Engl J Med 1991;325:293–302.
3. Cohn JN, Johnson G, Ziesche S, et al. A comparison of enalapril with hydralazine-isosorbide dinitrate in the treatment of chronic congestive heart failure. N Engl J Med 1991;325:303–310.
4. McCord JM, Fridovich I. Superoxide dismutase: an enzymatic function for erythrocuprein (hemecuprein). J Biol Chem 1969;244:6049–6055.
5. Myers ML, Bolli R, Lekich RF, et al. Enhancement of recovery of myocardial function by oxygen free radical scavengers after reversible myocardial ischemia. Circulation 1985;72:915–921.
6. Kloner RA, Przyklenk K. Deleterious effects of oxygen radicals in ischemia/reperfusion: resolved and unresolved issues. Circulation 1989;80:1115–1127.
7. Kobayashi A, Yamashita T, Kaneko M, et al. Effects of verapamil on experimental cardiomyopathy in the bio 14.6 Syrian hamster. J Am Coll Cardiol 1987;10:1128–1134.
8. Gupta M, Singal PK. Higher antioxidant capacity during chronic stable heart hypertrophy. Circ Res 1989;64:398–406.
9. Gupta M, Singal PK. Time course of structure, function, and metabolic changes due to an exogenous source of oxygen metabolites in rat heart. Can J Physiol Pharmacol 1989;67:1549–1559.
10. Singal PK, Kirsenbaum LA. A relative deficit in antioxidant reserve may contribute in cardiac failure. Can J Cardiol 1990;6:47–49.
11. Belch JJ, Bridges AB, Scott N, et al. Oxygen free radicals and congestive heart failure. Br Heart J 1991;65:245–248.
12. Sobotka PA, Brottman MD, Weitz Z, et al. Elevated breath pentane in heart failure reduced by free radical scavenger. Free Rad Biol Med 1993;14:643–647.
13. Weitz Z, Birnbaum AJ, Sobotka PA, et al. Elevated pentane levels during acute myocardial infarction. Lancet 1991;337:933–935.
14. McMurray J, McLay J, Chopra M, et al. Evidence for enhanced free radical activity in chronic congestive heart failure secondary to coronary artery disease. Am J Cardiol 1990;65:1261–1262.
15. Charney RH, Levy DK, Kalman J, et al. Free radical activity increases with NYHA class in congestive heart failure. J Am Coll Cardiol 1997;29(Suppl):102A.
16. Kukin ML, Kalman J, Charney RH, et al. Prospective randomized comparison of effect of long-term treatment with metoprolol or carvedilol on symp-

toms, exercise, ejection fraction, and oxidative stress in heart failure. Circulation 1999;20:2645–2651.

17. Preeta R, Nair RR. Stimulation of cardiac fibroblast proliferation by cerium: a superoxide anion-mediated response. J Mol Cell Cardiol 1999;31:1573–1580.

18. Cheng W, Li B, Kajstura J, Li P, et al. Stretch–induced programmed myocyte cell death. J Clin Invest 1995;96:2247–2259.

19. Griendling KK, Minieri CA, Ollershaw JD, et al. Angiotensin II stimulates NADH and NADPH oxidase activity in cultured vascular smooth muscle cells. Circ Res 1994;74:1141–1148.

20. Mohazzab KM, Kaminski PM, Wolin MS. NADH oxidoreductase is major source of superoxide anion in bovine coronary artery endothelium. Am J Physiol 1994;266:H2568–H2572.

21. Rajagopalan S, Kurz S, Munzel T, et al. Angiotensin II-mediated hypertension in the rat increases vascular superoxide production via membrane NADH/NADPH oxidase activation. J Clin Invest 1996;97:1916–1923.

22. Atarashi K, Takagi M, Minami M, et al. Effects of alacepril and amlodipine on the renal injury induced by a high-cholesterol diet in rats. J Hyperten 1999;17:1983–1986.

23. Maczewski M, Beresewicz A. The role of endothelin, protein kinase C and free radicals in the mechanism of the post-ischemic endothelial dysfunction in guinea pig hearts. J Mol Cell Cardiol 2000;32:297–310.

24. Prabba PS, Das UN, Koratkar R, et al. Free radical generation, lipid peroxidation and essential fatty acids in uncontrolled essential hypertension. Prostaglandins Leukot Essent Fatty Acids 1990;41:2–7.

25. Kumar KV, Das UN. Are free radicals involved in the pathobiology of human essential hypertension? Free Radic Res Commun 1993;19:59–66.

26. Ikemoto F, Song GB, Tominaga M, et al. Oxidation induced activity of angiotensin converting enzyme in the rat kidney. Biochem Biophys Res Commun 1988;153:1032–1037.

27. Ruiz-Munoz LM, Vidal-Vanaclocha F, Lampreabe I. Enalaprilat inhibits hydrogen peroxide production by murine mesangial cells exposed to high glucose concentrations. Nephrol Dial Transplant 1997;12:456–464.

28. Zahler S, Kupatt C, Mobert J, et al. Effects of ACE inhibition on redox status and expression of P-selectin of endothelial cells subjected to oxidative stress. J Mol Cell Cardiol 1998;29:2953–2960.

29. Ha H, Kim KH. Amelioration of diabetic microalbuminuria and lipid peroxidation by captopril. Yonsei Med J 1999;33:217–223.

30. Hayek T, Attias J, Smith J, et al. Antiatherosclerotic and antioxidative effects of captopril in apolipoprotein E-deficient mice. J Cardiovasc Pharmacol 1998; 31: 540–544.

31. Verbeelen DL, De Cramer D, Peters P, et al. Enalapril increases antioxidant enzyme activity in renal cortical tissue of five-sixths nephrectomized rats. Nephron 1999;80:214–219.

32. Sugimoto K, Tsuruoka S, Matsuhita K, et al. Enalapril on oxidative stress in 5/6 nephrectomized rats. Nephron 1999;83:282–283.

33. Kedziora-Kornatowska K. Effect of angiotensin convertase inhibitors and AT1 angiotensin receptor antagonists on the development of oxidative stress in the kidney of diabetic rats. Clin Chim Acta 1999;287:19–27.

34. Tesar V, Zima T, Jirsa M Jr, et al. Effect of losartan and enalapril on urinary excretion of 8-isoprostane in experimental nephritic syndrome. Cas lek Cesk 1997;138:560–564.

196 · Oxidative Stress and Cardiac Failure

35. De Cavanagh EM, Inserra F, Ferder L, et al. Enalapril and captopril enhance glutathione-dependent antioxidant defense in mouse tissues. Am J Physiol Regul Integr Comp Physiol 1998;278:R572–R577.
36. Pi XJ, Chen X. Captopril and ramiprilat protect against free radical injury in isolated working rat heart. J Mol Cell Cardiol 1989;21:1261–1271.
37. Schneider R, Iscovitz H, Ilan Z, et al. Oxygen free radical scavenger system intermediates in essential hypertensive patients before and immediately after sublingual captopril administration. Isr J Med Sci 1994;26:491–495.
38. De Cavanagh EM, Ferder L, Carrasquedo F, et al. Higher levels of antioxidant defenses in enalapril-treated versus non-enalapril-treated hemodialysis patients. Am J Kidney Dis 1999;34:445–455.
39. Chopra M, Scott N, McMurray J, et al. Captopril: a free radical scavenger. Br J Clin Pharmacol 1989;27:396–399.
40. Varin R, Mulder P, Tamion F, et al. Improvement of endothelial function by chronic angiotensin-converting enzyme inhibition in heart failure: role of nitric oxide, prostanoids, oxidant stress, and bradykinin. Circulation 2000;102:351–356.
41. Nlu XF, Smith W, Kubes P. Intracellular oxidative stress induced by nitric oxide synthesis inhibition increases endothelial cell adhesion to neutrophils. Circ Res 1994;74:1133–1140.
42. Inoue N, Ramasamy S, Fukai T, et al. Shear stress modulates expression of Cu/Zn superoxide dismutase in human aortic endothelial cells. Circ Res 1996;79:32–37.
43. Ruschitzka F, Noll G, Luscher TF. Angiotensin-converting enzyme inhibitors and vascular protection. J Cardiovasc Pharmacol 1999;34(Suppl 1):S3–S12.
44. Massoudy P, Becker BF, Gerlach E. Nitric oxide accounts for post-ischemic cardioprotection resulting from angiotensin-converting enzyme inhibition: indirect evidence for a radical scavenger effect in isolated guinea pig heart. J Cardiovasc Pharmacol 1995;25:440–447.
45. Barbagallo M, Dominguez LJ, Resnick LM. Protective effects of captopril against ischemic stress: role of cellular Mg. Hypertension 1999;34:958–63.
46. Engelman RM, Rousou JA, Iyengar J, et al. Captopril, an ACE inhibitor, for optimizing reperfusion after acute myocardial infarction. Ann Thorac Surg 1991;52:918–926.
47. Misik V, Mak IT, Stafford RE, et al. Reaction of captopril and epicaptopril with transition metal ions and hydroxyl radicals: an EPR spectroscopic study. Free Radic Biol Med 1993;15:611–619.
48. Suzuki S, Sato H, Shimada T, et al. Comparative free radical scavenging action of angiotensin-converting enzyme inhibitors with and without the sulfhydryl radical. Pharmacology 1993;47:61–65.
49. Mira ML, Silva MM, Queiroz MJ, et al. Angiotensin-converting enzyme inhibitors as oxygen free radical scavengers. Free Radic Res Commuun 1993;19:173–181.
50. Khaper N, Singal PK. Effects of afterload-reducing drugs on pathogenesis of antioxidant changes and congestive heart failure in rats. J Am Coll Cardiol 1997;29:856–861.
51. Lapenna D, De Gioia S, Ciofani G, et al. Captopril has no significant scavenging antioxidant activity in human plasma in vitro or in vivo. Br J Clin Pharmacol 1996;42:451–456.
52. Maczewski M, Beresewicz A. The role of endothelin, protein kinase C, and free radicals in the mechanism of the post-ischemic endothelial dysfunction in guinea pig hearts. J Mol Cell Cardiol 2000;32:297–310.

• 10 •

Angiotensin II Receptor Blockers and Oxidative Stress

Colin Berry, Mbchb, Phd, and
John McMurray, Bsc(Hons), Mbchb, MD

Introduction

Oxidative stress, a state of free radical (FR) activity in excess of normal cellular homeostatic antioxidant capacity, is a pathophysiological process that has been demonstrated in both animal models[1–13] of chronic heart failure and in humans with this syndrome.[14–25] Free radicals, such as superoxides ($\cdot O_2^-$), have a multiplicity of biological effects that are known to be involved in vascular disease. These effects include scavenging endothelium-derived nitric oxide (NO),[26] activation of tyrosine kinases and nuclear transcription factors,[27–29] regulation of cardiac and vascular cell growth,[30] and activation of vascular cell adhesion molecules (VCAM)[31] and matrix metalloproteinases.[32]

Furthermore, the pathogenesis of chronic heart failure involves a variety of pro-oxidant maladaptive processes.[33] For example, increased vascular FR activity is believed to lead to reduced endothelium-dependent vasorelaxation[34] and peripheral vasoconstriction, both of which are features of chronic heart failure.[35] Oxidative stress may also contribute to increased rates of cardiomyocyte apoptosis in chronic heart failure.[36]

One important source of FR in cardiovascular tissues is nicotinamide adenine dinucleotide phosphate (NAD(P)H) oxidase.[37] This enzyme may be activated by angiotensin II, stimulating NAD(P)H oxidase-dependent FR production.[37–39] This angiotensin type 1 receptor-dependent pathway

From: Kukin ML, Fuster V (eds). *Oxidative Stress and Cardiac Failure.* Armonk, NY: Futura Publishing Co., Inc. ©2003.

may contribute to the vasopressor effects of this hormone both in experimental animal models[39] and in humans.[37]

In this chapter, we will briefly review the evidence in support of oxidative stress in chronic heart failure, with particular emphasis on the pro-oxidant effects of the renin-angiotensin-aldosterone system (RAAS). We will consider how activation of the RAAS may promote FR production both in vascular diseases, which may precede and result in the development of chronic heart failure, and in chronic heart failure itself. We will subsequently then consider how angiotensin receptor blockers (ARBs) may attenuate vascular FR production and oxidative stress and how these actions may contribute to the therapeutic effects of these drugs in chronic heart failure.

Oxidative Stress in Chronic Cardiac Failure

Studies in Experimental Animals

How may oxidative stress be related to the pathophysiology of heart failure? One example is provided by a study in experimental mice that lacked the gene for manganese superoxide dismutase (SOD).[11] These mice had deficient mitochondrial scavenging of FR, such as superoxide ($\cdot O_2^-$), and enhanced oxidative FR activity resulted in myocyte damage and heart failure in these animals.

More recently, Bauersachs et al.[2] investigated the role of enhanced vascular $\cdot O_2^-$ production in a rat model of myocardial infarction. They found that there was enhanced NADH-dependent vascular $\cdot O_2^-$ production and impaired endothelium-dependent vasodilation, which could be improved by pretreatment with exogenous SOD. Taken together, these findings suggest that endothelial dysfunction in ischemic heart failure may, in part, be attributable to enhanced NADH oxidase-dependent FR production that, in turn, may result in a reduction in bioavailable nitric oxide (NO).

Enhanced myocardial FR activity may contribute to the pathogenesis of left ventricular dysfunction.[3–5,11] For example, Dhalla et al.,[3] in a guinea pig model of left ventricular dysfunction induced by aortic banding, demonstrated that early features of compensatory left ventricular hypertrophy were accompanied by a reduction in myocardial content of antioxidant enzymes such as SOD and catalase.[3] These animals were also randomized to receive either vitamin E or placebo. Treatment of these animals with vitamin E improved both myocardial and blood antioxidant enzyme concentrations and histological features of cardiomyocyte damage. Although antioxidant supplementation did not prevent left ventricular dysfunction in these animals, these data do suggest that oxidative stress may be an early process in the transition from cardiac hypertrophy to cardiac failure.

Studies in Humans That Demonstrate Evidence of Oxidative Stress in Chronic Heart Failure

Studies in humans with heart failure secondary to coronary artery disease have also demonstrated enhanced vascular FR activity.[23,40,41] Plasma malondialdehyde, a marker of lipid peroxidation, is elevated in chronic heart failure[42] and is related to exercise intolerance.[43] In other studies, increased plasma concentrations of malondialdehyde and decreased concentrations of glutathione, vitamin C, and E were correlated with both NYHA functional class[16,20] and plasma concentrations of the cytokine, tumor necrosis factor-alpha.[20]

Chronic heart failure is a state characterized by a number of processes that may promote reactive oxygen species (ROS) generation in vivo. Although a full discussion of these mechanisms is not within the scope of this chapter, these pro-oxidant pathways include cytokine activation,[33] mitochondrial dysfunction,[6] recurrent hypoxia-reperfusion,[36] and possibly genetic abnormalities.[44] There are a number of potential cellular sources implicated in enhanced ROS generation in chronic heart failure. It has recently been demonstrated, for example, that chronic heart failure patients may have increased leucocyte $\cdot O_2^-$ production,[45] which is related to severity of disease, as measured by NYHA functional class.[46] Other sources of enhanced ROS generation in human chronic heart failure are both the myocardium[19] and peripheral blood vessels.[18]

Angiotensin Type 1 (AT$_1$) Receptor: Physiological Effects

The cardiovascular effects of AT$_1$-receptor and AT$_2$-receptor activation are shown in Table 1.[47,48] AT$_1$-receptor activation mediates vasoconstriction, vascular cell hypertrophy and hyperplasia, and sodium retention. Other more recently described physiological effects of AT$_1$-receptor activation include stimulation of FR production,[37,39] and induction of inflammatory,[49] thrombotic,[50] and fibrotic processes.[51–53] Some of the pathophysiological effects of angiotensin II may be mediated through activation of the transcription factor nuclear factor-κB, (NF-κB),[54] which participates in a variety of inflammatory responses.[55] Many of these processes are implicated in the cardiac and vascular damage in chronic heart failure.[33,56]

Table 1
Physiological Effects of the Angiotensin Type 1 (AT_1)
and Angiotensin Type 2 (AT_2) Receptors

AT_1-Receptors	AT_2-Receptors
Vasoconstriction	Vasodilation
Cell proliferation	Apoptosis
Cell hypertrophy	Growth inhibition
Antinatriuresis	Natriuresis
Superoxide production	NO production
Endothelin release	
Lipid peroxidation	
Adhesion molecule expression	
Vascular matrix expansion	

Is Oxidative Stress in Vascular Disease Promoted by Activation of the Renin-Angiotensin System?

In Vitro Studies of ROS-Sensitive Intracellular Trophic Signaling Pathways

Cardiomyocyte and vascular smooth muscle cell (VSMC) hyperplasia and hypertrophy are redox-sensitive processes,[57] which are pathological features evident in the heart and blood vessels of patients with cardiovascular disease. There is evidence of tyrosine kinase activation in human chronic heart failure.[58] Tyrosine kinases are ROS-sensitive intracellular signaling pathways involved in cardiomyocyte and VSMC growth regulation.[59] For example, Frank et al.[60] have recently shown in cultured VSMC that the activity of the focal adhesion kinase, PYK2, is redox-sensitive, suggesting that ROS may regulate tyrosine kinase-induced trophic effects in these cells.

ROS may also be second messengers for AT_1-receptor activation. In rat VSMC studies, Frankl.[60] demonstrated that AT_1-receptor-induced ROS production stimulated Jun kinase (JNK) and p38 MAPK (mitogen-activated protein kinase), leading to an increase in activated protein-1 (AP-1) DNA binding. Interestingly, the involvement of ROS in non-receptor kinase activation[61] has raised the possibility that ROS may mediate other AT_1-receptor-induced tyrosine kinase-dependent growth-promoting pathways, such as epidermal growth factor receptor transactivation.[62]

Transcription factors, such as NF-κB and AP-1, are important upstream mediators of angiotensin II trophic effects.[49,63,64] Furthermore, the activity of the nuclear transcription factor, NF-κB, is also regulated by ROS activity.[49,65] These observations suggest the possibility that AT_1-receptor-induced ROS production may lead to activation of NF-κB. Studies by Pueyo et al.[66] in cultured endothelial cells recently confirmed this hypothesis and also demonstrated that AT_1-receptor-induced activation of NF-κB resulted in enhanced VCAM-1 expression.

Taken together, these findings suggest that AT_1-receptor activation stimulates the production of intracellular ROS, which may act as intracellular second messengers for the vasoactive effects of this hormone. Furthermore, these trophic cellular effects may be inhibited by treatment with an ARB.

Studies in Animal Models

In studies of a rat model of angiotensin II-induced hypertension, Rajagopalan et al.[39] investigated the importance of vascular ·O_2 production for the vasopressor effect of angiotensin II. In these studies, impaired acetylcholine-mediated vasorelaxation in aortic segments from rats that had been infused with both pressor and nonpressor doses of angiotensin for 4 days was attenuated by co-treatment with an ARB. In further studies by this group, co-treatment with liposome-encapsulated SOD also attenuated both angiotensin II-stimulated superoxide production and impaired endothelium-dependent vasorelaxation.[67] Taken together, these observations suggest that FR production contributes to the vasopressor effects of angiotensin II.

More recently, Zalba et al.[68] demonstrated in a rat model of hypertension that increased vascular ·O_2^- production in these animals is associated with enhanced expression of the transcripts of one of the subunits of NAD(P)H oxidase, p22phox, as determined by competitive rtPCR. Furthermore, both activation of vascular NAD(P)H oxidase and impaired endothelium-dependent responses in these animals could be normalized by co-treatment with an ARB.

Studies in Humans

Studies undertaken by Berry et al.[37] addressed the question of whether or not angiotensin II might stimulate ROS production in human blood vessels. Internal mammary arteries (IMAs) and subclavian veins (SVs), which were surplus to requirements after coronary revascularization surgery, were incubated with vehicle or angiotensin II. These studies demonstrated that angiotensin II stimulated ·O_2^- production in human arteries by an angiotensin type 1 receptor-dependent mechanism (Figure 1). These observations are corroborated by a report that the pressor effect of

·O$_2^-$ pmol/min/mg tissue

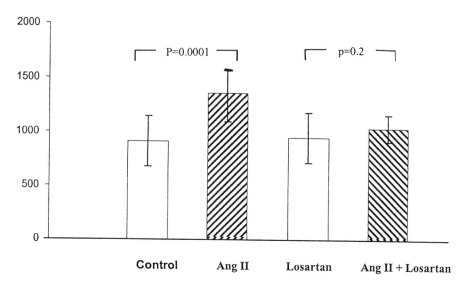

Figure 1. Effect of losartan, a specific AT$_1$-receptor antagonist, on angiotensin II-mediated increase in ·O$_2^-$ production. Internal mammary arteries (IMAs) were incubated in the presence or absence of angiotensin II 1 μmol/L (n=13), losartan 1 μmol/L or co-incubated with angiotensin II 1 μmol/L and losartan 1 μmol/L (n=15), for 4 hours. Results are expressed as pmol/min/mg tissue and shown as mean ±SEM. Open bars indicate control or losartan, atched bars indicate IMAs incubated with angiotensin II and/or losartan.[37]

intrabrachial artery infusion of angiotensin II in humans is attenuated by the co-infusion of vitamin C.[69]

Vascular NAD(P)H oxidase may be important in the pathogenesis of coronary heart disease. Using immunocytochemical techniques, Azumi et al. demonstrated that the expression of p22phox protein in atherosclerotic coronary arteries was more abundant than that in nonatherosclerotic arteries.[70] These observations suggest that vascular NAD(P)H oxidase-dependent FR production may be involved in the pathobiology of the atherosclerotic plaque.

There are now several reports that suggest a relationship between variation in the NAD(P)H oxidase gene and cardiovascular risk. Inoue et al. performed a case-control study in which an association was found between the C242T polymorphism of the p22phox gene, which encodes for one of the electron transport subunits of the NAD(P)H oxidase enzyme, and a reduced susceptibility to coronary artery disease.[71] In contrast, genotyping of the patients from the Lipoprotein and Coronary Artery Study

(LCAS) found an association between the C242T allele and the progression of coronary atherosclerosis.[72]

More recently, other studies have provided evidence of a functional effect of the C242T p22phox gene polymorphism in the blood vessels of patients with coronary heart disease. In studies in IMAs and SVs obtained from patients at the time of coronary artery bypass surgery, Guzik et al.[44] demonstrated that O_2^- production was reduced in the blood vessels of patients with the CT/TT genotype compared to those with other genotypes. More recently, Schachinger et al. investigated the vasodilator function of epicardial coronary arteries in patients with coronary heart disease in relation to the genotype for C242T polymorphism of the p22phox gene.[73] They found that patients with the C242T allele had enhanced coronary endothelium-dependent vasodilation compared to those with the CC genotype. These data suggest that the C242T mutation may lead to a functional inactivation of this protein, resulting in reduced vascular O_2^- production.

Taken together, these studies clearly demonstrate that vascular NAD(P)H oxidase is an important source of FR production in a variety of cardiovascular disease states. Angiotensin II stimulates NAD(P)H oxidase-dependent FR production, and this effect can be prevented by treatment with an ARB (Figure 1).[37] Activation of the RAAS in chronic heart failure,[74] with chronically increased concentrations of plasma angiotensin II, suggests that activation of NAD(P)H oxidase by angiotensin II may contribute to oxidative stress in chronic heart failure. We have recently demonstrated that in patients with CHD, vascular O_2^- concentrations are lower in those patients treated with either an angiotensin-converting enzyme (ACE) inhibitor or an ARB, compared to those who are not.[75]

It seems, therefore, that oxidative stress can be evident in a variety of cardiovascular disease states, such as hypertension and coronary artery disease, which are associated with activation of the RAAS. These diseases are risk factors for the development of, and may co-exist with, chronic heart failure. Given that chronic heart failure is also characterized by activation of the RAAS, angiotensin receptor inhibition may be an effective antioxidant strategy.

Oxidative Stress in Cardiac Failure: Potential Antioxidant Activity of ARBs

Antioxidant Properties of ARBs

The antioxidant properties of anti-ischemic drugs may be either direct, through FR scavenging effects, or indirect, through inhibition of FR bioactivity by either inhibiting the production of or increasing the removal of FR in the vasculature. In contrast to ACE inhibitors, which may scavenge FR directly,[76,77] there are no data to support a direct FR scavenging effect of ARBs. Alternatively, ARBs have been shown in both animal[39] and human[37] studies to reduce vascular FR concentrations by blockade of the angiotensin type 1 receptor, thereby preventing angiotensin II-stimulated FR production. These data suggest that ARBs may attenuate oxidative stress in vivo.

Are ARBs Cardioprotective in Patients at Risk of Developing Chronic Heart Failure?

Experimental studies in human cultured endothelial cells have demonstrated that treatment with an ARB may attenuate angiotensin II-induced recruitment of oxidized LDL[78] and its receptor,[79] and may also attenuate the activity of leucocyte chemoattractant factors,[80] thereby preventing leucocyte-endothelial cell interactions.[81] Angiotensin II is a leucocyte chemoattractant and local production of angiotensin II within vascular and cardiac tissues and may therefore lead to increased leucocyte migration, a process associated with atherosclerosis.[82] The observation that angiotensin II and its receptors are abundant within atherosclerotic plaques in the coronary arteries of patients with ischemic cardiomyopathy suggests that the RAAS is important in the development of coronary atherosclerosis and coronary heart disease.[83]

Studies in both healthy individuals[84] and in patients with coronary arteriosclerosis[85] have demonstrated that treatment with an ARB may enhance peripheral artery endothelium-dependent vasorelaxation. Taken together, these observations suggest that ARBs may protect the endothelium against the development of atherosclerosis and improve its function. Whether primary chronic ARB therapy may prevent chronic heart failure in high-risk patients, as is the case with ACE inhibitors,[86] is not known.

Effects of ARBs on Peripheral Hemodynamics

It is plausible that ARBs may also reduce vascular FR activity as a result of the vasodilator effects of these drugs.[8] In studies of a rat model of chronic heart failure induced by left anterior descending coronary artery ligation, chronic administration of either the ACE inhibitor, captopril, or the alpha-adrenoceptor antagonist, prazosin, reduced left ventricular end-diastolic pressure, this being ascribed to a reduction in total peripheral resistance by these drugs. Furthermore, the decreased plasma antioxidant enzyme activities observed in these animals and increased plasma concentrations of lipid peroxides, compared to sham controls, were improved by treatment with both of these drugs. These observations raise the possibility that vasoconstriction itself contributes to augmented vascular FR production in chronic heart failure, suggesting that ARBs, which reduce afterload, may attenuate oxidative stress promoted by this pathway.

Effects of ARBs on Cytokine Activation

Chronic heart failure is characterized by increased circulating concentrations of cytokines, such as TNF-α (or its soluble receptors) and interleukin-6.[87,88] Immune activation is an important process in the pathophysiology of chronic heart failure,[33] and increased concentrations of these cytokines are an adverse prognostic sign.[87,88] One deleterious effect of certain cytokines, such as TNF-α, is to stimulate ROS production in blood vessels by activation of vascular NAD(P)H oxidase.[89] The observation that ARB therapy may reduce increased circulating concentrations of TNF-α and IL-6[90] suggests that ARB therapy may have antioxidant effects by attenuating immune activation. This hypothesis merits further investigation.

Oxidative Stress in Cardiac Failure: A Proven Target for Angiotensin Receptor Blockade?

Effects of ARB on Endothelial Function in Chronic Heart Failure

Newby et al. recently demonstrated that angiotensin II directly contributes to impaired forearm blood flow in chronic heart failure.[91] They also demonstrated that treatment with the ARB, losartan, selectively improved peripheral vasoconstriction in these patients by causing arteriolar vasodilatation, whereas losartan had no such effect in healthy controls.

Watanabe et al.[25] recently studied the effects of losartan, or placebo, on markers of oxidative stress and endothelial function, when added to regular therapy, which included an ACE inhibitor, in 24 chronic heart failure patients. In this study, ARB adjunctive therapy for 6 months was associated with a reduction in plasma thiobarbituric acid reactive substances, markers of lipid peroxidation, and an improvement in endothelium-dependent flow-mediated brachial artery dilatation. Nitroglycerin-induced endothelium-independent vasodilation was not different in either losartan-treated or placebo-treated groups.

Conclusion

Oxidative stress is a feature of chronic heart failure and may contribute to the pathogenesis of both myocardial and vascular dysfunction. Chronic heart failure is characterized by chronic activation of the RAAS, and inhibitors of the RAAS, such as ACE inhibitors, are of proven benefit. Angiotensin II augments vascular ROS production, thereby promoting the trophic and pressor effects of this hormone. The role of ARBs in chronic heart failure continues to be investigated in large clinical trials. Studies in experimental animal models and in humans with both atherosclerosis and chronic heart failure have demonstrated, however, that ARBs may reduce cytokine activation and vascular ROS production. Consequently, ARB therapy has been associated with improved endothelium-dependent vasorelaxation.

References

1. Arimura K, Egashira K, Yamamoto M, et al. An oxygen free radical scavenger tiron improves coronary endothelial dysfunction in a canine model of tachycardia-induced heart failure. Circulation 1998;98(17):2127.
2. Bauersachs J, Bouloumie A, Fraccarollo D, et al. Endothelial dysfunction in chronic myocardial infarction despite increased vascular endothelial nitric oxide synthase and soluble guanylate cyclase expression: role of enhanced vascular superoxide production. Circulation 1999;100(3):292–298.
3. Dhalla AK, Hill MF, Singal PK. Role of oxidative stress in transition of hypertrophy to heart failure. J Am Coll Cardiol 1996;28(2):506–514.
4. Hill MF, Singal PK. Antioxidant and oxidative stress changes during heart failure subsequent to myocardial infarction in rats. Am J Pathol 1996;148(1): 291–300.
5. Hill MF, Singal PK. Right and left myocardial antioxidant responses during heart failure subsequent to myocardial infarction. Circulation 1997;96(7):2414–2420.
6. Ide T, Tsutsui H, Kinugawa S, et al. Mitochondrial electron transport complex I is a potential source of oxygen free radicals in the failing myocardium. Circ Res 1999;85:357–363.
7. Ide T, Tsutsui H, Kinugawa S, et al. Direct evidence for increased hydroxyl radicals originating from superoxide in the failing myocardium. Circ Res 2000; 86:152–157.
8. Khaper N, Singal PK. Effects of afterload-reducing drugs on pathogenesis of antioxidant changes and congestive heart failure in rats. J Am Coll Cardiol 1997;29(4):856–861.
9. Li RK, Sole MJ, Mickle DAG, et al. Vitamin E and oxidative stress in the heart of the cardiomyopathic Syrian hamster. Free Radical Biol Med 1998;24(2): 252–258.
10. Li X, Moody MR, Engel D, et al. Cardiac-specific overexpression of tumor necrosis factor-alpha causes oxidative stress and contractile dysfunction in mouse diaphragm. Circulation 2000;102(14):1690–1696.
11. Li YB, Huang TT, Carlson EJ, et al. Dilated cardiomyopathy and neonatal lethality in mutant mice lacking manganese superoxide-dismutase. Nature Genet 1995;11:376–381.
12. Oskarsson HJ, Coppey L, Weiss RM, et al. Antioxidants attenuate myocyte apoptosis in the remote non-infarcted myocardium following large myocardial infarction. Cardiovasc Res 2000;45:679–687.
13. Siwik DA, Tzortzis JD, Pimental DR, et al. Inhibition of copper-zinc super-

oxide dismutase induces cell growth, hypertrophic phenotype, and apoptosis in neonatal rat cardiac myocytes in vitro. Circ Res 1999;85(2):147–153.

14. Anderson RA, Ellis GR, Blackman DJ, et al. Primary platelet nitric oxide resistance and oxidative stress in patients with chronic heart failure. J Am Coll Cardiol 2000;35(2):222A–222A.

15. Baumer AT, Flesch M, Wang XK, et al. Antioxidative enzymes in human hearts with idiopathic dilated cardiomyopathy. J Mol Cell Cardiol 2000;32(1): 121–130.

16. Charney RH, Levy DK, Kalman J, et al. Free radical activity increases with NYHA class in congestive heart failure. J Am Coll Cardiol 1997;29(2):30159–30159.

17. De Vecchi E, Pala MG, Di Credico G, et al. Relation between left ventricular function and oxidative stress in patients undergoing bypass surgery. Heart 1998;79(3):242–247.

18. DiazVelez CR, GarciaCastineiras S, MendozaRamos E, et al. Increased malondialdehyde in peripheral blood of patients with congestive heart failure. Am Heart J 1996;131(1):146–152.

19. Dieterich S, Bieligk U, Beulich K, et al. Gene expression of antioxidative enzymes in the human heart: increased expression of catalase in the end-stage failing heart. Circulation 2000;101(1):33–39.

20. Keith M, Geranmayegan A, Sole MJ, et al. Increased oxidative stress in patients with congestive heart failure. J Am Coll Cardiol 1998;31(6):1352–1356.

21. Kukin ML, Kalman J, Charney RH, et al. Prospective, randomized comparison of effect of long-term treatment with metoprolol or carvedilol on symptoms, exercise, ejection fraction, and oxidative stress in heart failure. Circulation 1999;99:2645–2651.

22. Mallat Z, Philip I, Lebret M, et al. Elevated levels of 8-iso-prostaglandin F-2 alpha in pericardial fluid of patients with heart failure: a potential role for in vivo oxidant stress in ventricular dilatation and progression to heart failure. Circulation 1998;97(16):1536–1539.

23. McMurray JJV, McLay J, Chopra M, et al. Evidence for enhanced free adical activity in chronic congestive heart ailure secondary to coronary rtery disease. Am J Cardiol 1990;65:1261–1262.

24. Niebauer J, Webb-Peploe KM, Jourdan K, et al. Chronic exercise training modulates oxidative stress in patients with chronic heart failure. J Am Coll Cardiol 1998;31(2):509A–509A.

25. Watanabe H, Kakihana M. Effects of losartan on endothelium-dependent vasodilation in patients with chronic heart failure. J Am Coll Cardiol 2000; 35(2):254A–254A.

26. Moncada S, Higgs A. Mechanisms of disease: the L-arginine nitric oxide pathway. N Engl J Med 1993;329:2002–2012.

27. Frank GD, Motley ED, Inagami T, et al. PYK2/CAK beta represents a redox-sensitive tyrosine kinase in vascular smooth muscle cells. Biochem Biophys Res Comm 2000;270(3):761–765.

28. Muller DN, Dechend R, Mervaala EMA, et al. NF-κB inhibition ameliorates angiotensin II-induced inflammatory damage in rats. Hypertension 2000;35: 193–201.

29. Ruiz-Ortega M, Lorenzo O, Ruperez M, et al. Angiotensin II activates nuclear transcription factor kappa B through AT(1) and AT(2) in vascular smooth muscle cells: molecular mechanisms. Circ Res 2000;86(12):1266–1272.

30. Irani K. Oxidant signaling in vascular cell growth, death, and survival. Circ Res 2000;87:179–183.

208 · Oxidative Stress and Cardiac Failure

31. Marui N, Offermann MK, Swerlick R, et al. Vascular cell dhesion molecule-1 (VCAM-1) gene-transcription and expression are regulated through an antioxidant-ensitive mechanism in human vascular endothelial ells. J Clin Invest 1993;92:1866–1874.
32. Rajagopalan S, Meng XP, Ramasamy S, et al. Reactive oxygen species produced by macrophage-derived foam cells regulate the activity of vascular matrix metalloproteinases in vitro: mplications for atherosclerotic plaque stability. J Clin Invest 1996;98:2572–2579.
33. Berry C, Clark AL. Catabolism in chronic heart failure. Eur Heart J 2000; 21:521–532.
34. Gupte SA, Rupawalla T, Mohazzabh KM, et al. Regulation of NO-elicited pulmonary artery relaxation and guanylate cyclase activation by NADH oxidase and SOD. Am J Physiol-Heart Circ Physiol 1999;45:H1535–H1542.
35. Angus JA, Ferrier CP, Sudhir K, et al. Impaired contraction and relaxation in skin resistance arteries from patients with congestive heart failure. Cardiovasc Res 1993;27(2):204–210.
36. Ferrari R, Agnoletti L, Comini L, et al. Oxidative stress during myocardial ischaemia and heart failure. Eur Heart J 1998;19:B2–B11.
37. Berry C, Hamilton CA, Brosnan MJ, et al. An investigation into the sources of superoxide production in human blood vessels: angiotensin II increases superoxide production in human internal mammary arteries. Circulation 2000; 101:2206–2212.
38. Griendling KK, Minieri CA, Ollerenshaw JD, et al. Angiotensin I stimulates NADH and NADPH oxidase activity in cultured vascular smooth uscle cells. Circ Res 1994;74:1141–1148.
39. Rajagopalan S, Kurz S, Munzel T, et al. Angiotensin II-mediated hypertension in the rat increases vascular superoxide production via membrane NADH/NADPH oxidase activation: contribution to alterations of vasomotor tone. J Clin Invest 1996;97:1916–1923.
40. McMurray J, Chopra M, Reglinski J, et al. Disclosure of increased free rdical activity in heart filure by biochemical markers and proton nuclear-magnetic resonance spectroscopy. Br Heart J 1990;64(1):60–66.
41. McMurray J, Chopra M, Abdullah I, et al. Evidence of oxidative stress in chronic heart failure in humans. Eur Heart J 1993;14(11):1493–1498.
42. DiazVelez CR, GarciaCastineiras S, MendozaRamos E, et al. Increased malondialdehyde in peripheral blood of patients with congestive heart failure. Am Heart J 1996;131(1):146–152.
43. Nishiyama Y, Ikeda H, Haramaki N, et al. Oxidative stress is related to exercise intolerance in patients with heart failure. Am Heart J 1998;135(1):115–120.
44. Guzik TJ, West NEJ, Black E, et al. Functional effect of the C242T polymorphism in the NAD(P)H oxidase p22phox gene on vascular superoxide production in atherosclerosis. Circulation 2000;102:1744–1747.
45. Ellis GR, Anderson RA, Lang D, et al. Neutrophil superoxide anion-generating capacity, endothelial function and oxidative stress in chronic heart failure: effects of short- and long-term vitamin C therapy. J Am Coll Cardiol 2000;36(5):1474–1482.
46. Ellis GR, Lang D, Anderson RA, et al. Superoxide anion generation by neutrophils correlates with NYHA status in chronic heart failure. J Am Coll Cardiol 1998;31(2):248A–248A.
47. Ardaillou R. Angiotensin II receptors. J Am Soc Nephrol 1999;10:S30–S39.
48. Inagami T, Kitami Y. The tissue renin-angiotensin system in cardiovascular disease. Trends Cardiovasc Med 1992;2:94–99.

49. Muller DN, Dechend R, Mervaala EMA, et al. NF-κB inhibition ameliorates angiotensin II-induced inflammatory damage in rats. Hypertension 2000;35: 193–201.
50. Vaughan DE, Lazos SA, Tong K. Angiotensin I regulates the expression of plasminogen-activator inhibitor-1 in cultured endothelial ells: a potential link between the renin-angiotensin system and thrombosis. J Clin Invest 1995; 95:995–1001.
51. Boffa JJ, Tharaux PL, Placier S, et al. Angiotensin II activates collagen type I gene in the renal vasculature of transgenic mice during inhibition of nitric oxide synthesis: evidence for an endothelin-mediated mechanism. Circulation 1999;100(18):1901–1908.
52. Nakamura S, Nakamura S, Ma L, et al. Plasminogen activator inhibitor-1 expression is regulated by the angiotensin type 1 receptor in vivo. Kidney Int 2000;58:251–259.
53. Stanley AG, Williams B. Mechanical strain increases collagen I mRNA expression in cultured human vascular smooth muscle cells via an angiotensin II-dependent pathway. Am J Hypertens 1999;12(4):98A–98A.
54. Sadoshima J. Cytokine actions of angiotensin II. Circ Res 2000;86:1187.
55. Barnes PJ, Karin M. Nuclear factor-kB: a pivotal transcription factor in chronic inflammatory diseases. N Engl J Med 1997;336:1066–1071.
56. Givertz MM, Colucci WS. New targets for heart ailure therapy: endothelin, inflammatory cytokines, and oxidative stress. Lancet 1998;352:34–38.
57. Griendling KK, Sorescu D, Ushio Fukai M. NAD(P)H oxidase: role in cardiovascular biology and disease. Circ Res 2000;86:494–501.
58. Cook SA, Sugden PH, Clerk A. Activation of c-Jun N-terminal kinases and p38-mitogen-activated protein kinases in human heart failure secondary to ischemic heart disease. J Mol Cell Cardiol 1999;31(8):1429–1434.
59. Berk BC, Corson MA. Angiotensin II signal transduction in vascular smooth muscle: role of tyrosine kinases. Circ Res 1997;80(5):607–616.
60. Frank GD, Motley ED, Inagami T, et al. PYK2/CAK beta represents a redox-sensitive tyrosine kinase in vascular smooth muscle cells. Biochem Biophys Res Comm 2000;270(3):761–765.
61. Rao GN. Hydrogen peroxide induces complex formation of SHC-Grb2-SOS with receptor tyrosine kinases and activates Ras and extracellular signal-related protein kinase group of mitogen-activated protein kinases. Oncogene 1996;13: 713–719.
62. Eguchi S, Inagami T. Signal transduction of angiotensin II type 1 receptor through receptor tyrosine kinase. Regul Pept 2000;91:13–20.
63. Usui M, Egashira K, Tomita H, et al. Important role of local angiotensin II activity mediated via type 1 receptor in the pathogenesis of cardiovascular inflammatory changes induced by chronic blockade of nitric oxide synthesis in rats. Circulation 2000;101(3):305–310.
64. Kudoh S, Komuro I, Mizuno T, et al. Angiotensin II stimulates c-Jun NH_2-terminal kinase in cultured cardiac myocytes of neonatal rats. Circ Res 1997; 80:139–146.
65. Usui M, Egashira K, Tomita H, et al. Important role of local angiotensin II activity mediated via type 1 receptor in the pathogenesis of cardiovascular inflammatory changes induced by chronic blockade of nitric oxide synthesis in rats. Circulation 2000;101(3):305–310.
66. Pueyo ME, Gonzalez W, Nicoletti A, et al. Angiotensin II stimulates endothelial vascular cell adhesion molecule-1 via nuclear factor-kB activation induced by intracellular oxidative stress. Arterioscler Thromb Vasc Biol 2000;20:645–654.

67. Laursen JB, Rajagopalan S, Galis Z, et al. Role of superoxide in angiotensin II-induced but not catecholamine-induced hypertension. Circulation 1997;95: 588–593.
68. Zalba G, Beaumont FJ, SanJose G, et al. Vascular NADH/NADPH oxidase is involved in enhanced superoxide production in spontaneously hypertensive rats. Hypertension 2000;35:1055–1061.
69. DijkhorstOei LT, Stroes ESG, Koomans HA, et al. Acute simultaneous stimulation of nitric oxide and oxygen radicals by angiotensin II in humans in vivo. J Cardiovasc Pharmacol 1999;33:420–424.
70. Azumi H, Inoue N, Takeshita S, et al. Expression of NADH/NADPH oxidase p22(phox)in human coronary arteries. Circulation 1999;10014):1494–1498.
71. Inoue N, Kawashima S, Kanazawa K, et al. Polymorphism of the NADH/NADPH oxidase p22 phox gene in patients with coronary artery disease. Circulation 1998;97:135–137.
72. Cahilly C, Ballantyne CM, Lim DS, et al. A variant of p22(phox), involved in generation of reactive oxygen species in the vessel wall, is associated with progression of coronary atherosclerosis. Circ Res 2000;86(4):391–395.
73. Schachinger V, Britten MB, Dimmeler S, et al. NADH/NADPH oxidase p22 phox gene polymorphism is associated with improved coronary endothelial vasodilator function. Eur Heart J 2001;22:96–101.
74. Francis GS, Goldsmith SR, Levine TB, et al. The neurohumoral axis in congestive heart failure. Ann Intern Med 1984;101:370–377.
75. Berry C, Anderson N, Pathi V, et al. Renin-angiotensin system inhibition reduces free radical concentrations in arteries of patients with coronary heart disease. Circulation, in press.
76. McMurray JJV, Chopra M, McLay J, et al. Free adical activity in chronic heart ailure and effect of captopril. Br Heart J 1989;61:457–458.
77. Benzie IFF, Tomlinson B. Antioxidant power of angiotensin-converting enzyme inhibitors in vitro. Br J Clin Pharmacol 1998;45:168–169.
78. Li DY, Saldeen T, Romeo F, et al. Oxidized LDL upregulates angiotensin II type 1 receptor expression in cultured human coronary artery endothelial cells: the potential role of transcription factor NF-kappa B. Circulation 2000;102(16): 1970–1976.
79. Morawietz H, Rueckschloss U, Niemann B, et al. Angiotensin II induces LOX-1, the human endothelial receptor for oxidized low-density lipoprotein. Circulation 1999;100(9):899–902.
80. Pastore L, Tessitore A, Martinotti S, et al. Angiotensin II stimulates intercellular adhesion molecule-1 (ICAM-1) expression by human vascular endothelial cells and increases soluble ICAM-1 release in vivo. Circulation 1999; 100(15):1646–1652.
81. Piqueras L, Kubes P, Alvarez A, et al. Angiotensin II induces leukocyte-endothelial cell interactions in vivo via AT(1) and AT(2) receptor-mediated P-selectin upregulation. Circulation 2000;102(17):2118–2123.
82. Schmidt-Ott KM, Kagiyama S, Phillips MI. The multiple actions of angiotensin II in atherosclerosis. Regul Pept 2000;93(1–3):65–77.
83. Schieffer B, Schieffer E, Hilfiker-Kleiner D, et al. Expression of angiotensin II and interleukin 6 in human coronary atherosclerotic plaques: potential implications for inflammation and plaque instability. Circulation 2000;101(12): 1372–1378.
84. Komers R, Komersova K, Kazdova L, et al. Effect of ACE inhibition and angiotensin AT1 receptor blockade on renal and blood pressure response to L-arginine in humans. J Hypertension 2000;18(1):51–59.

85. Prasad A, Tupas-Habib T, Schenke WH, et al. Acute and chronic angiotensin-1 receptor antagonism reverses endothelial dysfunction in atherosclerosis. Circulation 2000;101(20):2349–2354.
86. Yusuf S, Phil D, Sleight P, et al. Effects of an angiotensin-converting-enzyme inhibitor, ramipril, on cardiovascular events in high-risk patients. N Engl J Med 2000;342:145–153.
87. Swedberg K, Eneroth P, Kjekshus J, et al. Effects of enalapril and neuroendocrine activation on prognosis in severe congestive heart failure (follow-up of CONSENSUS trial). Am J Cardiol 1990;66(11):D40–D45.
88. Tsutamoto T, Hisanaga T, Wada A, et al. Interleukin-6 spillover in the peripheral circulation increases with the severity of heart failure, and the high plasma level of interleukin-6 is an important prognostic predictor in patients with congestive heart failure. J Am Coll Cardiol 1998;31(2):391–398.
89. DeKeulenaer GW, Alexander RW, Ushio Fukai M, et al. Tumour necrosis factor alpha activates a p22(phox)-based NADH oxidase in vascular smooth muscle. Biochem J 1998;329:653–657.
90. Tsutamoto T, Wada A, Maeda K, et al. Angiotensin II type 1 receptor antagonist decreases plasma levels of tumor necrosis factor alpha, interleukin-6 and soluble adhesion molecules in patients with chronic heart failure. J Am Coll Cardiol 2000;35:714–721.
91. Newby DE, Goodfield NER, Flapan AD, et al. Regulation of peripheral vascular tone in patients with heart failure: contribution of angiotensin II. Heart 1998;80:134–140.

• 11 •

Microvasculature and Oxidative Stress
With Special Emphasis on the Acute Coronary Syndromes

Mardi Gomberg-Maitland, MD, MSc,
and Valentin Fuster, MD, PhD

Introduction: Atherothrombosis, the Microvasculature, and the Myocyte

Atherosclerosis relates to lipid-rich, thickened, hardened lesions of medium and large muscular and elastic arteries.[1] Early atherosclerotic plaques contain macrophage-derived foam cells, smooth muscle cells with extracellular lipid deposits, and fatty streaks that contain smooth muscle cells surrounded by extracellular connective tissue, fibrils, and lipid deposits.[2,3] These early lesions represent a dynamic balance of lipoprotein transport in and out of the cell.[1] As disease advances, thrombosis and organization of the thrombi significantly contribute to the process. For this reason, the term atherothrombosis is more accurate to describe the disease than the term atherosclerosis.

The molecular pathophysiology of acute coronary syndromes has unraveled, transforming earlier understandings and leading to new therapeutics. Chronic minimal injury to the arterial endothelium is physiological and leads to the accumulation of macrophages and lipids (usually in the form of low density lipoproteins, LDL).[4] Oxidation of LDL by the en-

From: Kukin ML, Fuster V (eds). *Oxidative Stress and Cardiac Failure.* Armonk, NY: Futura Publishing Co., Inc. ©2003.

213

dothelial cells is the main initiator of monocyte recruitment. Monocytes become macrophages. Macrophages may convert mildly oxidized LDL to highly oxidized LDL and become foam cells.[3] Plaque disruption usually produces asymptomatic mural thrombus. The thrombus organizes, the plaque enlarges, and thus atherothrombosis progresses. Acute occlusion or subocclusion of a disrupted plaque, usually lipid-rich and thus termed "vulnerable," by a thrombus, produces an acute coronary syndrome. The disruption of the plaque probably relates to its physical softness because of the high lipid content, and also to an inflammation with the release by monocytes of metalloproteinases. These enzymes contribute to the digestion and rupture of the plaque. Such acute complicated lesions manifest as either unstable angina or acute myocardial infarction.

Plaque disruption with acute thrombosis limits distal blood flow, creating an ischemic environment for the myocyte. Ischemia is oxygen deprivation accompanied by the accumulation of metabolites secondary to reduced perfusion.[5] This acute coronary syndrome progresses with molecular changes and interactions among the epicardial vessels, the microcirculation, and the myocytes. Molecular adaptations triggered as a result of these interactions allow cells to survive and even to generate new blood vessels during ischemic periods. Although it is not part of this chapter, intermittent ischemia in chronic coronary disease (i.e., in exertional stable angina) can lead to similar phenomena.

The disruption of the vessel wall during acute coronary syndromes or by iatrogenic manipulation in the setting of transcoronary revascularization results in embolization of plaque and vessel wall contents: lipid, matrix, endothelial cells, aggregated platelets, and thrombus into the microvasculature[6]; the larger the original clot burden, the higher the propensity for distal embolization.[7] The severity of plaque disruption appears to correlate with local platelet activation and epicardial occlusion.[7] Microembolization, once thought to be uncommon,[8–10] has received new validation, confirming previous pathological evidence (Figure 1).[4,8,11] Sometimes regional myocardial contractile dysfunction occurs in the absence of an atherosclerotic epicardial artery obstruction but has been associated with coronary microembolization. Therefore, inflamed arteries, even without obstruction, may embolize microparticulate atheromatous debris.

The goal of early treatment for acute coronary syndromes is restoration of epicardial blood flow in the infarct-related artery. However, successful reperfusion is no longer judged only by epicardial patency. Good patency of the microvasculature and myocardial tissue perfusion is part of this goal. This chapter will discuss the interactions of the myocyte, the epicardial vessel, and the microvasculature in acute coronary syndromes and the treatments aimed at improving myocardial perfusion.

Inflammation

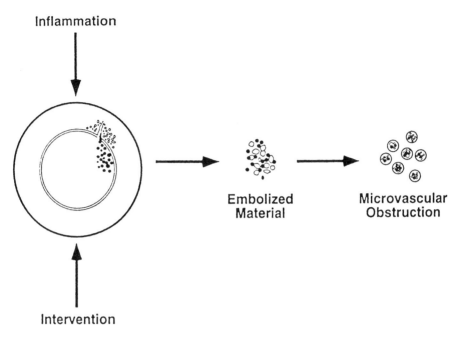

Embolized
Material

Microvascular
Obstruction

Intervention

Figure 1. Schematic of embolization. Inflammation, intervention, or both fissure the arterial wall. Small atherosclerotic (nano) particulate matter, sometimes including adherent platelet-thrombus, is embolized, leading to microvascular obstruction (represented in cross section). With permission from Topol et al.[6]

Pathogenesis: The Endothelium and Coronary Blood Flow

The endothelium is a single layer of cells between the vascular smooth muscle and the blood in the epicardial coronary arteries as well as in the microvasculature, which interacts with the circulating blood to maintain normal coronary flow. The endothelial cell separates the intravascular and extravascular spaces and thus regulates the transfer of nutrients to myocytes, the diapedesis of leukocytes, and the interaction between circulating vasoactive substances and smooth muscle.[12] The endothelial cell is antithrombogenic because it contains prostacyclin (PGI_2), heparin, antithrombin III, and thrombomodulin,[13] and it has powerful lytic properties (i.e., release of plasminogen activator).

Vascular tone is also modulated by factors secreted by the endothelium. The endothelium, via various receptors, regulates smooth muscle tone by interacting with acetylcholine, histamine, serotonin, catecholamines, bradykinin, and adenosine nucleotides.[13,14] Adenosine, released by the endothelial cells,[14,15] is a vasodilator and disaggregates platelets, inhibiting their release of thromboxane A_2.[16] Similarly, but more powerfully, endothelial secretion of prostacyclin (PGI_2)[17] and endothelial-derived relaxing factor (EDRF),[18-20] now known as nitric oxide (NO), significantly reduces vascular tone, increasing coronary flow.

Vasoconstriction is modulated by endothelin (ET). Endothelin, first isolated from bovine aortic and pulmonary endothelium, is a family of four 21-amino acid peptides, ET-1 through ET-4, with ET-1 being the predominant isoform.[21] Secretion of endothelin-1 causes vasoconstriction[22] and increases neutrophil and platelet adhesion, promoting lesion growth and thrombosis.[21] High levels of endothelin-1 are associated with atherosclerosis, congestive heart failure, and left ventricular dysfunction.[21] Prostacyclin counteracts endothelin-1 by limiting neutrophil adherence and platelet aggregation.[13,14,23,24]

Endothelial dysfunction leads to increased permeability to plasma lipoproteins, increased adhesion of blood leukocytes, and an imbalance of local thrombotic, growth, and vasoactive factors.[25] Clinically, endothelial dysfunction of the epicardial coronary arteries (depending on which of the two regions is affected) is demonstrated by impaired vasodilation of the microvasculature under stimulation (i.e., administration of acetylcholine). Significant damage of the endothelium exposes the vessel wall to platelets, leading to release of platelet-derived growth factor (PDGF) and transforming growth factor (TGF-β) with subsequent smooth muscle cell activation, and synthesis of extracellular matrix.[26] In addition, thromboxane A_2, released from activated platelets, monocytes, and damaged vasculature, contributes to ischemia and thrombosis by further promoting platelet aggregation, vasoconstriction, and hypertrophy of vascular smooth muscle.[27,28] Of interest, if the arterial region affected is not the epicardial coronary artery, but is the microvasculature, these pathological interactions of the endothelium, platelets, and monocytes play an important role in collateral vessel growth at sites of damaged vascular segments.[29] Thus, the impediment in blood flow tends to trigger a compensatory angiogenic response.

The Ischemic Environment: Oxidative Stress

Pathophysiology

Infarct size is directly related to duration of epicardial occlusion. Both the duration and severity of ischemia determine the amount of cell death and necrosis.[30,31] The subendocardium has the least collateral flow and the most oxygen consumption, and thus it is the most prone to ischemia.[5] In the absence of adequate collateral circulation, subendocardial necrosis occurs approximately 20 minutes after coronary occlusion, and is completed in the subepicardium after approximately 3 hours.[32]

Reperfusion Injury

Reperfusion, the restoration of blood flow, lessens ischemic damage.[33] Ironically, reperfusion can also damage the myocardial cell. Thus, reperfusion hastens necrosis of irreversibly injured myocytes, causes cell swelling and toxic calcium diffusion, and produces oxygen-derived free radicals. Reperfusion damages the microvasculature, resulting in endothelial biochemical and structural change, leading to growth factor induction. Platelet activation in the endothelium with leukocytes causes the no-reflow phenomenon and platelet extravasation produces hemorrhagic infarction.[14,19,33] Since early reperfusion is presently the most effective method to reduce infarct size, a better understanding of pathophysiology should allow the development of new therapeutics that will enhance the efficacy of early reperfusion techniques.

Ischemic Cell Swelling

Ischemic tissue injury impairs cell volume regulation.[34] Reperfusion increases cellular swelling in irreversibly injured cells and transiently in reversibly injured cells.[35–37] Myocyte "explosive" swelling may contribute to vascular compression, and swelling of endothelial cells may contribute to increased vascular resistance.[33]

Calcium Toxicity

Hearts exposed to calcium after perfusion in calcium-free media demonstrate massive tissue disruption, enzyme release, contraction, and reduction in phosphate stores.[33,38–40] This toxicity may be the result of disruption of the sarcolemmal bilayer, and the separation of the external lamina and the surface coat of the glycocalyx, leading to an influx of calcium.[39] The depletion in phosphate stores (adenosine triphosphate, ATP) interferes with transsarcolemmal Na^+/K^+ exchange. This leads to elevated intracellular Na^+ and, consequently, intracellular calcium because of the Na^+/Ca^+ exchange.[5] Calcium may enhance production of free radicals, activate phospholipases, or disrupt mitochondria, causing cell swelling and necrosis.[33] Calcium blockers diminish calcium influx by interfering with voltage-dependent channels, and beta-adrenoreceptor antagonists block recruitment of receptor-operated channels. Both medication classes delay ischemia-induced necrosis.[41,42]

Oxygen-Derived Free Radicals

Hearts exposed to oxygen after periods of anoxia demonstrate similar pathology to hearts exposed to calcium after perfusion in a calcium-free environment. Reperfusion causes contracture of myofibrils, disruption of the sarcolemma, and intramitochondrial calcium phosphate particles.[5] It is thought that the stimulation of the oxygen transport chain triggers uptake of calcium by the mitochondria. Oxygen activates xanthine oxidase (in the presence of necessary substrates, i.e., hypoxanthine) in the ischemic endothelial cell, producing superoxide free radicals.[43] Oxygen-derived free radicals are also produced by leukocytes.[44] Reactive oxidative species damage proteins and membrane structures and can activate apoptosis.[45,46] Diminished superoxide dismutase, catalase, and glutathione peroxidase during ischemia leaves a cell defenseless against free radicals.[14,47]

No-Reflow Phenomenon

Blood flow after reperfusion is more heterogeneous than prior to coronary obstruction and is called the no-reflow phenomenon.[35] Areas of reduced flow are caused by microvascular damage. Microvascular changes include endothelial cell swelling, "blebs," increased capillary permeability causing rouleaux of erythrocytes leading to stasis, and leukocyte adherence to endothelial cells, clogging capillaries and causing secretion of inflammatory mediators.[5,33,46] Platelet aggregates in capillaries may exacerbate no-reflow by release of thromboxane and platelet-activating factors.[14,48]

Reperfusion-Induced Hemorrhage

Damaged microvasculature allows extravasation of blood into the extravascular space, producing a hemorrhagic infarction.[33] Hemorrhage is confined to areas of myocardial necrosis.[49] In less ischemic areas, myocytes are irreversibly damaged but have an intact endothelium. This produces a bland infarct.[33] Myocardial hemorrhage does not appear to affect infarct size but may alter ventricular stiffness.[33]

Clinical Consequences of Reperfusion

Arrhythmia and Stunning

Reperfusion arrhythmias and myocardial "stunning" may be caused by free radical disruption of cellular membranes and promotion of reentrant circuits.[50,51] Reperfusion arrhythmias are benign, and occur within the first 2 days after myocardial infarction. These are typically accelerated idioventricular rhythms. Ventricular premature complexes also occur and are benign. Stunning is defined as prolonged left ventricular dysfunction and decreased ATP stores after ischemia.[33] Chronic stunning may persist over weeks. Stunning helps explain why, following reperfusion, patients may require prolonged pharmacological and/or mechanical support before functional recovery is achieved.

Cellular and Molecular Protective Responses Against Ischemic Injury/Oxidative Stress

Natural responses to an ischemic environment by the myocytes and the epicardial vessels help protect the heart from hypoxia-related damage.

Ischemic Preconditioning and Heat Shock Proteins

Damage from a sustained coronary occlusion is limited if the heart has been exposed to previous short episodes of ischemia. Preconditioning is the cytoprotective response to these episodes of ischemia and depends on posttranslational modification of preexisting cellular proteins[46] and changes in gene expression. Nitric oxide (NO) and hypoxia-inducible factor 1 (HIF-1, a heterodimer composed of α and β subunits)[52] can induce the preconditioning response.[53] HIF-1 activation promotes inducible NO synthase (iNOS)[54] and vascular endothelial growth factor (VEGF) production.[52] HIF-1 also stimulates expression of genes that enhance cellular anaerobic production of ATP and angiogenic growth factor release.[46]

Many forms of cell stress over time lead to increased concentration of heat shock proteins (HSP). Hsp70 is one of these proteins and directly protects against damage and limits infarct size in mouse hearts by improved metabolic and functional recovery.[55] Cells synthesize enzymes that detoxify reactive oxygen species (ROS), limiting protein and membrane structural damage.[46] The myocardial cell triggered by IGF-1, cardiotrophin-1, PDGF, or TNF-α protects mitochondrial function.[46,56] Induction of the sarcolemma Na^+/H^+ exchanger during ischemia also contributes to myocardial injury.[57] Canine hearts exposed to regional ischemia with reperfusion had smaller infarcts with inhibition of the sarcolemma Na^+/H^+ exchanger.[58]

Angiogenesis

A hypoxic environment often stimulates angiogenesis, the growth of new blood vessels from the preexisting vasculature. Angiogenesis is mediated by endothelial cell proliferation, migration, and remodeling.[59,60] Endothelial cell apoptosis appears to inhibit neovascularization.[61] Animal models of myocardial ischemia induced by coronary artery occlusion demonstrate induction of vascular endothelial-derived growth factor (VEGF) and formation of collateral blood vessels.[62,63] HIF-1 and VEGF induction appear to be some of the earliest responses to ischemia. Ventricular biopsies taken from coronary artery bypass patients with ischemia of less than 48 hours demonstrated elevated levels of both HIF-1α mRNA and VEGF.[64] Specimens taken from patients with chronic ischemia had undetectable levels of these factors.

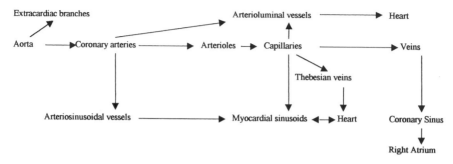

Figure 2. The microcirculation. Adapted with permission from Higano et al.[148]

Microvascular Obstruction

Experimental Pathophysiology

The coronary circulation consists of a network of large and small vessels linking the arterial and venous systems. The microvasculature refers to the arterioles, capillaries, and sinusoids (Figure 2). Microvascular ob-

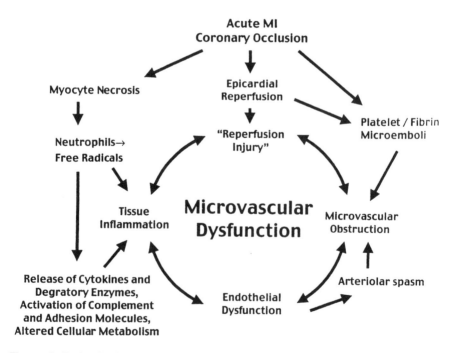

Figure 3. Pathophysiology of microvascular dysfunction after epicardial perfusion. With permission from Roe et al.[68]

struction reduces contractile function. Intracoronary injection of inert particles into the microvasculature produces regional contractile dysfunction proportionate to the number of injected particles.[65,66] Baseline blood flow in the microembolized area may be enhanced due to an adenosine-related hyperemia.[65,66] Multiple microinfarcts appear to alter contractility more than a single infarct of equivalent volume.[67] Injured myocytes and arterioles impede microvascular flow by increasing vascular resistance, stimulating spasm, and causing endothelial dysfunction.[68] Microvascular spasm after endothelial injury appears to be partially mediated by thromboxane A_2.[69] The inflammatory response appears to be more severe in response to microembolization compared to diminished flow from large vessel obstruction, and thus may contribute to the significant contractile dysfunction (Figures 3 and 4).[67]

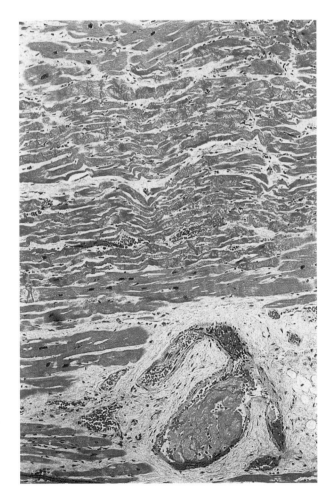

Figure 4. Autopsy specimen from a 53-year-old man with an acute myocardial infarction demonstrating myocardial necrosis and platelet aggregation/plugging of an arteriole. See color version of this figure between pages 236 and 237.

Clinical Evidence

Evaluation of myocardial perfusion by serum markers, electrocardiographic criteria, and new diagnostic modalities in the cardiac catheterization and noninvasive laboratories has complemented previous angiographic assessments of myocardial tissue perfusion.

Angiographic Markers

Use of coronary angiography to evaluate degree of epicardial coronary flow is the gold standard for determining successful reperfusion of the infarct-related vessel. The Thrombolysis In Myocardial Infarction (TIMI) investigators categorized flow on a scale from 0 to 3.[70] The definitions are: TIMI 0 = no antegrade flow, TIMI 1 = partial penetration of contrast past the point of occlusion, TIMI 2 = opacification but delayed filling of the distal vessel, and TIMI 3 = normal flow. Grades 0 and 1 are considered unsuccessful and grades 2 and 3 are considered successful. TIMI flow can be used as a surrogate endpoint for mortality after acute myocardial infarction.[71–73]

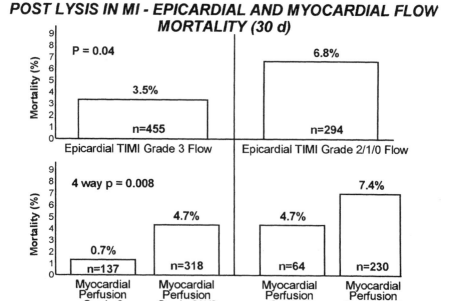

Figure 5. Post lysis in myocardial infarction: epicardial and myocardial flow mortality (30 days). Data from TIMI 10B with permission from Gibson et al.[75]

Evidence of frequent microvascular obstruction has been described by observing that distal coronary blood flow may vary and is often impaired in patients with TIMI grade 3 perfusion. Other risk stratification measures such as the corrected TIMI frame count (cTFC), the TIMI myocardial perfusion grade (TMP), and the myocardial blush score have helped characterized this flow.[74–76] TMP is an independent predictor of mortality and adds prognostic information to the epicardial TIMI flow grades and TIMI frame counts (measures of epicardial flow) in acute myocardial infarction patients post thrombolytic therapy.[75] Myocardial blush score predicts mortality in patients after primary angioplasty (Figure 5).[74]

Serum Markers

Serum levels of cardiac troponin T and troponin I, components of cardiac and skeletal muscle filament, can reflect small degrees of myocardial necrosis in unstable angina. Small levels of necrosis as evidenced by serum markers are more common in high-risk patients (ECG with ST depression, smokers, hypercholesterolemia, diabetes, and hypertension) with unstable angina.[77,78] High-risk angiographic findings such as complex lesions and presence of thrombus are common with elevated troponin levels.[79] This observation suggests that microvascular obstruction with focal necrosis is a result of microembolic may be frequently occurring in such high-risk patients.

Embolization of coronary thrombus mixed with plaque and inflammatory mediators may occur during and after coronary percutaneous intervention. Elevation of creatine kinase and troponin levels are common post intervention[80] and portend a worse prognosis.[81–84] Predictors of marker elevation are diffuse coronary disease, systemic atherosclerosis, stent usage, and absence of beta-blocker therapy.[85] Embolization is the likely mechanism for these elevations because other causes such as side-branch closure, abrupt closure, or long ischemic time are uncommon.[86]

The level of significant "threshold" CK release post intervention remains controversial. Many believe that levels ≥3 times normal is significant; however, most of the earlier studies used angioplasty (PTCA).[80,87] Initial studies also demonstrated higher levels post rotational atherectomy (PRCA).[88] Newer devices and improved techniques have limited microinfarctions. In 1675 patients, prospective studies post intervention did not demonstrate any statistically significant difference in CK release between PTCA and PRCA.[85] Patients with CK levels between one and five times normal had in-hospital events similar to patients without elevation, suggesting that these patients can be discharged home earlier than previously recommended.[85]

ST Segment Resolution

ST segment resolution is a validated predictor of better prognosis after fibrinolysis.[89,90] It may reflect improved myocardial tissue perfusion as a result of patency of both the epicardial coronary artery and the microvasculature. Indeed, early resolution improves ejection fraction, reduces infarct size, and improves survival.[91] This early ST segment resolution correlates with myocardial contrast echocardiography measures of microvascular reflow in the infarct territory.[92] Continuous monitoring of ST segments provides more information about speed and stability of reperfusion. The temporal pattern appears to estimate infarct size and left ventricular contractile recovery.[93,94]

Coronary Doppler Flow Wires

Assessment of microvascular dysfunction can be made by coronary Doppler flow wires during angiography. Wires measure coronary flow velocity and coronary flow reserve after epicardial reperfusion during angiography. Diminished flow velocity and reserve appear to predict recovery of regional left ventricular contractile reserve and function.[95]

Imaging

New imaging techniques have improved visualization of coronary plaque and the microvasculature. Angioscopy can detect intravascular thrombus[96,97] and intravascular ultrasound can distinguish between soft, fibrotic, and calcified plaques.[98–101] Myocardial contrast echocardiography allows visualization of microvascular obstruction. Myocardial contrast echocardiography used in patients with acute anterior wall myocardial infarction during cardiac catheterization and 25 days post procedure demonstrated epicardial flow without tissue level reperfusion. These patients had lower ejection fractions compared to patients with normal microvascular flow in long-term follow-up.[102,103]

Magnetic resonance (MR) imaging is a technique offering higher resolution and improved characterization of coronary plaque.[4,104] MR imaging after infarction has also demonstrated increased clinical events in patients with microvascular obstruction.[105] MR imaging post coronary revascularization appears to be a good perfusion measurement device.[106,107] However, technetium-99m (^{99}mTc)-sestamibi single photon emission computed tomography (SPECT) also appears to be a good noninvasive imaging technique to assess left ventricular dysfunction and amount of myocardial salvage after reperfusion, but it is also difficult to perform early during acute coronary syndromes.[108]

Therapeutic Strategies

Reperfusion with fibrinolytic agents is hindered by incomplete patency of the epicardial vessel and is not intended to directly improve microvascular perfusion. Despite recent intervention strategies of primary angioplasty and intracoronary stenting, survival rates have not improved.[109,110] New therapies aimed at improving microvascular perfusion and angiogenesis during oxidative stress should help improve patient outcomes.

Glycoprotein IIb/IIIa Inhibitors

A recent addition to therapy in acute coronary syndromes is the glycoprotein IIb/IIIa receptor inhibitors: the chimeric antibody abciximab and nonpeptide antagonists eptifibatide and tirofiban. These agents inhibit platelet aggregation by binding to the glycoprotein IIb/IIIa receptor, and are thought thereby to lessen the thromboembolic microvascular obstruction. Large-scale trials with IIb/IIIa inhibitors in high-risk patients during acute coronary syndromes,[111–113] acute myocardial infarction,[75,90,114–116] and percutaneous coronary revascularization[117–122] demonstrate improved clinical outcomes (Figure 6). Patients with elevated serum troponins or diabetes benefit most from glycoprotein IIb/IIIa therapy.[123–125]

New studies have combined interventional and medical therapies in acute coronary syndromes, an approach called facilitated percutaneous intervention (PCI), aimed at myocardial and microvasculature salvage. Neumann et al. were the first to demonstrate that improved microvascular perfusion in the setting of stent revascularization improves myocardial function.[126] Patients with acute coronary syndromes studied after coronary stenting, treated with abciximab and low-dose heparin, had improved intracoronary Doppler flow velocity versus those receiving standard-dose heparin alone. These patients also had improved ventricular function at 2 weeks post intervention.[126] The SPEED trial (GUSTO-V) is a large-scale multicenter trial evaluating the role of early PCI after reteplase (r-PA, a deletion mutant of t-PA, preferential binding of fibrin-bound plasminogen) with or without abciximab. The pilot trial SPEED (GUSTO IV AMI) data demonstrated an 86% TIMI flow grade 3 with early PCI and half-dose reteplase and abciximab and a trend toward fewer negative clinical outcomes.[127]

Although early clinical benefits from glycoprotein IIb/IIIa inhibitors appear to derive from prevention of thromboembolic microvascular obstruction, the explanation for late benefits is unclear. One mechanism may be prevention of remodeling, heart failure, and lethal arrhythmias.[67,86] Micronecrosis creates areas of slow conduction, increasing risk for ventricular arrhythmias by microreentrant circuits.[128] Benefits in diabetics may

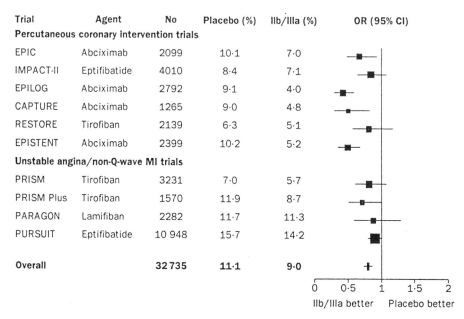

Trial	Agent	No	Placebo (%)	IIb/IIIa (%)	OR (95% CI)
Percutaneous coronary intervention trials					
EPIC	Abciximab	2099	10·1	7·0	
IMPACT-II	Eptifibatide	4010	8·4	7·1	
EPILOG	Abciximab	2792	9·1	4·0	
CAPTURE	Abciximab	1265	9·0	4·8	
RESTORE	Tirofiban	2139	6·3	5·1	
EPISTENT	Abciximab	2399	10·2	5·2	
Unstable angina/non-Q-wave MI trials					
PRISM	Tirofiban	3231	7·0	5·7	
PRISM Plus	Tirofiban	1570	11·9	8·7	
PARAGON	Lamifiban	2282	11·7	11·3	
PURSUIT	Eptifibatide	10 948	15·7	14·2	
Overall		32 735	11·1	9·0	

0   0·5   1   1·5   2
IIb/IIIa better   Placebo better

Figure 6. Death or nonfatal myocardial infarction outcomes at 30 days in 10 randomized, placebo-controlled trials of GPIIb-IIIa blockers. Risk ratio with 95% CI, size of RR box being proportional to total sample size. Frequency of death or nonfatal myocardial infarction in columns 4 and 5. Overall (all 10 trials) benefit of GPIIb-IIIa blockade highly significant (RR=0.79 (95% CI 0.73–0.85; $P<.10$) With permission from Topol et al.[113]

EPICARDIAL THROMBOSIS AND MICROCIRCULATION

plaque rupture

thrombosis

plaque erosion

microembolization

arrhythmias ← infarctions → dysfunction ← Coronary reserve↓

Figure 7. Epicardial thrombosis and microcirculation. Modified with permission from Erbel et al.[67]

be prevention of in-stent restenosis in addition to microvascular protection.[124] The myocardial cell's ability to increase blood flow during stress or ischemia is the coronary flow reserve (i.e., the difference between basal coronary blood flow and peak blood flow during reactive hyperemia). One of the clinical benefits of glycoprotein IIb/IIIa agents is improved coronary reserve (Figure 7).[67]

Mechanical Devices

New devices that prevent distal embolization appear to be effective. Two devices, the PercuSurge, a distal balloon that occludes the artery and aspirates debris with a catheter, and the Angioguard, a filter that traps particulate matter and then collapses for withdrawal, are the newest items.[6] PercuSurge, tested in patients having saphenous vein grafts and carotid interventions,[129] and the Angioguard, tested in renal, saphenous vein grafts and carotid interventions, both retrieve embolic material.[6] A few problems with the devices are: the devices are not yet easily deployed, the filters are unable to catch particles smaller than 50 μm, and the balloon devices do not allow angiography during inflation.[6] In the near future, with continued development, these devices will be easier to use and more safely protect the microvasculature.

Therapies Aimed at Improving Myocardial Perfusion: Creation of Microvasculature

Transmyocardial Revascularization

Patients with diffuse coronary disease unamenable to percutaneous or surgical revascularization have limited treatment options. Refractory angina is often not controlled with anti-ischemic medical therapy. Transmyocardial laser revascularization (TMLR) is a new technology aimed at improving myocardial perfusion in patients with intractable angina. The technique is modeled on the reptilian heart, an extensive sinusoidal network.[130,131] The theory is that ischemic myocardium might be revascularized by the creation of transmural channels between the left ventricular cavity and the myocardium, thus creating a sinusoidal network, a new microvasculature. TMLR trials use either a carbon dioxide or a homium: yttrium-aluminum-garnet laser to create transmyocardial channels to improve blood flow.

TMLR relieves refractory angina, increases exercise tolerance, and improves perceived quality of life in patients with refractory angina.[132–137] Survival after TMLR is slightly improved,[132,137,138] but operative mortality, however, is not insignificant in this high-risk patient population (Figures 8 and 9).[139,140] In a recent study, poor prognosis was associated with

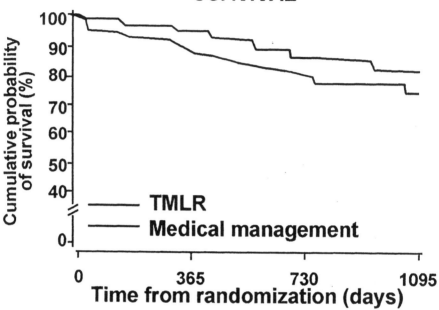

Figure 8. TMLR in refractory angina survival.[137,138,142]

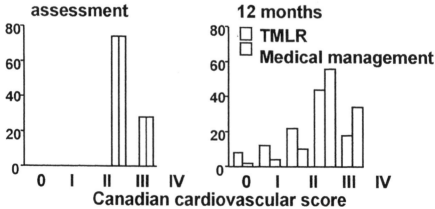

Figure 9. TMLR in refractory angina (N=188) symptoms (Canadian Score).[137,140,142,149]

the following risk factors: unprotected left main stenosis, diabetes, and class IV heart failure.[141] Operative mortality is reduced in patients with good blood flow in one native or vein graft territory.[142]

Despite clinical improvements, the long-term patency of the created channels and their theoretical ability to provide significant flow remains controversial.[143–145] Aaberge et al. demonstrated symptomatic improvement at 1 year without change in exercise tolerance.[134] However, in a recent study by Schneider et al. with longer follow-up time, TMLR statistically improved symptoms temporarily (up to 1.5 years of follow-up) at 3 years.[146] Clinical benefits may be caused by angiogenesis but remain unproved.[145]

TMLR with Revascularization and VEGF Administration

Not all studies had convincing results and investigators wondered if TMLR may be used as an adjuctive therapy to revascularization. In a recent prospective randomized trial comparing coronary artery bypass (CABG) patients plus TMLR versus CABG alone, those who received CABG plus TMLR had improved survival and less angina compared with patients receiving CABG alone (Figure 10).[133] Gene therapy techniques have also been tested in isolation and concurrent with CABG in patients with severe coronary artery disease. A recent phase 1 trial administered VEGF via an adenovirus vector during bypass surgery to an ischemic territory or it was inserted in isolation during a minimally invasive procedure.[147] CABG patients had improved angina and patients receiving VEGF only had improved exercise tolerance.[147]

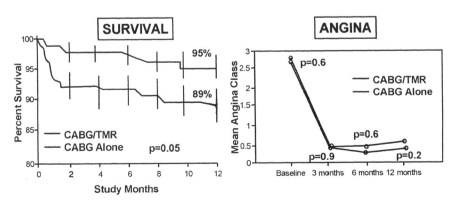

Figure 10. CABG and TMLR vs. CABG prospective trial (multicenter- N=263 patients). With permission from Allen et al.[133]

230 · Oxidative Stress and Cardiac Failure

MICROVASCULATURE, MYOCARDIAL CELL 2000

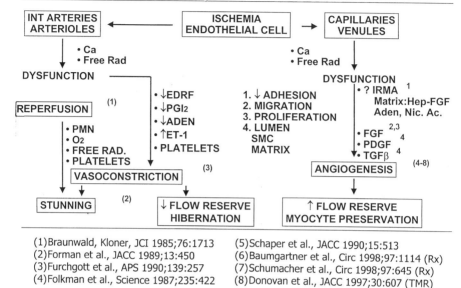

(1)Braunwald, Kloner, JCI 1985;76:1713
(2)Forman et al., JACC 1989;13:450
(3)Furchgott et al., APS 1990;139:257
(4)Folkman et al., Science 1987;235:422

(5)Schaper et al., JACC 1990;15:513
(6)Baumgartner et al., Circ 1998;97:1114 (Rx)
(7)Schumacher et al., Circ 1998;97:645 (Rx)
(8)Donovan et al., JACC 1997;30:607 (TMR)

Figure 11. Microvasculature, myocardial cell 2000.[14,19,20,29,33,150–152]

Conclusion (Figure 11)

The merging of basic science knowledge and clinical research has expanded our understanding of ischemia, reperfusion, and angiogenesis. With the help of improved laboratory and imaging techniques, microvasculature obstruction during oxidative stress is increasingly appreciated as an important consequence. Successful reperfusion now comprises normal blood flow in the epicardial vessels and adequate microvascular perfusion. Increasingly, acute coronary syndrome therapies will be directed toward improving the latter, and clinical investigations will determine the clinical significance of this approach.

References

1. Fuster V. Atherosclerosis-thrombosis and vascular biology. In: Goldman L, Bennett, JC, eds. Cecil's Textbook of Internal Medicine, Vol. 21. WB Saunders Co, Philadelphia, 2000; 291–296.
2. Stary HC, Chandler AB, Dinsmore RE, et al. A definition of advanced types of atherosclerotic lesions and a histological classification of atherosclerosis. A report from the Committee on Vascular Lesions of the Council on Arteriosclerosis, American Heart Association. Circulation 1995;92(5):1355–1374.

3. Fuster V. Lewis A. Conner Memorial Lecture. Mechanisms leading to myocardial infarction: insights from studies of vascular biology [published erratum appears in Circulation 1995 Jan 1;91(1):256]. Circulation 1994;90(4): 2126–2146.

4. Fuster V, Fayad, ZA, Badimon, JJ. Acute coronary syndromes: biology. Lancet 1999;353(Suppl II):5–9.

5. Ganz E. Coronary blood flow and myocardial ischemia. In: Braunwald E, ed. Heart Disease, Vol. 2. WB Saunders Co, Philadelphia, 1997; 1161–1183.

6. Topol EJ, Yadav JS. Recognition of the importance of embolization in atherosclerotic vascular disease. Circulation 2000;101(5):570–580.

7. Brener SJ, Topol EJ. Troponin, embolization and restoration of microvascular integrity. Eur Heart J 2000;21(14):1117–1119.

8. Frink RJ, Rooney PA Jr, Trowbridge JO, et al. Coronary thrombosis and platelet/fibrin microemboli in death associated with acute myocardial infarction. Br Heart J 1988;59(2):196–200.

9. Falk E. Unstable angina with fatal outcome: dynamic coronary thrombosis leading to infarction and/or sudden death. Autopsy evidence of recurrent mural thrombosis with peripheral embolization culminating in total vascular occlusion. Circulation 1985;71(4):699–708.

10. Davies MJ, Thomas AC, Knapman PA, et al. Intramyocardial platelet aggregation in patients with unstable angina suffering sudden ischemic cardiac death. Circulation 1986;73(3):418–427.

11. Falk E, Shah PK, Fuster V. Coronary plaque disruption. Circulation 1995; 92(3):657–671.

12. Kaiser L, Sparks HV Jr. Endothelial cells: not just a cellophane wrapper. Arch Intern Med 1987;147(3):569–573.

13. Gerlach E, Nees S, Becker BF. The vascular endothelium: a survey of some newly evolving biochemical and physiological features. Basic Res Cardiol 1985;80(5):459–474.

14. Forman MB, Puett DW, Virmani R. Endothelial and myocardial injury during ischemia and reperfusion: pathogenesis and therapeutic implications. J Am Coll Cardiol 1989;13(2):450–459.

15. Sparks HV Jr, Bardenheuer H. Regulation of adenosine formation by the heart. Circ Res 1986;58(2):193–201.

16. Tanabe M, Terashita Z, Nishikawa K, et al. Inhibition of coronary circulatory failure and thromboxane A2 release during coronary occlusion and reperfusion by 2-phenylaminoadenosine (CV-1808) in anesthetized dogs. J Cardiovasc Pharmacol 1984;6(3):442–448.

17. Moncada S, Gryglewski R, Bunting S, et al. An enzyme isolated from arteries transforms prostaglandin endoperoxides to an unstable substance that inhibits platelet aggregation. Nature 1976;263(5579):663–665.

18. Furchgott RF, Zawadzki JV. The obligatory role of endothelial cells in the relaxation of arterial smooth muscle by acetylcholine. Nature 1980;288(5789): 373–376.

19. Furchgott RF. The 1989 Ulf von Euler lecture. Studies on endothelium-dependent vasodilation and the endothelium-derived relaxing factor. Acta Physiol Scand 1990;139(2):257–270.

20. Folkman J, Klagsbrun M. Angiogenic factors. Science 1987;235(4787):442–447.

21. Luscher TF, Barton M. Endothelins and endothelin receptor antagonists: therapeutic considerations for a novel class of cardiovascular drugs. Circulation 2000;102(19):2434–2440.

232 · Oxidative Stress and Cardiac Failure

22. Yanagisawa M, Kurihara H, Kimura S, et al. A novel potent vasoconstrictor peptide produced by vascular endothelial cells. Nature 1988;332(6163):411–415.
23. Boxer LA, Allen JM, Schmidt M, et al. Inhibition of polymorphonuclear leukocyte adherence by prostacyclin. J Lab Clin Med 1980;95(5):672–678.
24. Aiken JW, Gorman RR, Shebuski RJ. Prevention of blockage of partially obstructed coronary arteries with prostacyclin correlates with inhibition of platelet aggregation. Prostaglandins 1979;17(4):483–494.
25. DiCorleto P, Gimbrone MA. Vascular endothelium. In: Fuster V, Ross R, Topol ES, eds. Atherosclerosis and Coronary Artery Disease, Vol. 1. Lippincott-Raven, Philadelphia, 1996; 387.
26. Ross R, Fuster V. The pathogenesis of atherosclerosis. In: Fuster V, Ross R, Topol E, eds. Arteriosclerosis and Coronary Artery Disease, Vol. 1. Lippincott-Raven, Philadelphia, 1996; 441–460.
27. Ali S, Davis MG, Becker MW, et al. Thromboxane A2 stimulates vascular smooth muscle hypertrophy by upregulating the synthesis and release of endogenous basic fibroblast growth factor. J Biol Chem 1993;268(23):17397–17403.
28. Gao Y, Yokota R, Tang S, et al. Reversal of angiogenesis in vitro, induction of apoptosis, and inhibition of akt phosphorylation in endothelial cells by thromboxane A(2). Circ Res 2000;87(9):739–745.
29. Schaper W, Sharma HS, Quinkler W, et al. Molecular biologic concepts of coronary anastomoses. J Am Coll Cardiol 1990;15(3):513–518.
30. DeBoer LW, Rude RE, Kloner RA, et al. A flow- and time-dependent index of ischemic injury after experimental coronary occlusion and reperfusion. Proc Natl Acad Sci USA 1983;80(18):5784–5788.
31. Reimer KA, Jennings RB. The wavefront phenomenon of myocardial ischemic cell death. II. Transmural progression of necrosis within the framework of ischemic bed size (myocardium at risk) and collateral flow. Lab Invest 1979; 40(6):633–644.
32. Jennings RB, Reimer KA. Factors involved in salvaging ischemic myocardium: effect of reperfusion of arterial blood. Circulation 1983;68(Pt 2):I25–36.
33. Braunwald E, Kloner RA. Myocardial reperfusion: a double-edged sword? J Clin Invest 1985;76(5):1713–1719.
34. Macknight AD, Leaf A. Regulation of cellular volume. Physiol Rev 1977; 57(3):510–573.
35. Kloner RA, Ganote CE, Jennings RB. The no-reflow phenomenon after temporary coronary occlusion in the dog. J Clin Invest 1974;54(6):1496–1508.
36. Kloner RA, Ellis SG, Carlson NV, et al. Coronary reperfusion for the treatment of acute myocardial infarction: postischemic ventricular dysfunction. Cardiology 1983;70(5):233–246.
37. Jennings RB, Schaper J, Hill ML, et al. Effect of reperfusion late in the phase of reversible ischemic injury: changes in cell volume, electrolytes, metabolites, and ultrastructure. Circ Res 1985;56(2):262–278.
38. Jennings RB, Reimer KA, Hill ML, et al. Total ischemia in dog hearts, in vitro. 1. Comparison of high-energy phosphate production, utilization, and depletion, and of adenine nucleotide catabolism in total ischemia in vitro versus severe ischemia in vivo. Circ Res 1981;49(4):892–900.
39. Hearse DJ, Humphrey SM, Feuvray D, et al. A biochemical and ultrastructural study of the species variation in myocardial cell damage. J Mol Cell Cardiol 1976;8(10):759–778.
40. Hearse DJ. Reperfusion of the ischemic myocardium. J Mol Cell Cardiol 1977;9(8):605–616.

41. Campbell CA, Kloner RA, Alker KJ, et al. Effect of verapamil on infarct size in dogs subjected to coronary artery occlusion with transient reperfusion. J Am Coll Cardiol 1986;8(5):1169–1174.
42. Braunwald E, Muller JE, Kloner RA, et al. Role of beta-adrenergic blockade in the therapy of patients with myocardial infarction. Am J Med 1983;74(1):113–123.
43. McCord JM. Oxygen-derived free radicals in postischemic tissue injury. N Engl J Med 1985;312(3):159–163.
44. Del Maestro R, Thaw HH, Bjork J, et al. Free radicals as mediators of tissue injury. Acta Physiol Scand Suppl 1980;492:43–57.
45. Semenza GL. Cellular and molecular dissection of reperfusion injury: ROS within and without. Circ Res 2000;86(2):117–118.
46. Williams RS, Benjamin IJ. Protective responses in the ischemic myocardium. J Clin Invest 2000;106(7):813–818.
47. McCord JM. Oxygen-derived radicals: a link between reperfusion injury and inflammation. Fed Proc 1987;46(7):2402–2406.
48. Forman MB, Puett DW, Bingham SE, et al. Preservation of endothelial cell structure and function by intracoronary perfluorochemical in a canine preparation of reperfusion. Circulation 1987;76(2):469–479.
49. Reimer KA, Lowe JE, Rasmussen MM, et al. The wavefront phenomenon of ischemic cell death: myocardial infarct size versus duration of coronary occlusion in dogs. Circulation 1977;56(5):786–794.
50. Bolli R. Oxygen-derived free radicals and postischemic myocardial dysfunction. J Am Coll Cardiol 1988;12(1):239–249.
51. Bernier M, Hearse DJ, Manning AS. Reperfusion-induced arrhythmias and oxygen-derived free radicals. Circ Res 1986;58(3):331–340.
52. Semenza GL. Surviving ischemia: adaptive responses mediated by hypoxia-inducible factor 1. J Clin Invest 2000;106(7):809–812.
53. Guo Y, Jones WK, Xuan YT, et al. The late phase of ischemic preconditioning is abrogated by targeted disruption of the inducible NO synthase gene. Proc Natl Acad Sci USA 1999;96(20):11507–11512.
54. Jung F, Palmer LA, Zhou N, et al. Hypoxic regulation of inducible nitric oxide synthase via hypoxia inducible factor-1 in cardiac myocytes. Circ Res 2000;86(3):319–325.
55. Martin JL, Mestril R, Hilal-Dandan R, et al. Small heat shock proteins and protection against ischemic injury in cardiac myocytes. Circulation 1997;96(12):4343–4348.
56. Kurrelmeyer KM, Michael LH, Baumgarten G, et al. Endogenous tumor necrosis factor protects the adult cardiac myocyte against ischemic-induced apoptosis in a murine model of acute myocardial infarction. Proc Natl Acad Sci USA 2000;97(10):5456–5461.
57. Lazdunski M, Frelin C, Vigne P. The sodium/hydrogen exchange system in cardiac cells: its biochemical and pharmacological properties and its role in regulating internal concentrations of sodium and internal pH. J Mol Cell Cardiol 1985;17(11):1029–1042.
58. Gumina RJ, Buerger E, Eickmeier C, et al. Inhibition of the Na(+)/H(+) exchanger confers greater cardioprotection against 90 minutes of myocardial ischemia than ischemic preconditioning in dogs. Circulation 1999;100(25):2519–2526; discussion 2469–2472.
59. Klagsbrun M, D'Amore PA. Regulators of angiogenesis. Ann Rev Physiol 1991;53:217–239.
60. Folkman J, D'Amore PA. Blood vessel formation: what is its molecular basis? Cell 1996;87(7):1153–1155.

234 · Oxidative Stress and Cardiac Failure

61. Dimmeler S, Zeiher AM. Endothelial cell apoptosis in angiogenesis and vessel regression. Circ Res 2000;87(6):434–439.
62. Banai S, Shweiki D, Pinson A, et al. Upregulation of vascular endothelial growth factor expression induced by myocardial ischemia: implications for coronary angiogenesis. Cardiovasc Res 1994;28(8):1176–1179.
63. Banai S, Jaklitsch MT, Shou M, et al. Angiogenic-induced enhancement of collateral blood flow to ischemic myocardium by vascular endothelial growth factor in dogs. Circulation 1994;89(5):2183–2189.
64. Lee SH, Wolf PL, Escudero R, et al. Early expression of angiogenesis factors in acute myocardial ischemia and infarction. N Engl J Med 2000;342:626–633.
65. Hori M, Gotoh K, Kitakaze M, et al. Role of oxygen-derived free radicals in myocardial edema and ischemia in coronary microvascular embolization. Circulation 1991;84(2):828–840.
66. Hori M, Inoue M, Kitakaze M, et al. Role of adenosine in hyperemic response of coronary blood flow in microembolization. Am J Physiol 1986;250(3 Pt 2): H509–518.
67. Erbel R, Heusch G. Coronary microembolization. J Am Coll Cardiol 2000;36: 22–24.
68. Roe MT, Ohman EM, Maas AC, et al. Shifting the open-artery hypothesis downstream: the quest for optimal reperfusion. J Am Coll Cardiol 2001;37(1): 9–18.
69. Saitoh S, Onogi F, Aikawa K, et al. Multiple endothelial injury in epicardial coronary artery induces downstream microvascular spasm as well as remodeling partly via thromboxane A2. J Am Coll Cardiol 2001;37(1):308–315.
70. The Thrombolysis in Myocardial Infarction (TIMI) trial. Phase I findings. TIMI Study Group. N Engl J Med 1985;312(14):932–936.
71. The effects of tissue plasminogen activator, streptokinase, or both on coronary artery patency, ventricular function, and survival after acute myocardial infarction. The GUSTO Angiographic Investigators. N Engl J Med 1993;329(22): 1615–1622.
72. Ross AM, Coyne KS, Moreyra E, et al. Extended mortality benefit of early postinfarction reperfusion. GUSTO-I Angiographic Investigators. Global Utilization of Streptokinase and Tissue Plasminogen Activator for Occluded Coronary Arteries Trial. Circulation 1998;97(16):1549–1556.
73. Simes RJ, Topol EJ, Holmes DR Jr, et al. Link between the angiographic substudy and mortality outcomes in a large randomized trial of myocardial reperfusion: importance of early and complete infarct artery reperfusion. GUSTO-I Investigators. Circulation 1995;91(7):1923–1928.
74. van't Hof AW, Liem A, et al. Angiographic assessment of myocardial reperfusion in patients treated with primary angioplasty for acute myocardial infarction: myocardial blush grade. Zwolle Myocardial Infarction Study Group. Circulation 1998;97(23):2302–2306.
75. Gibson CM, Cannon CP, Murphy SA, et al. Relationship of TIMI myocardial perfusion grade to mortality after administration of thrombolytic drugs. Circulation 2000;101(2):125–130.
76. Gibson CM, Cannon CP, Daley WL, et al. TIMI frame count: a quantitative method of assessing coronary artery flow. Circulation 1996;93(5):879–888.
77. Heeschen C, Goldmann BU, Terres W, et al. Cardiovascular risk and therapeutic benefit of coronary interventions for patients with unstable angina according to the troponin T status. Eur Heart J 2000;21(14):1159–1166.
78. Hamm CW, Ravkilde J, Gerhardt W, et al. The prognostic value of serum troponin T in unstable angina. N Engl J Med 1992;327(3):146–150.

79. Heeschen C, van Den Brand MJ, et al. Angiographic findings in patients with refractory unstable angina according to troponin T status. Circulation 1999; 100(14):1509–1514.

80. Califf RM, Abdelmeguid AE, Kuntz RE, et al. Myonecrosis after revascularization procedures. J Am Coll Cardiol 1998;31(2):241–251.

81. Kong TQ, Davidson CJ, Meyers SN, et al. Prognostic implication of creatine kinase elevation following elective coronary artery interventions. JAMA 1997;277(6):461–466.

82. Adgey AA, Mathew TP, Harbinson MT. Periprocedural creatine kinase-MB elevations: long-term impact and clinical implications. Clin Cardiol 1999;22(4): 257–265.

83. Bertinchant JP, Polge A, Ledermann B, et al. Relation of minor cardiac troponin I elevation to late cardiac events after uncomplicated elective successful percutaneous transluminal coronary angioplasty for angina pectoris. Am J Cardiol 1999;84(1):51–57.

84. Garbarz E, Iung B, Lefevre G, et al. Frequency and prognostic value of cardiac troponin I elevation after coronary stenting. Am J Cardiol 1999;84(5): 515–518.

85. Kini A, Marmur JD, Kini S, et al. Creatine kinase-MB elevation after coronary intervention correlates with diffuse atherosclerosis, and low-to-medium level elevation has a benign clinical course: implications for early discharge after coronary intervention. J Am Coll Cardiol 1999;34(3):663–671.

86. Yamada DM, Topol EJ. Importance of microembolization and inflammation in atherosclerotic heart disease. Am Heart J 2000;140(6 Suppl):S90–S102.

87. Abdelmeguid AE, Topol EJ, Whitlow PL, et al. Significance of mild transient release of creatine kinase-MB fraction after percutaneous coronary interventions. Circulation 1996;94(7):1528–1536.

88. Kugelmass AD, Cohen DJ, Moscucci M, et al. Elevation of the creatine kinase myocardial isoform following otherwise successful directional coronary atherectomy and stenting. Am J Cardiol 1994;74(8):748–754.

89. Schroder R, Dissmann R, Bruggemann T, et al. Extent of early ST segment elevation resolution: a simple but strong predictor of outcome in patients with acute myocardial infarction. J Am Coll Cardiol 1994;24(2):384–391.

90. de Lemos JA, Antman EM, Gibson CM, et al. Abciximab improves both epicardial flow and myocardial reperfusion in ST-elevation myocardial infarction. Observations from the TIMI 14 trial. Circulation 2000;101(3):239–243.

91. Matetzky S, Novikov M, Gruberg L, et al. The significance of persistent ST elevation versus early resolution of ST segment elevation after primary PTCA. J Am Coll Cardiol 1999;34(7):1932–1938.

92. Santoro GM, Valenti R, Buonamici P, et al. Relation between ST-segment changes and myocardial perfusion evaluated by myocardial contrast echocardiography in patients with acute myocardial infarction treated with direct angioplasty. Am J Cardiol 1998;82(8):932–937.

93. Moons KG, Klootwijk P, Meij SH, et al. Continuous ST-segment monitoring associated with infarct size and left ventricular function in the GUSTO-I trial. Am Heart J 1999;138(Pt 1):525–532.

94. Andrews J, Straznicky IT, French JK, et al. ST-Segment recovery adds to the assessment of TIMI 2 and 3 flow in predicting infarct wall motion after thrombolytic therapy. Circulation 2000;101(18):2138–2143.

95. Tsunoda T, Nakamura M, Wakatsuki T, et al. The pattern of alteration in flow velocity in the recanalized artery is related to left ventricular recovery in pa-

tients with acute infarction and successful direct balloon angioplasty. J Am Coll Cardiol 1998;32(2):338–344.

96. Uchida Y, Nakamura F, Tomaru T, et al. Prediction of acute coronary syndromes by percutaneous coronary angioscopy in patients with stable angina. Am Heart J 1995;130(2):195–203.

97. Thieme T, Wernecke KD, Meyer R, et al. Angioscopic evaluation of atherosclerotic plaques: validation by histomorphologic analysis and association with stable and unstable coronary syndromes. J Am Coll Cardiol 1996;28(1): 1–6.

98. Ge J, Chirillo F, Schwedtmann J, et al. Screening of ruptured plaques in patients with coronary artery disease by intravascular ultrasound. Heart 1999; 81(6):621–627.

99. Nissen SE, De Franco AC, Tuzcu EM, et al. Coronary intravascular ultrasound: diagnostic and interventional applications. Coron Artery Dis 1995; 6(5): 355–367.

100. Weinberger J, Ramos L, Ambrose JA, et al. Morphologic and dynamic changes of atherosclerotic plaque at the carotid artery bifurcation: sequential imaging by real time B-mode ultrasonography. J Am Coll Cardiol 1988; 12(6):1515–1521.

101. Weinberger J, Azhar S, Danisi F, et al. A new noninvasive technique for imaging atherosclerotic plaque in the aortic arch of stroke patients by transcutaneous real-time B-mode ultrasonography: an initial report. Stroke 1998;29(3):673–676.

102. Ito H, Maruyama A, Iwakura K, et al. Clinical implications of the 'no reflow' phenomenon: a predictor of complications and left ventricular remodeling in reperfused anterior wall myocardial infarction. Circulation 1996;93(2):223–228.

103. Ito H, Okamura A, Iwakura K, et al. Myocardial perfusion patterns related to thrombolysis in myocardial infarction perfusion grades after coronary angioplasty in patients with acute anterior wall myocardial infarction. Circulation 1996;93(11):1993–1999.

104. Fayad Z, Fuster, V. Characterization of atherosclerotic plaques by magnetic resonance imaging. Ann NY Acad Sci 2000;902:173–186.

105. Wu KC, Zerhouni EA, Judd RM, et al. Prognostic significance of microvascular obstruction by magnetic resonance imaging in patients with acute myocardial infarction. Circulation 1998;97(8):765–772.

106. Al-Saadi N, Nagel E, Gross M, et al. Improvement of myocardial perfusion reserve early after coronary intervention: assessment with cardiac magnetic resonance imaging. J Am Coll Cardiol 2000;36(5):1557–1564.

107. Al-Saadi N, Nagel E, Gross M, et al. Noninvasive detection of myocardial ischemia from perfusion reserve based on cardiovascular magnetic resonance. Circulation 2000;101(12):1379–1383.

108. Gibbons RJ, Miller TD, Christian TF. Infarct size measured by single photon emission computed tomographic imaging with (99m)Tc-sestamibi: a measure of the efficacy of therapy in acute myocardial infarction. Circulation 2000; 101(1):101–108.

109. White HD. Future of reperfusion therapy for acute myocardial infarction. Lancet 1999;354(9180):695–697.

110. Topol EJ. Toward a new frontier in myocardial reperfusion therapy: emerging platelet preeminence. Circulation 1998;97(2):211–218.

111. A comparison of aspirin plus tirofiban with aspirin plus heparin for unstable angina. Platelet Receptor Inhibition in Ischemic Syndrome Management (PRISM) Study Investigators. N Engl J Med 1998;338(21):1498–1505.

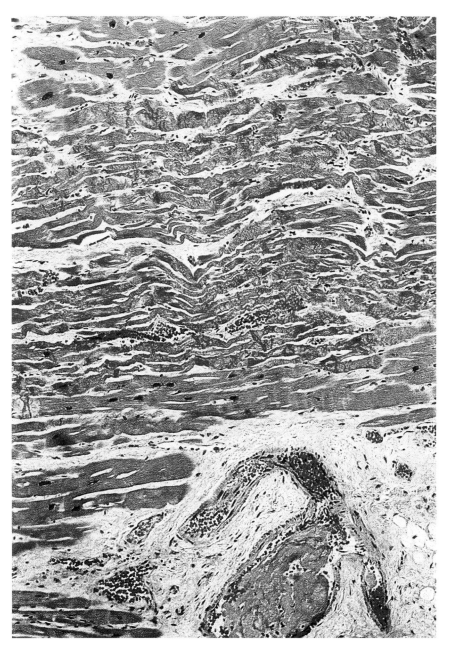

Figure 11-4. Autopsy specimen from a 53-year-old man with an acute myocardial in-farction demonstrating myocardial necrosis and platelet aggregation/plugging of an arteriole.

112. Inhibition of the platelet glycoprotein IIb/IIIa receptor with tirofiban in unstable angina and non-Q-wave myocardial infarction. Platelet Receptor Inhibition in Ischemic Syndrome Management in Patients Limited by Unstable Signs and Symptoms (PRISM-PLUS) Study Investigators. N Engl J Med 1998;338(21):1488–1497.

113. Topol EJ, Byzova TV, Plow EF. Platelet GPIIb-IIIa blockers. Lancet 1999; 353(9148):227–231.

114. Trial of abciximab with and without low-dose reteplase for acute myocardial infarction. Strategies for Patency Enhancement in the Emergency Department (SPEED) Group. Circulation 2000;101(24):2788–2794.

115. Ohman EM, Kleiman NS, Gacioch G, et al. Combined accelerated tissue-plasminogen activator and platelet glycoprotein IIb/IIIa integrin receptor blockade with integrilin in acute myocardial infarction. Results of a randomized, placebo-controlled, dose-ranging trial. IMPACT-AMI Investigators. Circulation 1997;95(4):846–854.

116. Antman EM, Giugliano RP, Gibson CM, et al. Abciximab facilitates the rate and extent of thrombolysis: results of the thrombolysis in myocardial infarction (TIMI) 14 trial. The TIMI 14 Investigators. Circulation 1999;99(21): 2720–2732.

117. Platelet glycoprotein IIb/IIIa receptor blockade and low-dose heparin during percutaneous coronary revascularization. The EPILOG Investigators. N Engl J Med 1997;336(24):1689–1696.

118. Randomised placebo-controlled and balloon-angioplasty-controlled trial to assess safety of coronary stenting with use of platelet glycoprotein-IIb/IIIa blockade. The EPISTENT Investigators. Evaluation of Platelet IIb/IIIa Inhibitor for Stenting. Lancet 1998;352(9122):87–92.

119. Randomised placebo-controlled trial of abciximab before and during coronary intervention in refractory unstable angina: the CAPTURE Study. Lancet 1997;349:1429–1435.

120. Platelet glycoprotein IIb/IIIa receptor blockade and low-dose heparin during percutaneous coronary revascularization. The EPILOG Investigators. N Engl J Med 1997;336(24):1689–1696.

121. Use of a monoclonal antibody directed against the platelet glycoprotein IIb/IIIa receptor in high-risk coronary angioplasty. The EPIC Investigation. N Engl J Med 1994;330(14):956–961.

122. Topol EJ, Mark DB, Lincoff AM, et al. Outcomes at 1 year and economic implications of platelet glycoprotein IIb/IIIa blockade in patients undergoing coronary stenting: results from a multicentre randomised trial. EPISTENT Investigators. Evaluation of Platelet IIb/IIIa Inhibitor for Stenting. Lancet 1999;354(9195):2019–2024.

123. King SB, 3rd, Mahmud E. Will blocking the platelet save the diabetic? Circulation 1999;100(25):2466–2468.

124. Marso SP, Lincoff AM, Ellis SG, et al. Optimizing the percutaneous interventional outcomes for patients with diabetes mellitus: results of the EPISTENT (Evaluation of Platelet IIb/IIIa Inhibitor for Stenting trial) diabetic substudy. Circulation 1999;100(25):2477–2484.

125. Theroux P, Alexander J Jr, Pharand C, et al. Glycoprotein IIb/IIIa receptor blockade improves outcomes in diabetic patients presenting with unstable angina/non-ST-elevation myocardial infarction: results from the Platelet Receptor Inhibition in Ischemic Syndrome Management In Patients Limited by Unstable Signs and Symptoms (PRISM-PLUS) study. Circulation 2000; 102(20):2466–2472.

126. Neumann FJ, Blasini R, Schmitt C, et al. Effect of glycoprotein IIb/IIIa re-

ceptor blockade on recovery of coronary flow and left ventricular function after the placement of coronary artery stents in acute myocardial infarction. Circulation 1998;98(24):2695–2701.

127. Herrmann HC, Moliterno DJ, Ohman EM, et al. Facilitation of early percutaneous coronary intervention after reteplase with or without abciximab in acute myocardial infarction: results from the SPEED (GUSTO-4 Pilot) Trial. J Am Coll Cardiol 2000;36(5):1489–1496.

128. Euler DE, Prood CE, Spear JF, et al. The interruption of collateral blood flow to the ischemic canine myocardium by embolization of a coronary artery with latex: effects on conduction delay and ventricular arrhythmias. Circ Res 1981;49(1):97–108.

129. Carlino M, De Gregorio J, Di Mario C, et al. Prevention of distal embolization during saphenous vein graft lesion angioplasty: experience with a new temporary occlusion and aspiration system. Circulation 1999;99(25):3221–3223.

130. Sen P, Udwadia, TE, Kinare SG, et al. Transmyocardial acupuncture. J Thorac Cardiovasc Surg 1965;50:151–189.

131. Mirhoseini M, Cayton MM. Revascularization of the heart by laser. J Microsurg 1981;2(4):253–260.

132. Burkhoff D, Schmidt S, Schulman SP, et al. Transmyocardial laser revascularisation compared with continued medical therapy for treatment of refractory angina pectoris: a prospective randomised trial. ATLANTIC Investigators. Lancet 1999;354(9182):885–890.

133. Allen KB, Dowling RD, DelRossi AJ, et al. Transmyocardial laser revascularization combined with coronary artery bypass grafting: a multicenter, blinded, prospective, randomized, controlled trial. J Thorac Cardiovasc Surg 2000;119(3):540–549.

134. Aaberge L, Nordstrand K, Dragsund M, et al. Transmyocardial revascularization with CO_2 laser in patients with refractory angina pectoris: clinical results from the Norwegian randomized trial. J Am Coll Cardiol 2000;35(5):1170–1177.

135. Frazier OH, March RJ, Horvath KA. Transmyocardial revascularization with a carbon dioxide laser in patients with end-stage coronary artery disease. N Engl J Med 1999;341(14):1021–1028.

136. Landolfo CK, Landolfo KP, Hughes GC, et al. Intermediate-term clinical outcome following transmyocardial laser revascularization in patients with refractory angina pectoris. Circulation 1999;100(Suppl):II128–133.

137. Schofield PM, Sharples LD, Caine N, et al. Transmyocardial laser revascularisation in patients with refractory angina: a randomised controlled trial. Lancet 1999;353(9152):519–524.

138. Dowling RD, Petracek MR, Selinger SL, et al. Transmyocardial revascularization in patients with refractory, unstable angina. Circulation 1998;98 (Suppl):II73–75; discussion II75–76.

139. Hughes GC, Landolfo KP, Lowe JE, et al. Perioperative morbidity and mortality after transmyocardial laser revascularization: incidence and risk factors for adverse events. J Am Coll Cardiol 1999;33(4):1021–1026.

140. Burns SM, Sharples LD, Tait S, et al. The transmyocardial laser revascularization international registry report. Eur Heart J 1999;20(1):31–37.

141. Tjomsland O, Aaberge L, Almdahl SM, et al. Perioperative cardiac function and predictors for adverse events after transmyocardial laser treatment. Ann Thorac Surg 2000;69(4):1098–1103.

142. Burkhoff D, Wesley MN, Resar JR, et al. Factors correlating with risk of

mortality after transmyocardial revascularization. J Am Coll Cardiol 1999; 34(1):55–61.

143. Gassler N, Wintzer HO, Stubbe HM, et al. Transmyocardial laser revascularization: histological features in human nonresponder myocardium. Circulation 1997;95(2):371–375.

144. Cooley DA, Frazier OH, Kadipasaoglu KA, et al. Transmyocardial laser revascularization: anatomic evidence of long-term channel patency. Texas Heart Inst J 1994;21(3):220–224.

145. Kohmoto T, Fisher PE, Gu A, et al. Does blood flow through holmium:YAG transmyocardial laser channels? Ann Thorac Surg 1996;61(3):861–868.

146. Schneider J, Diegeler A, Krakor R, et al. Transmyocardial laser revascularization with the holmium:YAG laser: loss of symptomatic improvement after 2 years. Eur J Cardiothorac Surg 2001;19(2):164–169.

147. Rosengart TK, Lee LY, Patel SR, et al. Angiogenesis gene therapy: phase I assessment of direct intramyocardial administration of an adenovirus vector expressing VEGF121 cDNA to individuals with clinically significant severe coronary artery disease. Circulation 1999;100(5):468–474.

148. Higano S. Coronary artery physiology: intracoronary ultrasonography, Doppler and pressure tracings. In: Murphy J, ed. Mayo Clinic Cardiology Review. Lippincott Williams & Wilkins, Philadelphia, 2000; 909.

149. Kantor B, McKenna CJ, Caccitolo JA, et al. Transmyocardial and percutaneous myocardial revascularization: current and future role in the treatment of coronary artery disease. Mayo Clin Proc 1999;74(6):585–592.

150. Baumgartner I, Pieczek A, Manor O, et al. Constitutive expression of phVEGF165 after intramuscular gene transfer promotes collateral vessel development in patients with critical limb ischemia. Circulation 1998;97(12): 1114–1123.

151. Schumacher B, Pecher P, von Specht BU, et al. Induction of neoangiogenesis in ischemic myocardium by human growth factors: first clinical results of a new treatment of coronary heart disease. Circulation 1998;97(7):645–650.

152. Donovan CL, Landolfo KP, Lowe JE, et al. Improvement in inducible ischemia during dobutamine stress echocardiography after transmyocardial laser revascularization in patients with refractory angina pectoris. J Am Coll Cardiol 1997;30(3):607–612.

• 12 •

The Role of Reactive Oxygen Species in the Pathogenesis of Endothelial Dysfunction in Patients with Chronic Heart Failure

Haoyi Zheng, MD, Henry Krum, MBBS, PhD, and Stuart D. Katz, MD

Introduction

Accumulating evidence from numerous investigators suggests that endothelial dysfunction plays an important role in the progression of many cardiovascular diseases, including chronic heart failure. This chapter will review experimental and clinical studies related to the potential role of endothelial dysfunction in the pathogenesis of heart failure, possible mechanisms of endothelial dysfunction in heart failure, evidence of increased production of reactive oxygen species (ROS) in heart failure, potential vascular sources of ROS in heart failure, cellular effects of ROS that may impact on endothelial function, and the potential effects of specific antioxidant therapeutic interventions on vascular function in heart failure.

Endothelial Dysfunction in the Pathogenesis of Heart Failure

The pathogenesis of congestive heart failure is related to the myocardial and peripheral vascular responses to myocellular injury (Figure 1).[1]

From: Kukin ML, Fuster V (eds). *Oxidative Stress and Cardiac Failure.* Armonk, NY: Futura Publishing Co., Inc. ©2003.

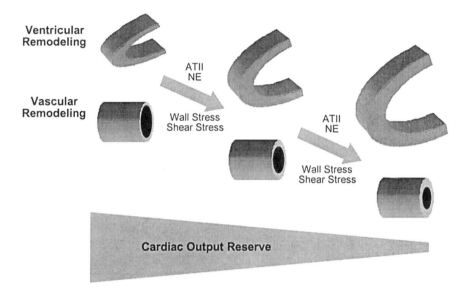

Figure 1. Pathophysiology of heart failure. Chronic changes in cardiovascular structure and function related to neurohormonal activation (ATII, NE) and altered hemodynamic forces (wall stress, shear stress) lead to gradual reduction of cardiac output reserve and progressive symptoms of heart failure. ATII = angiotensin II; NE = norepinephrine.

The myocardial response is characterized by progressive hypertrophy and dilatation of the ventricle and is not closely correlated with clinical symptoms in many patients.[2,3] The peripheral vascular response is characterized by increased peripheral vasomotor tone at rest and in response to vasodilating stimuli and is closely correlated to the degree of exercise intolerance in patients with symptomatic congestive heart failure.[4,5] Exercise intolerance in heart failure is attributable to reduction in maximal cardiac output reserve and vascular abnormalities that alter regional distribution of cardiac output.[6] Decreased vasodilatory reserve in the skeletal muscle circulation during exercise limits skeletal muscle hyperemia, reduces peripheral oxygen delivery, and is thereby an important determinant of reduced peak aerobic capacity in patients with heart failure.[7-10]

The vascular endothelium produces numerous biologically active substances that are important in the normal regulation of vascular structure and function, thrombosis and fibrinolysis, and inflammation in the vessel wall.[11] Furchgott and colleagues first described the obligatory role of the vascular endothelium in mediating the vasodilation response to acetylcholine in isolated rabbit descending thoracic aorta.[12] The "endothelium-derived relaxing factor" proposed by Furchgott was subsequently identified to be chemically indistinguishable from nitric oxide (NO).[13] Vascular endothelial cells synthesize NO from the guanidino nitrogen of L-arginine, by the action of a constitutively expressed reductase enzyme, nitric oxide synthase (eNOS), in response to a diverse array of hormonal agonists, physiochemical, and physical stimuli.[14]

Abnormal function of the vascular endothelium may contribute to the pathogenesis of chronic heart failure via several potential mechanisms (Figure 2). Endothelium-derived NO regulates skeletal muscle blood flow as part of a coordinated system that preferentially supplies blood flow to muscles with high oxidative capacity during submaximal exercise.[15] Endothelium-dependent NO-mediated vasodilation in response to hormonal agonists is impaired in experimental and clinical heart failure.[16–22] Exercise-induced NO-mediated vasodilation is impaired in the intact skeletal muscle circulation of rats with heart failure due to experimental

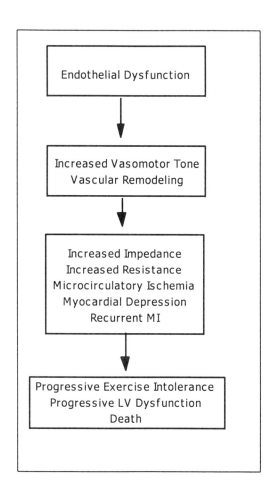

Figure 2. Potential mechanisms of endothelial dysfunction in the progression of chronic heart failure.

myocardial infarction,[23] and in the forearm circulation of patients with heart failure.[24] In patients with congestive heart failure, exercise capacity and functional class correlate with the severity of impairment of NO-mediated vasodilation.[24-28]

Endothelium-dependent changes in vascular structure may also limit exercise-induced hyperemia in skeletal muscle.[29-34] In patients with heart failure, subintimal hyalinosis and basement membrane thickening have been described in resistance arterioles and capillaries of the skeletal muscle and skin circulation.[35,36] The vascular endothelium plays an important role as an autocrine/paracrine organ in the regulation of vascular structure.[37-40] Decreased synthesis of NO and increased synthesis of endothelin-1 and angiotensin II may result in the reduction of the caliber of resistance arterioles and/or rarefaction of arterioles, which limits maximal skeletal muscle perfusion (and thus peak oxygen uptake) during exercise.[41]

Abnormal endothelium-dependent vasomotion in the coronary circulation may also directly contribute to progression of heart failure.[20,42] In dogs with progressive heart failure induced by repeated coronary embolization, endothelial dysfunction in the nonembolized artery preceded the onset of left ventricular hemodynamic dysfunction.[43] Early onset of endothelial dysfunction suggests a possible etiological role in progression of myopathic changes remote from infarcted myocardium. In clinical studies, endothelial dysfunction has been reported in the coronary circulation of patients with recent onset heart failure due to idiopathic dilated cardiomyopathy.[44]

Mechanisms of Endothelial Dysfunction

The mechanisms that contribute to endothelial dysfunction in patients with heart failure have not been fully characterized. Widespread distribution of endothelial dysfunction in vascular beds subjected to diverse hemodynamic forces suggests that circulating factors in serum may contribute to endothelial dysfunction in patients with heart failure.[45] Circulating factors have been implicated in the pathogenesis of endothelial dysfunction in patients with advanced renal disease and patients with preeclampsia.[46-48] Autocrine/paracrine factors that are increased in the serum of heart failure patients, including (but not limited to) norepinephrine,[49-53] angiotensin II,[52,54-58] and endothelin-1[59,60] may contribute to endothelial dysfunction in heart failure.

Both agonist-induced and shear stress-induced endothelium-dependent vasodilation are impaired in patients with heart failure.[22,24] Impaired endothelium-dependent vasodilation in heart failure is at least partly attributable to decreased synthesis of NO.[61] As the upstream signaling

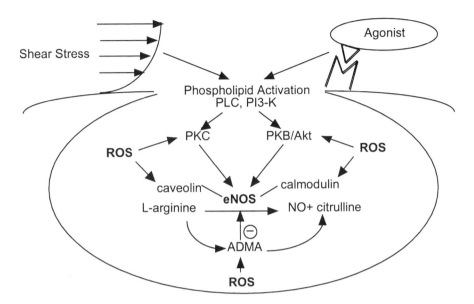

Figure 3. Possible pathways of endothelial dysfunction in heart failure. ROS may have an impact on signal transduction pathways, expression, and/or regulation of eNOS, and production of ADMA, an endogenous inhibitor of eNOS. ADMA = asymmetric dimethyl arginine; eNOS = endothelial nitric oxide synthase; NO = nitric oxide; PKC = protein kinase C; PKB = protein kinase B; PLC = phospholipase C; PI3-K = phosphatidylinositol 3-kinase; ROS = reactive oxygen species.

pathways of agonist receptor binding and shear stress are distinct, these observations indicate that impaired endothelium-dependent vasodilation in patients with congestive heart failure may be caused by: (1) alterations in a critical downstream signal transduction pathway that is common to both agonist-induced and shear stress-induced activation of eNOS; (2) alterations in the expression of eNOS and/or other key regulatory proteins; (3) alterations in availability of eNOS substrate and/or NO bioavailability.

This chapter will focus on the potential role of ROS in relation to each of these proposed mechanisms of endothelial dysfunction in patients with heart failure (Figure 3).

Evidence of Increased Oxidative Stress in Heart Failure

Evidence of increased production of ROS is reviewed in greater detail elsewhere in this book. Evidence of increased free radical formation has been reported in animal models of heart failure induced by pressure or volume overload and myocardial infarction.[62] Adriamycin-induced and catecholamine-induced cardiomyopathy appear to be mediated by excess production of oxygen free radicals and can be prevented in animal models with specific antioxidant therapy.[62] Indirect evidence of increased oxidative stress (via measurement of products of lipid peroxidation) has been reported in patients with heart failure secondary to coronary artery disease, rheumatic heart disease, or idiopathic dilated cardiomyopathy.[63–66] Of interest, evidence of sympathetic activation, cytokine activation, and increased free radical formation has been reported early in the disease process, even in patients with early left ventricular dysfunction with minimal or no symptoms.[64,67] Increased blood levels of lipid peroxidation products are associated with increased cytokine activation and worsening functional class in patients with heart failure.[68]

Potential Vascular Sources of Reactive Oxygen Species

Endothelial cells, vascular smooth muscle, myocytes, macrophages, and neutrophils are potential cellular sources of ROS that may impact vascular endothelial function.[62,69–72] However, vascular smooth muscle cells and fibroblasts appear to be the predominant sources of ROS in the vessel wall.[73] Increased formation of free radicals in heart failure may be related to activation of cytokines such as tumor necrosis factor, interleukin-1, and interleukin-2, increased activity of the cyclooxygenase pathway, or due to increased concentrations of norepinephrine and angiotensin II.[58,69,74,75] In addition, changes in regional flow and pressure patterns present in patients with heart failure may contribute to increased free radical production.[76,77]

Cultured endothelial cells and vascular smooth muscle cells produce superoxide anion and hydrogen peroxide.[78–80] Potential sources of superoxide production include mitochondrial respiration, arachadonic acid pathway enzymes lipoxygenase and cyclooxygenase, xanthine oxidase, NO synthase, and membrane-bound NAD(P)H oxidase.[81–83]

The predominant source of ROS in vascular tissue is the membrane-bound NADH/NADPH oxidase.[73,84] The vascular NAD(P)H oxidase shares some structural homology with the neutrophil NADPH oxidase. The p22phox subunit appears to play an important role for maintenance of enzyme activity in both vascular and neutrophil isozymes.[85] However, vascular NAD(P)H oxidase differs from the neutrophil form in several important aspects. Vascular NAD(P)H oxidase is a low-output, slow-release enzyme that appears to release superoxide in the intracellular space.[73] The enzyme is constitutively present with continuous basal production of superoxide. The activity of this enzyme is regulated by hormonal agonists and physical forces that appear to be important in the normal regulation of vascular structure and function and progression of vascular diseases. Angiotensin II, tumor necrosis factor alpha, platelet-derived growth factor, and shear stress increase activity of NAD(P)H oxidase in vascular smooth muscle cells. In cultured endothelial cells, continuous laminar shear stress induces a transient increase in activity whereas cyclical shear stress induces a sustained increase in activity.[77] In isolated human saphenous vein, NAD(P)H oxidase activity is directly associated with impaired NO-mediated vasodilation and presence of clinical risk factors for atherosclerosis.[86,87] Genetic variants in the p22phox component of NAD(P)H oxidase may be linked to endothelial dysfunction and increased risk of clinical vascular events.[88–91]

Xanthine oxidoreductase is a cytosolic molybdoenzyme that may exist in two forms as xanthine reductase and xanthine oxidase. The oxidase form catalyzes oxidation of hypoxanthine and xanthine, leading to the production of superoxide and hydrogen peroxide.[81] While xanthine oxidase activity has been detected in cultured rat pulmonary endothelial cells, the importance of this enzyme as a source of ROS in the intact circulation is uncertain.[92] Xanthine oxidase has been identified as a vascular source of superoxide generation in cultured human endothelial cells exposed to anoxia and reoxygenation.[82] Inhibition of xanthine oxidase has been reported to reduce blood pressure in the spontaneously hypertensive rat, and acutely improve endothelium-dependent vasodilation in patients with hypertension and hypercholesterolemia.[93–95] The potential role of xanthine oxidase has not been studied in experimental or clinical congestive heart failure.

In the absence of adequate concentrations of L-arginine as substrate, or adequate concentrations of the essential cofactor tetrahydrobiopterin, NO synthase can produce superoxide anion and hydrogen peroxide.[70,71] While uncoupling of NO synthase has been demonstrated in purified enzyme preparations in the absence of its normal regulatory proteins, the role of this phenomenon in the intact cell under physiological and pathophysiological conditions is uncertain. Tetrahydrobiopterin administration improved endothelium-dependent vasodilation in insulin-resistant rats and in human subjects with endothelial dysfunction related to smoking.[96–99]

Cellular Effects of ROS

ROS appear to play an important role in regulation of cell signal transduction pathways, gene expression, cell growth, and apoptosis. Whether ROS act primarily as physiological mediators of normal vascular function or pathological mediators of disease appears to be dependent on several factors.[100,101] The proportion of different ROS present is likely an important factor. Highly reactive species such as peroxynitrite and hydroxyl anion may primarily mediate cytotoxic effects whereas a more stable species such as hydrogen peroxide appears to be important in cellular signaling.[102–106] Superoxide anion specifically inhibits cGMP-associated vasorelaxation in isolated bovine pulmonary artery segments.[107] Subcellular localization of production, kinetics, and amplitude of ROS production, and interaction with endogenous antioxidant enzymes are also likely to play an important role in determining the net effect of ROS on cellular function. In experimental and clinical heart failure, the net effect of ROS production appears to be an altered endothelial phenotype that contributes to progression of disease. The potential role of ROS on the three proposed mechanisms of endothelial dysfunction in heart failure are discussed below.

Alterations in Cellular Signaling

Binding of hormonal agonists to specific receptors on the endothelial cell membrane increases NO synthesis by a calcium-dependent process that involves hydrolysis of membrane phospholipids (regulated by heterotrimeric G-proteins), inositol triphosphate-dependent release of calcium from intracellular stores, and subsequent activation of an energy-requiring capacitive calcium influx.[6] Shear stress increases NO synthesis via a calcium-independent process that involves hydrolysis of membrane phospholipids (regulated by the ras G-protein), and subsequent phosphorylation eNOS and other regulatory proteins, notably caveolin-1.[7–10] Shear stress activation of eNOS is partly dependent on activation of receptor tyrosine kinases but also involves activation of serine/threonine protein kinases.[108,109] ROS may alter eNOS activity through their effects on calcium signaling, alterations in protein phosphorylation involving tyrosine kinases, protein kinase C, and protein kinase B signaling cascades, and/or alterations in protein phosphatase activity. Detailed consideration of the effects of ROS on these signal transduction pathways is beyond the scope of this discussion and has been the subject of recent reviews.[101,110,111]

Alterations in Expression of eNOS and/or Key Regulatory Proteins

The presence of AP-1, AP-2, nuclear factor 1, p53, sterol regulatory, and shear stress response elements in the eNOS gene suggests that many factors can influence eNOS expression.[112] In experimental congestive heart failure models, eNOS mRNA and protein content in aortic endothelial cells are decreased when compared with control animals.[113–115] Activity of eNOS protein is regulated by post-translational modification

(N-myristoylation and palmitoylation), protein phosphorylation, and by binding to calcium-calmodulin, hsp90, and caveolin-1.[112,116–120] Sera from patients with hypercholesterolemia upregulates caveolin-1 expression, increases inhibitory caveolin-1-eNOS interactions, and decreases basal and stimulated NO release in endothelial cells.[121] ROS appear to play an important role in the regulation of gene expression in the endothelial cell.[122] Expression of inflammatory cell adhesion molecules in response to cytokine stimulation or other proinflammatory stimuli occurs by activation of the NF-κB. Activity of transcription factors AP-1 and NF-κB are highly regulated by the redox state of the cell. ROS produced in response to cyclic strain or shear stress increase c-fos and ICAM gene expression in cultured HUVEC.[123–125] Hydrogen peroxide generated from xanthine oxidase increases c-jun expression and promotes vascular smooth muscle growth in cultured rat cells.[126] Incubation of cultured human endothelial cells with serum from patients with heart failure for 48 hours leads to downregulation of eNOS protein, which is partially reversed by immunological blockade of TNF-α effects.[127]

Alterations in Availability of eNOS Substrate and/or NO Bioavailability

Decreased availability of L-arginine as substrate for eNOS is a controversial hypothesis as normal plasma and tissue levels of arginine (1–2 mM) greatly exceed the K_m for eNOS (5 μM).[128] This "arginine paradox" may be attributable to intracellular compartmentalization of eNOS, or competition for eNOS binding sites from endogenous inhibitors of NO synthase such as asymmetric dimethyl arginine (ADMA) and L-NMMA.[46,129] ADMA and L-NMMA are synthesized from L-arginine by the action of methylase I, a ubiquitous enzyme that catalyzes methylation of arginine at its guanidino nitrogens.[130] Dimethylarginine dimethylaminohydrolase (DDAH) is a widely distributed redox-sensitive enzyme present in human endothelial cells that hydrolyzes ADMA and L-NMMA to citrulline and dimethylamine.[131] DDAH is co-localized with eNOS on the cell surface membrane and appears to regulate eNOS activity by altering intracellular ADMA concentrations.[132,133] In ECV304 human endothelial cell culture, incubation with oxidized LDL and TNF-α for 48 hours increases ADMA in the conditioned medium and decreases DDAH activity without change in DDAH protein abundance.[134] In patients with type II diabetes mellitus, decreased endothelium-dependent vasodilation after ingestion of a high-fat meal is associated with acute increases in plasma ADMA.[135] Plasma ADMA levels are increased in patients with heart failure when compared with normal subjects.[136]

ROS may reduce NO bioavailability and/or attenuate the effects of NO in vascular smooth muscle. Depletion of the essential cofactor tetrahydrobiopterin induces purified eNOS enzyme to produce superoxide and hydrogen peroxide instead of NO. In the presence of large amounts of superoxide, NO is rapidly converted to the highly reactive ROS peroxynitrite. The rapid kinetics of this reaction effectively shortens the half-life of bioavailable NO and reduces interaction with its target enzyme soluble guanylyl cyclase in vascular smooth muscle.[101] Peryoxinitrite may have direct cytotoxic effects that further reduce NO synthesis and may possibly regulate protein kinase signaling cascades via protein nitrosylation.[101] ROS may also attenuate NO-mediated vasodilation through direct inhibition of soluble guanylate cyclase activation in vascular smooth muscle, alterations in tyrosine kinase signaling in smooth muscle, or via direct effects on sarcoplasmic reticulum activity in smooth muscle.[106,137–139]

Therapeutic Implications

As the specific stimulus and source for increased oxygen free radical production in heart failure is unknown, nonspecific antioxidant therapy is the most feasible interventional strategy. Normal host defenses against cellular damage from ROS include the endogenous antioxidant proteins (superoxide dismutase, catalase, and glutathione peroxidase, metal-binding proteins), water-soluble antioxidants (ascorbic acid, urate, glutathione), and lipid-soluble antioxidants (α-tocopherol and β-carotene).[140] The water-soluble ascorbate (vitamin C), and lipid-soluble α-tocopherol (vitamin E) are the most easily modifiable, and therefore have been the most frequent subject of investigation. Both decrease superoxide anion production in balloon-injured porcine coronary arteries.[141]

Ascorbic acid (vitamin C) is the most abundant and important inhibitor of free oxygen radical damage in extracellular fluid.[142] Vitamin C potently inhibits initiation and propagation of free radical production in aqueous solutions and inhibits lipid peroxidation. Vitamin C also alters intracellular redox state through interactions with glutathione.[143,144] Short-term administration of intravenous and oral vitamin C enhances endothelium-dependent vasodilation in the forearm circulation of patients with hypercholesterolemia, diabetes mellitus, and atherosclerosis.[145–147] In a small uncontrolled trial, short-term therapy with vitamin C improved endothelium-dependent vasodilation in the radial arteries of patients with chronic heart failure.[148]

Alpha-tocopherol (vitamin E) is incorporated into the plasma membrane lipid bilayer and functions as a chain-breaking antioxidant that prevents the propagation of free radical damage in biological membranes.[149] Vitamin E is a potent peroxyl radical scavenger that protects polyunsaturated fatty acids within the phospholipid cell membrane and plasma lipoproteins from oxidation. In cultured human endothelial cells, vitamin E reduces oxidative injury and reduces hydrogen peroxide production after hypoxia/reoxygenation.[150–152] Vitamin E prevents endothelial dysfunction in response to oxidized LDL by inhibiting activation of PKC and increases resistance to free radical damage in human aortic endothelial cell culture.[153] In cholesterol-fed rabbits, vitamin E enhanced endothelium-dependent vasodilation in isolated aortic and carotid artery rings, and in the isolated perfused coronary circulation.[154–156] In a small clinical trial, 3 months of therapy with vitamin E did not alter endothelium-dependent vasodilation in the forearm circulation of 12 patients postmyocardial infarction.[157] In patients with heart failure, 4 weeks of therapy with vitamin E (400 mg daily) was associated with reduced serum malonyldialdehyde levels and increased activity of superoxide dismutase and catalase.[158] Retrospective epidemiological studies have demonstrated reduced risk of coronary events in persons with greater daily dietary intake of vitamin E, but prospective studies of vitamin E therapy have reported mixed findings.[159–162]

Antioxidant vitamins act primarily in the extracellular space or in the cell membrane lipid bilayer, whereas the detrimental effects of oxygen free radicals in endothelial cells occur primarily in the cytosol.[81] Accordingly, development of an antioxidant therapy that acts within the cell may provide better protection against the damaging effects of oxygen free radicals than antioxidant vitamins. Dexrazoxane, a membrane-permeable cyclic derivative of the chelating agent edetic acid (EDTA), is currently approved for the prevention of anthracycline cardiotoxicity.[163,164] The cardioprotective action of dexrazoxane is believed to be attributable to its binding of intracellular free iron, thereby reducing the formation of anthracycline-iron complexes and the subsequent generation of ROS which are toxic to cardiac myocytes.[164,165] Free intracellular iron is an essential cofactor in the Fenton reaction, which nonenzymatically converts hydrogen peroxide to the highly reactive hydroxyl anion.[163] Whether binding of free intracellular iron by dexrazoxane can reduce oxygen free radical cell injury in states of increased oxidant stress unrelated to anthracyclines in cell types other than myocytes is unknown.

Intracoronary infusion of the cell-permeable oxygen free radical scavenger tiron inhibited oxygen free radical formation and improved coronary endothelium-dependent vasodilation in dogs with pacing-induced chronic heart failure, but not in control animals.[166] Endothelium-dependent vasodilation was tested in this model by assessment of vascular responses to intracoronary acetylcholine infusion. Moreover, L-NMMA diminished the beneficial effect of tiron in chronic heart failure dogs, suggesting a NO-dependent mechanism of benefit of this agent. Tiron infusion had no acute effects on hemodynamic parameters or myocardial metabolic status, suggesting that the observed changes in endothelial function were not related to overall improvements in cardiovascular status secondary to improvements in myocardial function.

Since angiotensin II is known to increase activity of vascular NAD(P)H oxidase, angiotensin-converting enzyme (ACE) inhibitors may mediate some of their clinical benefits in heart failure via reduction in vascular production of ROS. In rats with heart failure after LAD ligation, chronic treatment with captopril was associated with increased activity of SOD, glutathione peroxidase, and catalase as well as decreased lipid peroxidation when compared with placebo.[167] The improvement in endothelial function associated with ACE inhibition in the postmyocardial infarction heart failure model of the rat is partly attributable to decreased effects of ROS.[168] In clinical studies, ACE inhibition therapy is associated with improved endothelial function and reduced risk for myocardial infarction.[169,170]

The sympathetic nervous system is a major stimulus for oxygen free radical production and thus may be one of the important mechanisms by which endothelial dysfunction occurs in chronic heart failure. Carvedilol is a nonselective beta-blocker and α_1-receptor antagonist that has powerful antioxidant properties in vitro.[171] Carvedilol has been shown to reduce nitrate tolerance, which is thought to be due, at least in part, to inactivation of guanylate cyclase via an increase in superoxide anion production. Watanabe and colleagues demonstrated that carvedilol, but neither a β_1-selective beta-blocker (metoprolol) nor an alpha-1 antagonist (doxazosin), attenuated nitrate tolerance in patients with chronic heart failure.[172] It is uncertain whether these presumed antioxidant effects of carvedilol occur because of more comprehensive adrenergic blockade or via a distinct direct antioxidant property of the drug. In support of a class effect are the data presented by Kukin and colleagues, in which therapy with both carvedilol and metoprolol was associated with decreased serum levels of lipid peroxidation products.[173] A preliminary report indicates that beta-blocker therapy does not enhance endothelium-dependent vasodilation in patients with heart failure.[174]

Physical training has been shown to enhance endothelium-dependent vasodilation in patients with chronic heart failure.[175,176] However, it remains uncertain whether exercise training results in enhanced NO production or reduced NO degradation via enhanced clearance of ROS. The portion of flow-dependent dilatation reduced by the NO synthase inhibitor L,N-monomethylarginine (L-NMMA) is higher following physical training, suggesting that a major contribution comes from enhancement of NO release.[177] However, data from animal studies suggest that exercise may also reduce the degradation of NO from ROS.[178,179] The free radical scavenger N-(2-mercaptopropionyl)-glycine (MPG) improved flow-mediated vasodilation to a greater extent in nontrained rats when compared to trained rats with experimental heart failure. These observations sug-

ROS and Endothelial Dysfunction · 253

gest that exercise training reduces the contribution of ROS to reductions in NO-dependent, flow-mediated dilatation in the setting of chronic heart failure.[115] Thus, reduction in the contribution of ROS to endothelial dysfunction may, at least in part, contribute to the improvement in endothelium-dependent vasodilation observed following exercise training.

Conclusion

Increased production of ROS within the vasculature contributes to vascular endothelial and smooth muscle dysfunction in patients with chronic heart failure. Much additional work is needed to determine the primary stimuli and sources of ROS, as greater understanding of the genesis of oxidative stress in heart failure may lead to novel approaches to therapy.

References

1. Mancini DM, LeJemtel TH, Factor S, et al. Central and peripheral components of cardiac failure. Am J Med 1986;80:2–13.
2. Pfeffer MA, Braunwald E. Ventricular remodleing after myocardial infarction: experimental observations and clinical implications. Circulation 1990;81:1161–1172.
3. Franciosa JA, Park M, Levine TB. Lack of correlation between exercise capacity and indexes of resting left ventricular performance in heart failure. Am J Cardiol 1981;47:33–39.
4. Zelis R, Mason DT, Braunwald E. A comparison of the effects of vasodilator stimuli on peripheral resistance vessels in normal subjects and in patients with congestive heart failure. J Clin Invest 1968;47:960–970.
5. Jondeau G, Katz SD, Toussaint JF, et al. Regional specificity of peak hyperemic response in patients with congestive heart failure: correlation with peak aerobic capacity. J Am Coll Cardiol 1993;22:1399–1402.
6. Davis MJ, Sharma NR. Calcium-release-activated calcium influx in endothelium. J Vasc Res 1997;34:186–195.
7. Takahashi M, Ishida T, Traub O, et al. Mechanotransduction in endothelial cells: temporal signaling events in response to shear stress. J Vasc Res 1997;34:212–219.
8. Fleming I, Bauersachs J, Fisslthaler B, et al. Calcium-independent activation of the endothelial nitric oxide synthase in response to tyrosine phosphatase inhibitors and fluid shear stress. Circ Res 1998;82:686–695.
9. Bredt DS, Ferris CD, Snyder SH. Nitric oxide synthase regulatory sites. J Biol Chem 1992;267:10976–10981.
10. Tang ZL, Scherer PE, Lisanti MP. The primary sequence of murine caveolin reveals a conserved consensus site for phosphorylation by protein kinase C. Gene 1994;147:299–300.
11. Vane JR, Anggard EE, Botting RM. Regulatory functions of the vascular endothelium. N Engl J Med 1990;323:27–36.
12. Furchgott RF, Zawadzki JV. The obligatory role of endothelial cells in the re-

laxation of arterial smooth muscle by acetylcholine. Nature 1980;288:374–376.

13. Palmer RMJ, Ferrige AG, Moncada S. Nitric oxide release accounts for the biological activity of endothelium-derived relaxing factor. Nature 1987;327:524–526.

14. Moncada S, Palmer RMJ, Higgs EA. Nitric oxide: physiology, pathophysiology, and pharmacology. Pharmacol Rev 1991;43:109–142.

15. Hirai T, Visneski MD, Kearns KJ, et al. Effects of NO synthase inhibition on the muscular blood flow response to treadmill exercise in rats. J Applied Physiol 1994;77:1288–1293.

16. Kaiser L, Spickard RC, Olivier NB. Heart failure depresses endothelium-dependent responses in canine femoral artery. Am J Physiol 1989;256:H962–H967.

17. Ontkean M, Gay R, Greenberg B. Diminished endothelium-derived relaxing factor activity in an experimental model of chronic congestive heart failure. Circ Res 1991;69:1088–1096.

18. Elsner D, Muntze A, Kromer EP, et al. Systemic vasoconstriction induced by inhibition of nitric oxide synthesis is attenuated in conscious dogs with heart failure. Cardiovasc Res 1991;25:438–440.

19. Drexler H, Lu W. Endothelial dysfunction of hindquarter resistance vessels in experimental heart failure. Am J Physiol 1992;262:H1640–H1645.

20. Treasure CB, Vita JA, Cox DA, et al. Endothelium-dependent dilation of the coronary microvasculature is impaired in dilated cardiomyopathy. Circulation 1990;81:772–779.

21. Kubo SH, Rector TS, Bank AJ, et al. Endothelium-dependent vasodilation is attenuated in patients with heart failure. Circulation 1991;84:1589–1596.

22. Katz SD, Biasucci L, Sabba C, et al. Impaired endothelium-mediated vasodilation in the peripheral vasculature of patients with congestive heart failure. J Am Coll Cardiol 1992;19:918–925.

23. Hirai T, Zelis R, Musch TI. Effects of nitric oxide synthase inhibition on the muscle blood flow response to exercise in rats with heart failure. Cardiovasc Res 1995;30:469–476.

24. Katz SD, Krum H, Khan T, et al. Exercise-induced vasodilation in forearm circulation of normal subjects and patients with congestive heart failure: role of endothelium-derived nitric oxide. J Am Coll Cardiol 1996;28:585–590.

25. Lindsay DC, Holdright DR, Clarke D, et al. Endothelial control of lower limb blood flow in chronic heart failure. Heart 1996;75:469–476.

26. Nakamura M, Ishikawa M, Funakoshi T, et al. Attenuated endothelium-dependent peripheral vasodilation and clinical characteristics in patients with chronic heart failure. Am Heart J 1994;128:1164–1169.

27. Nakamura M, Chiba M, Ueshima K, et al. Effects of mitral and/or aortic valve replacement or repair on endothelium-dependent peripheral vasorelaxation and its relation to improvement in exercise capacity. Am J Cardiol 1996;77:98–102.

28. Carville C, Adnot S, Sediame S, et al. Relation between impairment in nitric oxide pathway and clinical status in patients with congestive heart failure. J Cardiovasc Pharmacol 1998;32:562–570.

29. Gaballa MA, Raya TE, Goldman S. Large artery remodeling after myocardial infarction. Am J Physiol 1995;268:H2092–H2103.

30. Schieffer B, Wollert KC, Berchtold M, et al. Development and prevention of skeletal muscle structural alterations after experimental myocardial infarction. Am J Physiol 1995;269:H1507–H1513.

31. Heeneman S, Leenders PJ, Aarts PJ, et al. Peripheral vascular alterations during experimental heart failure in the rat. Do they exist? Arterioscler Thromb Vasc Biol 1995;15:1503–1511.
32. Heeneman S, Smits JF, Leenders PJ, et al. Effects of angiotensin II on cardiac function and peripheral vascular structure during compensated heart failure in the rat. Arterioscler Thromb Vasc Biol 1997;17:1985–1994.
33. Mulder P, Elfertak L, Richard V, et al. Peripheral artery structure and endothelial function in heart failure: effect of ACE inhibition. Am J Physiol 1996;271:H469–477.
34. Buus NH, Kahr O, Mulvany MJ. Effect of short- and long-term heart failure on small artery morphology and endothelial function in the rat. J Cardiovasc Pharmacol 1999;34:34–40.
35. Lindsay DC, Anand IS, Bennett JG, et al. Ultrastructural analysis of skeletal muscle: microvascular dimensions and basement membrane thickness in chronic heart failure. Eur Heart J 1994;15:1470–1476.
36. Wroblewski H, Sindrup JH, Nørgaard T, et al. Effects of orthotopic cardiac transplantation on structural microangiopathy and abnormal hemodynamics in idopathic dilated cardiomyopathy. Am J Cardiol 1996;77:281–285.
37. Langille BL, O'Donnell F. Reductions in arterial diameter produced by chronic decreases in blood flow are endothelium-dependent. Science 1986;231:405–407.
38. Numaguchi K, Egashira K, Takemoto M, et al. Chronic inhibition of nitric oxide synthesis causes coronary microvascular remodeling in rats. Hypertension 1995;26:957–962.
39. Rudic RD, Shesely EG, Maeda N, et al. Direct evidence for the importance of endothelium-derived nitric oxide in vascular remodeling. J Clin Invest 1998;101:731–736.
40. Pollman MJ, Naumovski L, Gibbons GH. Vascular cell apoptosis: cell type-specific modulation by transforming growth factor-beta1 in endothelial cells versus smooth muscle cells. Circulation 1999;99:2019–2026.
41. Pollman MJ, Yamada T, Horiuchi M, et al. Vasoactive substances regulate vascular smooth muscle cell apoptosis: countervailing influences of nitric oxide and angiotensin II. Circ Res 1996;79:748–756.
42. Mohri M, Egashira K, Tagawa T, et al. Basal release of nitric oxide is decreased in the coronary circulation in patients with heart failure. Hypertension 1997;30:50–56.
43. Knecht M, Burkhoff D, Yi GH, et al. Coronary endothelial dysfunction precedes heart failure and reduction of coronary reserve in awake dogs. J Mol Cell Cardiol 1997;29:217–227.
44. Mathier MA, Rose GA, Fifer MA, et al. Coronary endothelial dysfunction in patients with acute-onset idiopathic dilated cardiomyopathy. J Am Coll Cardiol 1998;32:216–224.
45. Katz SD. The role of endothelium-derived vasoactive substances in the pathophysiology of exercise intolerance in patients with congestive heart failure. Prog Cardiovasc Dis 1995;28:23–50.
46. Vallance P, Leone A, Calver A, et al. Accumulation of an endogenous inhibitor of nitric oxide synthesis in chronic renal failure. Lancet 1992;339:572–575.
47. Prabhakar SS, Zeballos GA, Montoya-Zavala M, et al. Urea inhibits inducible nitric oxide synthase in macrophage cell line. Am J Physiol 1997;273:C1882–C1888.
48. Haller H, Hempel A, Homuth V, et al. Endothelial cell permeability and protein kinase C in pre-eclampsia. Lancet 1998;351:945–949.

256 • Oxidative Stress and Cardiac Failure

49. Steinberg SF, Jaffe EA, Bilezikian JP. Endothelial cells contain beta adreno-ceptors. Naunyn Schmiedebergs Arch Pharmacol 1984;325:310–313.
50. Bachetti T, Comini L, Agnoletti L, et al. Effects of chronic noradrenaline on the nitric oxide pathway in human endothelial cells. Basic Res Cardiol 1998; 93:250–256.
51. Bacic F, McCarron RM, Uematsu S, et al. Adrenergic receptors coupled to adenylate cyclase in human cerebromicrovascular endothelium. Metab Brain Dis 1992;7:125–137.
52. Schena M, Mulatero P, Schiavone D, et al. Vasoactive hormones induce nitric oxide synthase mRNA expression and nitric oxide production in human en-dothelial cells and monocytes. Am J Hypertens 1999;12:388–397.
53. Yamazaki T, Komuro I, Zou Y, et al. Norepinephrine induces the raf-1 kinase/mitogen-activated protein kinase cascade through both alpha 1- and beta-adrenoceptors. Circulation 1997;95:1260–1268.
54. Pueyo ME, Arnal JF, Rami J, et al. Angiotensin II stimulates the production of NO and peroxynitrite in endothelial cells. Am J Physiol 1998;274:C214–220.
55. Li D, Yang B, Philips MI, et al. Proapoptotic effects of ANG II in human coro-nary artery endothelial cells: role of AT1 receptor and PKC activation. Am J Physiol 1999;276:H786–92.
56. Li D, Tomson K, Yang B, et al. Modulation of constitutive nitric oxide syn-thase, bcl-2 and Fas expression in cultured human coronary endothelial cells exposed to anoxia-reoxygenation and angiotensin II: role of AT1 receptor ac-tivation. Cardiovasc Res 1999;41:109–115.
57. Ardaillou R. Angiotensin II receptors. J Am Soc Nephrol 1999;10(Suppl)11: S30–39.
58. Rajagopalan S, Kurz S, Münzel T, et al. Angiotensin II-mediated hyperten-sion in the rat increases vascular superoxide production via membrane NADH/NADPH oxidase activation: contribution to alterations of vasomotor tone. J Clin Invest 1996;97:1916–1923.
59. Hagar JM. Endogenous endothelin-1 impairs endothelium-dependent relax-ation after myocardial ischemia and reperfusion. Am J Physiol 1994;267: H1833–841.
60. Stanimirovic DB, Yamamoto T, Uematsu S, et al. Endothelin-1 receptor bind-ing and cellular signal transduction in cultured human brain endothelial cells. J Neurochem 1994;62:592–601.
61. Katz SD, Khan T, Zeballos GA, et al. Decreased activity of the L-arginine-nitric oxide metabolic pathway in patients with congestive heart failure. Cir-culation 1999;99:2113–2117.
62. Singh N, Dhalla AK, Seneviratne C, et al. Oxidative stress and heart failure. Molec Cell Biochem 1995;147:77–81.
63. Belch JJF, Bridges AB, Scott N, et al. Oxygen free radicals and congestive heart failure. Br Heart J 1991;65:245–248.
64. Diaz-Velez CR, Garcia-Castineiras S, Mendoza-Ramos E, et al. Increased malondialdehyde in peripheral blood of patients with congestive heart fail-ure. Am Heart J 1996;131:146–152.
65. McMurray J, McLay J, Chopra M, et al. Evidence for enhanced free radical activity in chronic congestive heart failure secondary to coronary artery dis-ease. Am J Cardiol 1990;65:1261–1262.
66. Sobotka PA, Brottman MD, Weitz Z, et al. Elevated breath pentane in heart failure reduced by free radical scavenger. Free Radical Biol Med 1993;14: 643–647.

67. Torre-Amione G, Kapadia S, Benedict C, et al. Proinflammatory cytokine levels in patients with depressed left ventricular ejection fraction: a report from the Studies of Left Ventricular Dysfunction (SOLVD). J Am Coll Cardiol 1996;27:1201–1206.
68. Keith M, Geranmayegan A, Sole MJ, et al. Increased oxidative stress in patients with congestive heart failure. J Am Coll Cardiol 1998;31:1352–1356.
69. Mann DL, Young JB. Basic mechanisms in congestive heart failure: recognizing the role of proinflammatory cytokines. Chest 1994;105:897–904.
70. Pou S, Pou WS, Bredt DS, et al. Generation of superoxide by purified brain nitric oxide synthase. J Biol Chem 1992;267:24173–24176.
71. Heinzel B, John M, Klatt P, et al. Calcium/calmodulin-dependent formation of hydrogen peroxide by brain nitric oxide synthase. Biochem J 1992;281:627–630.
72. Bauersachs J, Bouloumie A, Fraccarollo D, et al. Endothelial dysfunction in chronic myocardial infarction despite increased vascular endothelial nitric oxide synthase and soluble guanylate cyclase expression: role of enhanced vascular superoxide production. Circulation 1999;100:292–298.
73. Griendling KK, Sorescu D, Ushio-Fukai M. NAD(P)H oxidase: role in cardiovascular biology and disease. Circ Res 2000;86:494–501.
74. Dzau VJ, Packer M, Lilly LS, et al. Prostaglandins in severe congestive heart failure: relation to activation of the renin-angiotensin system and hyponatremia. N Engl J Med 1984;310:347–352.
75. Matsubara T, Ziff M. Increased superoxide anion release from human endothelial cells in response to cytokines. J Immunol 1986;137:3295–3298.
76. Laurindo FR, Pedro MDA, Barbeiro HV, et al. Vascular free radical release: ex vivo and in vivo evidence for a flow-dependent endothelial mechanism. Circ Res 1994;74:700–709.
77. De Keulenaer GW, Chappell DC, Ishizaka N, et al. Oscillatory and steady laminar shear stress differentially affect human endothelial redox state: role of a superoxide-producing NADH oxidase. Circ Res 1998;82:1094–1101.
78. Miller FJ Jr, Gutterman DD, Rios CD, et al. Superoxide production in vascular smooth muscle contributes to oxidative stress and impaired relaxation in atherosclerosis. Circ Res 1998;82:1298–1305.
79. Rosen GM, Freeman BA. Detection of superoxide generated by endothelial cells. Proc Natl Acad Sci USA 1984;81:7269–7273.
80. Thannickal VJ, Hassoun PM, White AC, et al. Enhanced rate of H_2O_2 release from bovine pulmonary artery endothelial cells induced by TGF-beta 1. Am J Physiol 1993;265:L622–626.
81. Cai H, Harrison DG. Endothelial dysfunction in cardiovascular diseases: the role of oxidant stress. Circ Res 2000;87:840–844.
82. Zweier JL, Broderick R, Kuppusamy P, et al. Determination of the mechanism of free radical generation in human aortic endothelial cells exposed to anoxia and reoxygenation. J Biol Chem 1994;269:24156–24162.
83. Holland JA, Pritchard KA, Pappolla MA, et al. Bradykinin induces superoxide anion release from human endothelial cells. J Cell Physiol 1990;143:21–25.
84. Mohazzab KM, Kaminski PM, Wolin MS. NADH oxidoreductase is a major source of superoxide anion in bovine coronary artery endothelium. Am J Physiol 1994;266:H2568–2572.
85. Ushio-Fukai M, Zafari AM, Fukui T, et al. p22phox is a critical component of the superoxide-generating NADH/NADPH oxidase system and regulates angiotensin II-induced hypertrophy in vascular smooth muscle cells. J Biol Chem 1996;271:23317–23321.

86. Guzik TJ, West NE, Black E, et al. Vascular superoxide production by NAD(P)H oxidase: association with endothelial dysfunction and clinical risk factors. Circ Res 2000;86:E85–90.
87. Guzik TJ, West NE, Black E, et al. Functional effect of the C242T polymorphism in the NAD(P)H oxidase p22phox gene on vascular superoxide production in atherosclerosis. Circulation 2000;102:1744–1747.
88. Cahilly C, Ballantyne CM, Lim DS, et al. A variant of p22(phox), involved in generation of ROS in the vessel wall, is associated with progression of coronary atherosclerosis. Circ Res 2000;86:391–395.
89. Inoue N, Kawashima S, Kanazawa K, et al. Polymorphism of the NADH/NADPH oxidase p22phox gene in patients with coronary artery disease. Circulation 1998;97:135–137.
90. Schachinger VV, Britten MB, Dimmeler S, et al. NADH/NADPH oxidase p22phox gene polymorphism is associated with improved coronary endothelial vasodilator function. Eur Heart J 2001;22:96–101.
91. Wolin MS. How could a genetic variant of the p22(phox) component of NAD(P)H oxidases contribute to the progression of coronary atherosclerosis? Circ Res 2000;86:365–366.
92. Dupont GP, Huecksteadt TP, Marshall BC, et al. Regulation of xanthine dehydrogenase and xanthine oxidase activity and gene expression in cultured rat pulmonary endothelial cells. J Clin Invest 1992;89:197–202.
93. Suzuki H, DeLano FA, Parks DA, et al. Xanthine oxidase activity associated with arterial blood pressure in spontaneously hypertensive rats. Proc Natl Acad Sci USA 1998;95:4754–4759.
94. Butler R, Morris AD, Belch JJ, et al. Allopurinol normalizes endothelial dysfunction in type 2 diabetics with mild hypertension. Hypertension 2000;35:746–751.
95. Cardillo C, Kilcoyne CM, Cannon RO 3rd, et al. Xanthine oxidase inhibition with oxypurinol improves endothelial vasodilator function in hypercholesterolemic but not in hypertensive patients. Hypertension 1997;30:57–63.
96. Shinozaki K, Nishio Y, Okamura T, et al. Oral administration of tetrahydrobiopterin prevents endothelial dysfunction and vascular oxidative stress in the aortas of insulin-resistant rats. Circ Res 2000;87:566–573.
97. Shinozaki K, Kashiwagi A, Nishio Y, et al. Abnormal biopterin metabolism is a major cause of impaired endothelium-dependent relaxation through nitric oxide/O_2 imbalance in insulin-resistant rat aorta. Diabetes 1999;48:2437–2445.
98. Heitzer T, Brockhoff C, Mayer B, et al. Tetrahydrobiopterin improves endothelium-dependent vasodilation in chronic smokers: evidence for a dysfunctional nitric oxide synthase. Circ Res 2000;86:E36–41.
99. Ueda S, Matsuoka H, Miyazaki H, et al. Tetrahydrobiopterin restores endothelial function in long-term smokers. J Am Coll Cardiol 2000;35:71–75.
100. Irani K. Oxidant signaling in vascular cell growth, death, and survival: a review of the roles of reactive oxygen species in smooth muscle and endothelial cell mitogenic and apoptotic signaling. Circ Res 2000;87:179–183.
101. Wolin MS. Interactions of oxidants with vascular signaling systems. Arterioscler Thromb Vasc Biol 2000;20:1430–1442.
102. Burke TM, Wolin MS. Hydrogen peroxide elicits pulmonary arterial relaxation and guanylate cyclase activation. Am J Physiol 1987;252:H721–732.
103. Burke-Wolin T, Abate CJ, Wolin MS, et al. Hydrogen peroxide-induced pulmonary vasodilation: role of guanosine 3′,5′-cyclic monophosphate. Am J Physiol 1991;261:L393–398.

104. Drummond GR, Cai H, Davis ME, et al. Transcriptional and posttranscriptional regulation of endothelial nitric oxide synthase expression by hydrogen peroxide. Circ Res 2000;86:347–354.
105. Roebuck KA, Rahman A, Lakshminarayanan V, et al. H_2O_2 and tumor necrosis factor-alpha activate intercellular adhesion molecule 1 (ICAM-1) gene transcription through distinct cis-regulatory elements within the ICAM-1 promoter. J Biol Chem 1995;270:18966–18974.
106. Wu L, de Champlain J. Effects of superoxide on signaling pathways in smooth muscle cells from rats. Hypertension 1999;34:1247–1253.
107. Cherry PD, Omar HA, Farrell KA, et al. Superoxide anion inhibits cGMP-associated bovine pulmonary arterial relaxation. Am J Physiol 1990;259: H1056–1062.
108. Corson MA, James NL, Latta SE, et al. Phosphorylation of endothelial nitric oxide synthase in response to fluid shear stress. Circ Res 1996;79:984–991.
109. Michel T, Li GK, Busconi L. Phosphorylation and subcellular translocation of endothelial nitric oxide synthase. Proc Natl Acad Sci USA 1993;90:6252–6256.
110. Lander HM. An essential role for free radicals and derived species in signal transduction. FASEB J 1997;11:118–124.
111. Wolin MS, Davidson CA, Kaminski PM, et al. Oxidant-nitric oxide signalling mechanisms in vascular tissue. Biochemistry (Mosc) 1998;63:810–816.
112. Sessa WC. The nitric oxide synthase family of proteins. J Vasc Res 1994;31: 131–143.
113. Comini L, Bachetti T, Gaia G, et al. Aorta and skeletal muscle NO synthase expression in experimental heart failure. J Mol Cell Cardiol 1996;28:2241–2248.
114. Smith CJ, Sun D, Hoegler C, et al. Reduced gene expression of vascular endothelial NO synthase and cyclooxygenase-1 in heart failure. Circ Res 1996; 78:58–64.
115. Varin R, Mulder P, Richard V, et al. Exercise improves flow-mediated vasodilatation of skeletal muscle arteries in rats with chronic heart failure: role of nitric oxide, prostanoids, and oxidant stress. Circulation 1999;99: 2951–2957.
116. Garcia-Cardena G, Martasek P, Masters BS, et al. Dissecting the interaction between nitric oxide synthase (NOS) and caveolin: functional significance of the nos caveolin binding domain in vivo. J Biol Chem 1997;272: 25437–25440.
117. Ju H, Zou R, Venema VJ, et al. Direct interaction of endothelial nitric-oxide synthase and caveolin-1 inhibits synthase activity. J Biol Chem 1997;272: 18522–18525.
118. Werner-Felmayer G, Werner ER, Fuchs D, et al. Pteridine biosynthesis in human endothelial cells. J Biol Chem 1993;268:1842–1846.
119. Garcia-Cardena G, Fan R, Shah V, et al. Dynamic activation of endothelial nitric oxide synthase by Hsp90. Nature 1998;392:821–824.
120. Michel JB, Feron O, Sacks D, et al. Reciprocal regulation of endothelial nitric-oxide synthase by Ca^{2+}-calmodulin and caveolin. J Biol Chem 1997;272: 15583–15586.
121. Feron O, Dessy C, Moniotte S, et al. Hypercholesterolemia decreases nitric oxide production by promoting the interaction of caveolin and endothelial nitric oxide synthase. J Clin Invest 1999;103:897–905.
122. Kunsch C, Medford RM. Oxidative stress as a regulator of gene expression in the vasculature. Circ Res 1999;85:753–766.

123. Cheng JJ, Wung BS, Chao YJ, et al. Cyclic strain-induced reactive oxygen species involved in ICAM-1 gene induction in endothelial cells. Hypertension 1998;31:125–130.
124. Chiu JJ, Wung BS, Shyy JY, et al. Reactive oxygen species are involved in shear stress-induced intercellular adhesion molecule-1 expression in endothelial cells. Arterioscler Thromb Vasc Biol 1997;17:3570–3577.
125. Hsieh HJ, Cheng CC, Wu ST, et al. Increase of reactive oxygen species (ROS) in endothelial cells by shear flow and involvement of ROS in shear-induced c-fos expression. J Cell Physiol 1998;175:156–162.
126. Rao GN, Berk BC. Active oxygen species stimulate vascular smooth muscle cell growth and proto-oncogene expression. Circ Res 1992;70:593–599.
127. Agnoletti L, Curello S, Bachetti T, et al. Serum from patients with severe heart failure downregulates eNOS and is proapoptotic: role of tumor necrosis factor-alpha. Circulation 1999;100:1983–1991.
128. Cooke JP, Tsao PS. Arginine: a new therapy for atherosclerosis? Circulation 1997;95:311–312.
129. Arnal JF, Munzel T, Venema RC, et al. Interactions between L-arginine and L-glutamine change endothelial NO production. J Clin Invest 1995;95:2565–2572.
130. Rawal N, Rajpurohit R, Paik WK, et al. Purification and characterization of S-adenosylmethionine-protein-arginine N-methyltransferase from rat liver. Biochem J 1994;300:483–489.
131. Kimoto M, Miyatake S, Sasagawa T, et al. Purification, cDNA cloning and expression of human NG,NG-dimethylarginine dimethylaminohydrolase. Eur J Biochem 1998;258:863–868.
132. Tojo A, Welch WJ, Bremer V, et al. Colocalization of demethylating enzymes and NOS and functional effects of methylarginines in rat kidney. Kidney Int 1997;52:1593–1601.
133. MacAllister RJ, Parry H, Kimoto M, et al. Regulation of nitric oxide synthesis by dimethylarginine dimethylaminohydrolase. Br J Pharmacol 1996;119:1533–1540.
134. Ito A, Tsao PS, Adimoolam S, et al. Novel mechanism for endothelial dysfunction: dysregulation of dimethylarginine dimethylaminohydrolase. Circulation 1999;99:3092–3095.
135. Fard A, Tuck CH, Donis JA, et al. Acute elevations of plasma asymmetric dimethylarginine and impaired endothelial function in response to a high-fat meal in patients with type 2 diabetes. Arterioscler Thromb Vasc Biol 2000;20:2039–2044.
136. Hanssen H, Brunini TM, Conway M, et al. Increased L-arginine transport in human erythrocytes in chronic heart failure. [Clin Sci 1998 Mar;94(3):333]. Clin Sci (Colch) 1998;94:43–48.
137. Omar HA, Cherry PD, Mortelliti MP, et al. Inhibition of coronary artery superoxide dismutase attenuates endothelium-dependent and -independent nitrovasodilator relaxation. Circ Res 1991;69:601–608.
138. Jin N, Rhoades RA. Activation of tyrosine kinases in H_2O_2-induced contraction in pulmonary artery. Am J Physiol 1997;272.II2686–2692.
139. Grover AK, Samson SE, Fomin VP, et al. Effects of peroxide and superoxide on coronary artery: ANG II response and sarcoplasmic reticulum Ca2+ pump. Am J Physiol 1995;269:C546–553.
140. Frei B. Reactive oxygen species and antioxidant vitamins: mechanisms of action. Am J Med 1994;97:5S–13S; discussion 22S–28S.

141. Nunes GL, Robinson K, Kalynych A, et al. Vitamins C and E inhibit O_2 production in the pig coronary artery. Circulation 1997;96:3593–3601.
142. Frei B, England L, Ames BN. Ascorbate is an outstanding antioxidant in human blood plasma. Proc Natl Acad Sci 1989;86:6377–6381.
143. Winkler BS, Orselli SM, Rex TS. The redox couple between glutathione and ascorbic acid: a chemical and physiological perspective. Free Rad Biol Med 1994;17:333–349.
144. Meister A. Glutathione-ascorbic acid antioxidant system in animals. J Biol Chem 1994;269:9397–9400.
145. Ting HH, Timimi FK, Haley EA, et al. Vitamin C improves endothelium-dependent vasodilation in forearm resistance vessels of humans with hypercholesterolemia. Circulation 1997;95:2617–2622.
146. Ting HH, Timimi FK, Boles KS, et al. Vitamin C improves endothelium-dependent vasodilation in patients with non-insulin-dependent diabetes mellitus. J Clin Invest 1996;97:22–28.
147. Levine GN, Frei B, Koulouris SN, et al. Ascorbic acid reverses endothelial vasomotor dysfunction in patients with coronary artery disease. Circulation 1996;93:1107–1113.
148. Hornig B, Arakawa N, Kohler C, et al. Vitamin C improves endothelial function of conduit arteries in patients with chronic heart failure. Circulation 1998;97:363–368.
149. Traber MG. Cellular and molecular mechanisms of oxidants and antioxidants. Miner Electrolyte Metab 1997;23:135–139.
150. Martin A, Wu D, Baur W, et al. Effect of vitamin E on human aortic endothelial cell responses to oxidative injury. Free Radic Biol Med 1996;21:505–511.
151. Kaneko T, Nakano S-I, Matsuo M. Protective effect of vitamin E on linoleic acid hydroperoxide-induced injury to human endothelial cells. Lipids 1991;26:345–348.
152. Martin A, Zulueta J, Hassoun P, et al. Effect of vitamin E on hydrogen peroxide production by human vascular endothelial cells after hypoxia/reoxygenation. Free Radic Biol Med 1996;20:99–105.
153. Keaney JF, Jr., Guo Y, Cunningham D, et al. Vascular incorporation of alpha-tocopherol prevents endothelial dysfunction due to oxidized LDL by inhibiting protein kinase C stimulation. J Clin Invest 1996;98:386–394.
154. Keaney JF, Gaziano JM, Xu A, et al. Dietary antioxidants preserve endothelium-dependent vessel relaxation in cholesterol-fed rabbits. Proc Natl Acad Sci 1993;90:11880–11884.
155. Stewart-Lee AL, Forster LA, Nourooz-Zadeh J, et al. Vitamin E protects against impairment of endothelium-mediated relaxations in cholesterol-fed rabbits. Arterioscler Thromb 1994;14:494–499.
156. Andersson TL, Matz J, Ferns GA, et al. Vitamin E reverses cholesterol-induced endothelial dysfunction in the rabbit coronary circulation. Atherosclerosis 1994;111:39–45.
157. Elliott TG, Barth JD, Mancini GB. Effects of vitamin E on endothelial function in men after myocardial infarction. Am J Cardiol 1995;76:1188–1190.
158. Ghatak A, Brar MJ, Agarwal A, et al. Oxy free radical system in heart failure and therapeutic role of oral vitamin E. Int J Cardiol 1996;57:119–127.
159. Diaz MN, Frei B, Vita JA, et al. Antioxidants and atherosclerotic heart disease. N Engl J Med 1997;337:408–416.
160. Stephens NG, Parsons A, Schofield PM, et al. Randomised controlled trial of

vitamin E in patients with coronary disease: Cambridge Heart Antioxidant Study (CHAOS). Lancet 1996;347:781–786.

161. Rapola JM, Virtamo J, Ripatti S, et al. Randomised trial of alpha-tocopherol and beta-carotene supplements on incidence of major coronary events in men with previous myocardial infarction. Lancet 1997;349:1715–1720.

162. Yusuf S, Dagenais G, Pogue J, et al. Vitamin E supplementation and cardiovascular events in high-risk patients. The Heart Outcomes Prevention Evaluation Study Investigators. N Engl J Med 2000;342:154–160.

163. Hasinoff BB. Chemistry of dexrazoxane and analogues. Semin Oncol 1998; 25:3–9.

164. Wiseman LR, Spencer CM. Dexrazoxane: a review of its use as a cardioprotective agent in patients receiving anthracycline-based chemotherapy. Drugs 1998;56:385–403.

165. Sawyer DB, Fukazawa R, Arstall MA, et al. Daunorubicin-induced apoptosis in rat cardiac myocytes is inhibited by dexrazoxane. Circ Res 1999;84: 257–265.

166. Arimura K, Egashira K, Nakamura R, et al. Increased inactivation of nitric oxide is involved in coronary endothelial dysfunction in heart failure. Am J Physiol Heart Circ Physiol. 2001;280:H68–75.

167. Khaper N, Singal PK. Effects of afterload-reducing drugs on pathogenesis of antioxidant changes and congestive heart failure in rats. J Am Coll Cardiol 1997;29:856–861.

168. Varin R, Mulder P, Tamion F, et al. Improvement of endothelial function by chronic angiotensin-converting enzyme inhibition in heart failure: role of nitric oxide, prostanoids, oxidant stress, and bradykinin. Circulation 2000; 102:351–356.

169. Mancini GB. Role of angiotensin-converting enzyme inhibition in reversal of endothelial dysfunction in coronary artery disease. Am J Med 1998;105: 40S–47S.

170. The SOLVD Investigators. Effect of enalapril on survival in patients with reduced left ventricular ejection fractions and congestive heart failure. N Engl J Med 1991;325:293–302.

171. Feuerstein G, Yue TL, Ma X, et al. Novel mechanisms in the treatment of heart failure: inhibition of oxygen radicals and apoptosis by carvedilol. Prog Cardiovasc Dis 1998;41:17–24.

172. Watanabe H, Kakihana M, Ohtsuka S, et al. Randomized, double-blind, placebo-controlled study of carvedilol on the prevention of nitrate tolerance in patients with chronic heart failure. J Am Coll Cardiol 1998;32:1194–1200.

173. Kukin ML, Kalman J, Charney RH, et al. Prospective, randomized comparison of effect of long-term treatment with metoprolol or carvedilol on symptoms, exercise, ejection fraction, and oxidative stress in heart failure. Circulation 1999;99:2645–2651.

174. Schoene N, Keicher C, Erbs S, et al. Prospective randomized double-blind comparison of the effects of carvedilol versus metoprolol on endothelial dysfunction and hemodynamic parameters in chronic heart failure. J Am Coll Cardiol 2001; presented at the 50th Scientific Sessions of the American College of Cardiology.

175. Hornig B, Maier V, Drexler H. Physical training improves endothelial function in patients with chronic heart failure. Circulation 1996;93:212–214.

176. Katz SD, Yuen JL, Bijou R, et al. Physical training specifically improves endothelium-dependent control of vascular reactivity in resistance vessels of patients with congestive heart failure. Circulation 1997;182:1488–1492.

177. Hambrecht R, Fiehn E, Weigl C, et al. Regular physical exercise corrects endothelial dysfunction and improves exercise capacity in patients with chronic heart failure. Circulation 1998;98:2709–2715.
178. Bauersachs J, Bouloumie A, Fraccarollo D, et al. Endothelial dysfunction in chronic myocardial infarction despite increased vascular endothelial nitric oxide synthase and soluble guanylate cyclase expression: role of enhanced vascular superoxide production. Circulation 1999;100:292–298.
179. Wang J, Yi GH, Knecht M, et al. Physical training alters the pathogenesis of pacing-induced heart failure through endothelium-mediated mechanisms in awake dogs. Circulation 1997;96:2683–2692.

Antioxidant Vitamins and Apoptosis

Fuzhong Qin, MD, PhD, and
Chang-seng Liang, MD, PhD

Introduction

Apoptosis is a cellular process that is accurately orchestrated and organized inside the cell by gene products.[1] It is characterized by cell shrinkage, membrane blebs, chromatin condensation, lack of inflammatory response, and internucleosomal DNA fragmentation.[2,3] Apoptosis has been shown to play an important role in a variety of physiological and pathological processes.[4] As such, apoptosis has been recognized as a common component of many cardiovascular disorders, such as hypertension, atherosclerosis, aging, ischemic-reperfusion injury, myocardial infarction, and cardiomyopathies.[5–7] Apoptosis also has been shown to be an important feature in chronic heart failure.[8] There is a significant correlation between apoptosis and progression of heart failure.[9,10]

Recent studies suggest that reactive oxygen species (ROS) are important inducers of myocyte apoptosis.[11] The ROS, such as superoxide anion, hydrogen peroxide, hydroxyl free radical, single oxygen, and peroxynitrite, are produced either as a consequence of normal metabolic processes or by a toxic insult to the cells.[12] ROS may saturate the cell's natural antioxidant defense system and cause a shift of the cellular redox balance to a prooxidant state, known as oxidative stress.[13] As such, ROS will react with

The work was supported in part by an American Heart Association grant, USPHS Grant #HL-68151, and the Paul N. Yu Fellowship, University of Rochester Medical Center.
From: Kukin ML, Fuster V (eds). *Oxidative Stress and Cardiac Failure.* Armonk, NY: Futura Publishing Co., Inc. ©2003.

various cellular biological macromolecules, including nucleic acid, protein, carbohydrates, and lipids,[14] and cause oxidative damage.[15,16]

The purposes of this chapter are to address the effects of antioxidant therapy with vitamins on myocyte apoptosis, discuss the possible mechanisms involved in this process, and address the association between the inhibition by antioxidant vitamins of apoptosis and the improvement of cardiac function in heart failure. Also, we briefly review oxidative stress in heart failure, apoptosis in heart failure, effects of oxidative stress on apoptosis, and the protection by antioxidant vitamins against heart failure.

Oxidative Stress in Heart Failure

Increases in malondialdehyde and superoxide anion and a decrease in the ratio of reduced to oxidized glutathione (GSH/GSSG) have been used to indicate oxidative stress.[17] Considerable evidence exists that increased oxidative stress occurs in chronic heart failure.[18] Cardiac malondialdehyde has been shown to increase and antioxidant reserve has been shown to decrease in chronic volume overload-induced heart failure.[15] Similarly, in a rat myocardial infarction model of heart failure, there is an increase in lipid peroxidation and a decrease in antioxidant enzyme activities such as superoxide dismutase, glutathione peroxidase and catalase, and antioxidant vitamin E.[18] Changes in oxidative stress and antioxidant defense mechanisms correlate significantly with the development of cardiac dysfunction in the different stages of heart failure induced by myocardial infarction.[19] Superoxide production has also been shown to increase in pacing-induced dog heart failure.[20] Decreased myocardial glutathione peroxidase activity and increased lipid peroxidation correlate significantly with ventricular dysfunction in Adriamycin-induced congestive heart failure in rats.[21,22] Furthermore, studies have shown that plasma superoxide anion and malondialdehyde are increased and the levels of antioxidant enzymes are decreased in human heart failure.[23–26]

More recently, using mitochondrial DNA 8-hydroxy-7,8 dihydro-2'-deoxyguanosine (8-oxo-dG), a sensitive stable marker of oxidative stress in cellular DNA,[27] we found myocardial mitochondrial DNA 8-oxo-dG was increased along with increased GSSG in rapid pacing-induced cardiomyopathy.[28] A direct linkage between ROS generation, mitochrondrial dysfunction, and contractile defects has been demonstrated, suggesting that oxidative stress is of importance to the pathogenesis of congestive heart failure.[20] Likewise, we have shown that oxidative stress is increased in norepinephrine (NE)-induced cardiomyopathy.[29] These data suggest that NE is an important inducer for oxidative stress and both elevated NE and oxidative stress are predictors for prognosis of heart failure.

Apoptosis in Heart Failure

Myocyte apoptosis is a common feature in cardiomyopathy.[30,31] It has been shown to increase during the transition from cardiac hypertrophy to heart failure in spontaneously hypertensive rats,[31,32] in animals with chronic heart failure induced by rapid pacing,[33] multiple intracoronary microembolizations,[34] myocardial infarction,[35] and chronic pressure overload.[36] Furthermore, apoptosis is increased in human failing hearts.[37–42]

However, the significance of myocyte apoptosis in the development of cardiomyopathy remains controversial.[9,30] Several investigators have reported that the rate of apoptosis is variable and in many instances it is very low (0.1–0.4%), and they speculate that apoptosis is an epiphenomenon in heart failure that lacks any mechanistic significance.[10,43] However, it appears intuitive that progressive loss of myocytes by apoptosis may lead to deterioration of cardiac function.[44] A study in dogs with heart failure produced by intracoronary microembolization[45] showed that cardiomyocyte apoptosis, evaluated by terminal deoxynucleotidyl transferase-mediated dUTP nick end-labeling (TUNEL) assay, was associated with progressive left ventricular dysfunction. There is also a correlation between the degree of cardiomyocyte apoptosis and the severity of left ventricular dilation and systolic dysfunction in acromegalic cardiomyopathy in humans.[46] The improvement after enalapril treatment in ventricular systolic function in dogs with heart failure was associated with attenuation of cardiomyocyte apoptosis.[47] The increase of apoptotic cells during the transition from left ventricular hypertrophy to left ventricular dilation and systolic dysfunction also supports a functional significant role of myocyte apoptosis in heart failure.[36]

More recently, transgenic technology has been utilized to study the functional role of apoptosis in heart failure.[30] In an elegant study with cardiac-selective overexpression of caspase-8, Wencker et al.[48] showed that the transgenic animals developed cardiomyocyte apoptosis, and over a period of time developed a lethal dilated cardiomyopathy. In another murine model of heart failure, cardiac-specific knockout of gp 130, a subunit of the interleukin-6 family of cytokine receptors, promotes cell survival in the face of conditions that otherwise induce apoptosis.[30,49,50] In addition, overexpression of heterotrimeric G protein, such as Gqα or Gsα, in transgenic animals promotes myocyte apoptosis.[30,51,52] These findings suggest that Gsα stimulation plays a role in the pathogenesis of cardiomyopathy and that cardiomyocyte apoptosis is important for the progressive cardiac dysfunction in chronic heart failure.

Oxidative Stress and Apoptosis

Oxidative stress has been shown to induce apoptosis in a variety of cell types.[12,53] Direct exposure of cultured rat cardiomyocytes to H_2O_2 and

O_2^- induces myocyte apoptosis.[54,55] Mechanical stretch of the myocytes can also induce myocyte apoptosis via the increased production of ROS[56]; this change can be abolished by a free radical scavenging nitric oxide donor. Oxygen free radicals also have been implicated as a mediator for myocyte apoptosis induced by daunorubicin[57] and cytokine.[58] The antiapoptotic effect of carvedilol in myocardial ischemia and reperfusion is probably mediated via its antioxidant action.[59] Moreover, increased production of lipid peroxidation contributes to myocyte apoptosis in rats after a large myocardial infarction.[44] Norepinephrine-derived oxidative stress also has been demonstrated to induce myocyte apoptosis.[60]

Antioxidant Vitamins and Heart Failure

Since oxidative stress has been shown to trigger myocyte apoptosis and may play an important role in the progression of heart failure, we speculate that antioxidant vitamins such as vitamin A (β-carotene), vitamin C (ascorbic acid), and vitamin E (α-tocopherol) may be beneficial in the treatment of heart failure.

Alpha-tocopherol and β-carotene are lipid soluble and are capable of inhibiting lipid peroxidation of the cell membrane. Alpha-tocopherol reacts with a variety of oxygen free radicals, including single oxygen, lipid peroxide products, and superoxide radical, to form a relatively innocuous tocopherol radical, whereas β-carotene is an efficient "quencher" of single oxygen.[61] Ascorbic acid, on the other hand, is water soluble. It reacts with superoxide, hydroxyl radical, single oxygen, and hydrochlorous acid[62] in both intracellular and extracellular fluid, and potentiates the effects of α-tocopherol by regenerating α-tocopherol from its radical.[63]

Although the use of antioxidants (e.g., vitamin E) in cardiovascular diseases remains divergent,[64] studies have shown an inverse association between antioxidant intake or body status and the risk of cardiovascular diseases.[65,66] Vitamin E has been shown to reduce risk for cardiovascular disease and to improve immune function in the elderly.[67] Dietary supplementation with vitamin E and α-lipoic acid also protects the aged heart against ischemia-reperfusion-induced lipid peroxidation by scavenging ROS. This beneficial action on lipid peroxidation is associated with improved cardiac performance after ischemia and reperfusion injury.[68] Vitamin E administration also has been shown to increase myocardial content of the vitamin and myocardial GSH/GSSG ratio and to decrease lipid peroxidation in the transition from compensatory hypertrophy to heart failure in guinea pigs.[69] The potential role of vitamin E in protecting against oxidative stress and cardiovascular events is a subject of a recent critical review.[70]

Vitamin C has a beneficial effect on endothelium-dependent vasodilation in individuals with coronary artery disease.[71] Vitamin C improves endothelial function of conduit arteries in patients with chronic heart failure, as a result of increased availability of nitric oxide.[72] Vitamin C can prevent the development of nitrate tolerance, which is related to the cGMP reduction caused by increased superoxide, during continuous nitrate therapy in patients with chronic heart failure.[73]

Furthermore, a combination of vitamins C and E has been shown to protect against the development of atherosclerosis.[66] We have demonstrated that vitamins A, C, and E attenuate cardiac sympathetic nerve terminal abnormalities[29] and myocyte apoptosis against NE-derived oxidative stress.[60]

Antioxidant Vitamins, Apoptosis, and Cardiac Function

Evidence has accumulated that antioxidant vitamins can attenuate or prevent apoptosis mediated by oxidative stress and that this mechanism may be involved in the regulation of cardiac function in chronic heart failure.

Effects of Antioxidant Vitamins on Apoptosis

A number of antioxidant vitamins have been shown to reduce myocyte apoptosis in cardiomyopathy. Kumar et al.[74] showed that trolox, a water-soluble vitamin E analog,[75] reduced apoptosis in isolated adult cardiomyocytes exposed to Adriamycin. Administration of antioxidants N-acetylcysteine and dithiothreitol also has been shown to attenuate cardiomyocyte apoptosis induced by cytokines, such as interleukin-1β, interleukin-γ, and tumor necrosis factor-α.[58] Likewise, carvedilol inhibits myocyte apoptosis mediated by oxidative stress in myocardial ischemia and reperfusion.[14,59] In a recent report, antioxidants probucol and pyrrolidine dithiocarbamate were found to attenuate oxidative stress and myocyte apoptosis in the remote noninfarcted myocardium following myocardial infarction.[44]

Significant evidence on antioxidant vitamin-inhibited apoptosis in other cell types also has been gathered. For example, antioxidant vitamins C and E attenuate oxidative stress-induced apoptosis in endothelial cells,[76,77] smooth muscle cells,[78] and neurons.[79,80]

Possible Mechanisms of Antioxidant Vitamin-Inhibited Apoptosis

Recent studies have shown that oxidative stress triggers apoptosis through multiple signal pathways; they include the Bcl-2 family proteins, mitogen-activated protein kinase (MAPK) pathways, and mitochondrial-mediated caspase pathway.[10,53] The protective effects of antioxidant vitamins against oxidative stress-induced apoptosis may involve one or several of these processes.

Bcl-2 Family

The Bcl-2 family contains several members of oncoproteins that can either inhibit or promote apoptosis. The net effect is determined by the relative expression of the proapoptotic Bax and the antiapoptotic Bcl-2.[81] The Bcl-2 gene product has been shown to prevent programmed cell death of ventricular myocytes.[82] Studies have shown that the Bcl-2 protein is located in mitochondia, endoplasmic reticula, and nuclear membranes where most of the oxygen free radicals are generated and where the free radicals exert their effects.[83]

In our recent study, NE decreases Bcl-2 protein expression (Figure 1) and increases Bax expression (Figure 2), leading to a marked reduction of the Bcl-2 to Bax ratio in favor of cell apoptosis. A decrease in the Bcl-2 to Bax ratio by NE also has been reported in cultured myocytes.[84] The changes are abolished by antioxidant vitamins A, C, and E. The results suggest that NE-derived oxygen free radicals are involved in the regulation of Bcl-2 and Bax protein expression.

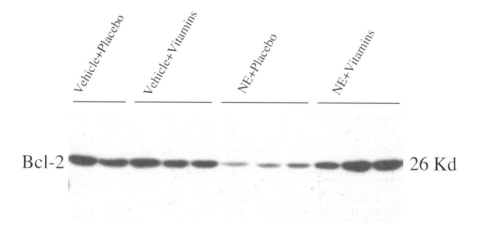

Figure 1. A representative blot of Bcl-2 protein showing the decrease produced by norepinephrine (NE) and return to control by antioxidant vitamin administration in ferrets.

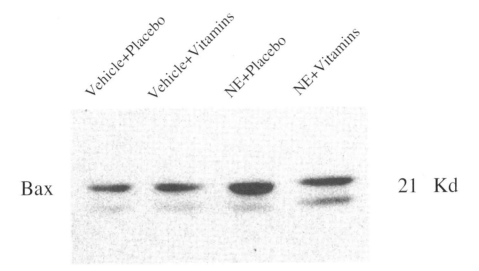

Figure 2. A representative blot of Bax protein showing the increase produced by norepinephrine and return to control by antioxidant vitamin administration in ferrets.

MAPK Pathways

The mitogen-activated protein kinases (MAPKs) belong to a family of serine-threonine kinases. Three major MAPK signal pathways, including extracellular signal-regulated protein kinase (ERK), p38 MAPK (p38), and stress-activated protein kinase (SAPK)/c-Jun NH_2-terminal kinase (JNK), have been demonstrated in myocytes.[85,86] Recently, oxidative stress has been shown to activate ERK, JNK, and p38 pathways in cultured myocytes, suggesting that MAPK activation is involved in the regulation of cell growth and apoptosis.[87,88] Studies in the isolated perfused heart showed that oxidative stress activated JNK and p38 pathways with minimal activation of ERK.[89] Similar changes occurred in myocardial ischemia and reperfusion,[85,86] pacing-induced cardiomyopathy,[90] and in human heart failure secondary to ischemic heart disease.[91] Oxidative stress and activation of JNK also occurred in rat failing hearts with myocyte apoptosis.[92] In addition, there exists a close structural and functional correlation between Bcl-2 and JNK in neuronal apoptosis.[93] Overexpression of Bcl-2 has been shown to suppress JNK activity in PC12.[94] The observations in cultured cells suggest that dopamine induces apoptosis through an oxidation-involved SAPK/JNK activation pathway.[95] Similarly, activa-

tion of JNK/SAPK and the decreased ratio of Bcl-2 to Bax appear to be associated with the auto-oxidized dopamine-induced apoptosis.[96]
Our recent study[90] has further shown that antioxidant vitamins reduced JNK activity and augmented ERK and p38 activity in chronic heart failure (Figure 3). These findings suggest that JNK stimulates myocyte apoptosis while ERK protects myocytes against apoptosis.

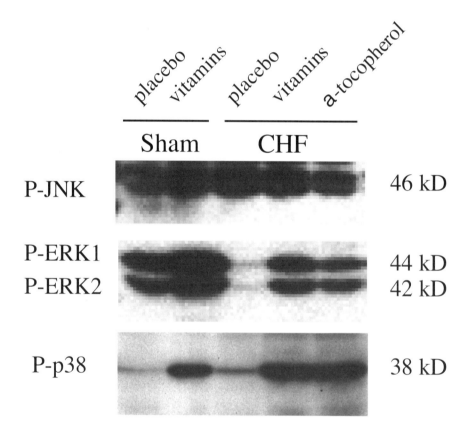

Figure 3. A representative blot of phospho-JNK (p-JNK), phospho-ERK1 (p-ERK1)/ phospho-ERK2 (p-ERK2), and phospho-p38 (p-p38), in Sham and congestive heart failure (CHF) animals with and without antioxidant vitamins or α-tocopherol alone.

Mitochondrial-Mediated Caspase Pathway

Recently, activation of caspases, a family of protease, which participates in a cascade and ultimately cleaves a set of proteins, has been shown to cause apoptosis.[97] Caspase 3, representing the final common pathway of the caspase cascade, has been found in neonatal and adult cardiomyocytes.[97] The activation of caspase is regulated by a variety of other factors, such as MAPKs and the Bcl-2 family. Several studies have shown that apoptosis is associated with the loss of cytochrome *c* from the intermembrane space of mitochondria and subsequent release into cytosol.[97–99] This change has been shown to occur in the failing heart.[41] Cytochrome *c* binds to apoptosis-activating factor 1 to form a complex with caspase 9. Activated caspase 9 cleaves caspase 3 to cause its activation and result in apoptosis.[97] The loss of cytochrome *c* is related to mitochondrial membrane potential.[100,101] Thus, it is possible that oxidative stress triggers the loss of mitochondrial membrane potential, thus releasing cytochrome *c* to cytosol, to activate caspase 3 and finally cause cardiomyocyte apoptosis.[55] In contrast, Bcl-2 inhibits mitochondrial cytochrome *c* release, caspase activation, and apoptosis.[55] Therefore, the regulation of Bcl-2 and mitochondrial function is of importance to oxidative stress-induced cardiomyocyte apoptosis. Additionally, JNK has been implicated in oxidative stress-induced caspase activation.[87] The apoptotic effects of probucol and pyrrolidine dithiocarbamate in heart failure probably are also mediated via the caspase-3 pathway.[44] Likewise, antioxidant vitamins may act to prevent the loss of mitochondrial transmembrane potential and cytosolic release of cytochrome c for their antiapoptotic effects.[102,103]

Involvement of Antioxidant Vitamin-Inhibited Apoptosis in the Improvement of Cardiac Function in Chronic Heart Failure

We have recently shown that antioxidant vitamins attenuate myocyte apoptosis produced by NE infusion[60] and pacing-induced heart failure,[90] and that the attenuation of apoptosis is functionally important. The antiapoptotic effects of antioxidant vitamins are shared by trolox and superoxide dismutase (Figure 4).[104] Furthermore, we have shown in heart failure that the reduction of apoptosis by antioxidant vitamins is associated with the improvement of cardiac function (Figure 5).[28,90]

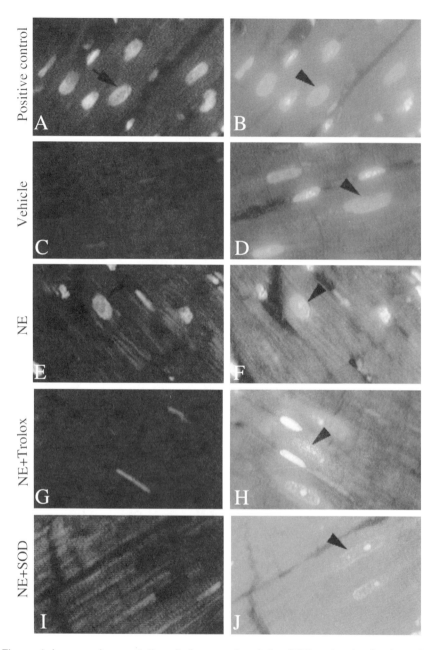

Figure 4. Increase in apoptotic cells by norepinephrine (NE) and reduction by trolox and superoxide dismutase (SOD) in NE-treated ferrets. Apoptotic nuclei (arrow) are shown by green fluorescence in the left panels. The localization of nuclei is documented by propidium iodide staining (arrowhead) and peripheral distribution of myosin antibody labeling of myocyte cytoplasm is illustrated by red fluorescence in the right panels. Panels A-J represent positive control, vehicle, NE, NE plus trolox, and NE plus SOD groups, respectively. See color version of this figure between pages 276 and 277.

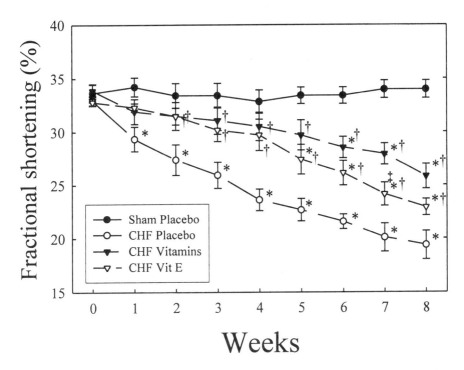

Figure 5. Effects of antioxidant vitamins on left ventricular (LV) fractional shortening in rapid pacing-induced congestive heart failure (CHF). Bars denote SEM. *$P<0.05$ versus the sham-operated animals. †$P<0.05$ versus the CHF placebo group. Figure taken from ref. 28.

Conclusion

Oxidative stress is increased in chronic heart failure and correlates with the progression of cardiac dysfunction in chronic heart failure. The exact mechanism by which oxidative stress causes cardiac dysfunction is not known, but myocyte apoptosis is most likely involved. The effects of oxidative stress may involve several signal transduction pathways, such as Bcl-2 family, mitochondrial-mediated caspase, MAPK, and other pathways. Evidence suggests that these pathways may be interrelated, leading to cytosolic release of cytochrome c, myocyte apoptosis, and progressive cardiac dysfunction. Antioxidant vitamin administration increases antioxidant reserve and reduces tissue oxidative stress. As a result, antioxidant vitamins are expected to deactivate the ROS-induced apoptotic transduction pathways and improve cardiac function in heart failure (Figure 6). Antioxidant therapy may be beneficial in the treatment of human heart failure.

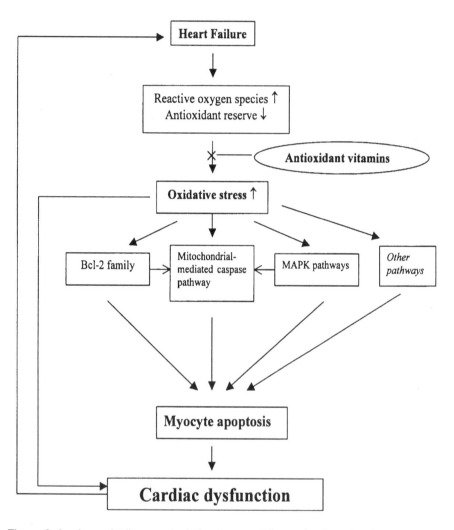

Figure 6. A schematic diagram depicting the possible mechanisms involved in oxidative stress-induced myocyte apoptosis and subsequent cardiac dysfunction in heart failure, and the intervention by antioxidant vitamins.

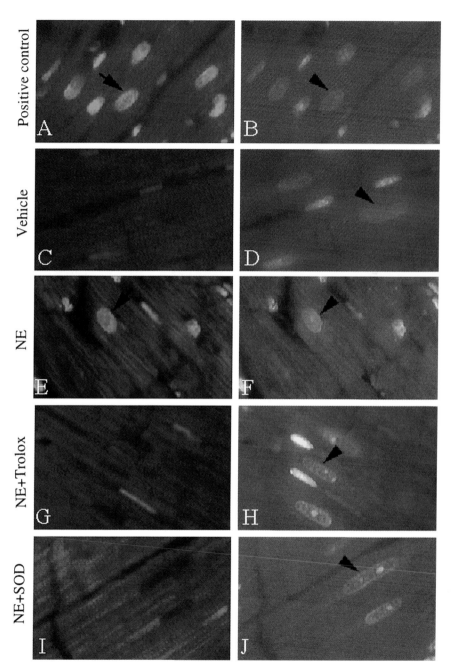

Figure 13-4. Increase in apoptotic cells by norepinephrine (NE) and reduction by trolox and superoxide dismutase (SOD) in NE-treated ferrets. Apoptotic nuclei (arrow) are shown by green fluorescence in the left panels. The localization of nuclei is documented by propidium iodide staining (arrowhead) and peripheral distribution of myosin antibody labeling of myocyte cytoplasm is illustrated by red fluorescence in the right panels. Panels A-J represent positive control, vehicle, NE, NE plus trolox, and NE plus SOD groups, respectively.

References

1. Van Heerde WL, Robert-Offerman S, Dumont E, et al. Markers of apoptosis in cardiovascular tissues: focus on annexin V. Cardiovasc Res 2000;45:549–559.
2. Weiland U, Haendeler J, Ihling C, et al. Inhibition of endogenous nitric oxide synthase potentiates ischemia-reperfusion-induced myocardial apoptosis via a caspase-3 dependent pathway. Cardiovasc Res 2000;45:671–678.
3. James TN. Apoptosis in cardiac disease. Am J Med 1999;107:606–620.
4. Teiger E, Dam TV, Richard L, et al. Apoptosis in pressure overload-induced heart hypertrophy in the rat. J Clin Invest 1996;97:2891–2897.
5. Anversa P. Myocyte apoptosis and heart failure. Eur Heart J 1998;19:359–360.
6. Aukrust P, Gullestad L, Frøland SS. Is apoptosis an important pathogenic factor in cardiovascular disease? Eur J Clin Invest 1999;29:369–371.
7. Fox JC, Patel VV. Apoptosis and the cardiovascular system. ACC Curr J Rev 1998;March–April:13–15.
8. Sanders WR. Apoptosis and heart failure. N Engl J Med 1999;341:759–760.
9. Guerra S, Leri A, Wang XW, et al. Myocyte death in the failing human heart is gender dependent. Circ Res 1999;85:856–866.
10. Haunstetter A, Izumo S. Apoptosis: basic mechanisms and implications for cardiovascular disease. Circ Res 1998;82:1111–1129.
11. Ferrari R, Agnoletti L, Comini L, et al. Oxidative stress during myocardial ischemia and heart failure. Eur Heart J 1998;19(Suppl B):B2–B11.
12. Anderson KM, Seed T, Ou D, et al. Free radicals and reactive oxygen species in programmed cell death. Med Hypotheses 1999;52:451–463.
13. Chandra J, Samall A, Orrenius S. Triggering and modulation of apoptosis by oxidative stress. Free Radic Biol Med 2000;29:323–333.
14. Feuerstein G, Yue TL, Ma XL, et al. Novel mechanisms in the treatment of heart failure: inhibition of oxygen radicals and apoptosis by carvedilol. Prog Cardiovasc Dis 1998;41(Suppl 1):17–24.
15. Prasad K, Gupta JB, Kalra J, et al. Oxidative stress as a mechanism of cardiac failure in chronic volume overload in canine model. J Mol Cell Cardiol 1996;28:375–385.
16. Dhalla NS, Temsah RM, Netticadan T. Role of oxidative stress in cardiovascular diseases. J Hypertens 2000;18:655–673.
17. Devi BG, Chan AW. Effect of cocaine on cardiac biochemical functions. J Cardiovasc Pharmacol 1999;33:1–6.
18. Hill MF, Singal PK. Antioxidant and oxidative stress changes during heart failure subsequent to myocardial infarction in rats. Am J Pathol 1996;148:291–300.
19. Hill MF, Singal PK. Right and left myocardial antioxidant responses during heart failure subsequent to myocardial infarction. Circulation 1997;96:2414–2420.
20. Ide T, Tsutsui H, Kinugawa S, et al. Mitochondrial electron transport complex I is a potential source of oxygen free radicals in the failing myocardium. Circ Res 1999;85:357–363.
21. Siveski-Iliskovic N, Kaul N, Singal PK. Probucol promotes endogenous antioxidants and provides protection against Adriamycin-induced cardiomyopathy in rats. Circulation 1994;89:2829–2835.
22. Siveski-Iliskovic N, Hill M, Chow DA, et al. Probucol protects against Adriamycin cardiomyopathy without interfering with its antitumor effect. Circulation 1995;91:10–15.

278 · Oxidative Stress and Cardiac Failure

23. Chen L, Zang Y, Bai B, et al. Electron spin resonance determination and superoxide dismutase activity in polymorphonuclear leukocytes in congestive heart failure. Can J Cardiol 1992;8:756–760.
24. Ghatak A, Brar MJS, Agarwal A, et al. Oxy free radical system in heart failure and therapeutic role of oral vitamin E. Int J Cardiol 1996;57:119–127.
25. Diaz-Velez CR, Garcia-Castineiras S, Mendoza-Ramos E, et al. Increased malondialdehyde in peripheral blood of patients with congestive heart failure. Am Heart J 1996;131:146–152.
26. Keith M, Geranmayegan A, Sole MJ, et al. Increased oxidative stress in patients with congestive heart failure. J Am Coll Cardiol 1998;31:1352–1356.
27. Shigenaga MK, Ames BN: Assays for 8-hydroxy-2'-deoxyguanosine: a biomarker of in vivo oxidative DNA damage. Free Radic Biol Med 1991;10:211–216.
28. Shite J, Qin FZ, Mao WK, et al. Antioxidant vitamins attenuate oxidative stress and cardiac dysfunction in tachycardia-induced cardiomyopathy. J Am Coll Cardiol 2001;38:1734–1740.
29. Liang CS, Rounds NK, Dong ED, et al. Alterations by norepinephrine of cardiac sympathetic nerve terminal function and myocardial β-adrenergic receptor sensitivity in the ferret: normalization by antioxidant vitamins. Circulation 2000;102:96–103.
30. Kang PM, Izumo S. Apoptosis and heart failure: a critical review of the literature. Circ Res 2000;86:1107–1113.
31. Boluyt MO, Bing OH, Lakatta EG. The aging spontaneously hypertensive rat as a model of the transition from stable compensated hypertrophy to heart failure. Eur Heart J 1995;16 (Suppl N):19–30.
32. Li Z, Bing OH, Long X, et al. Increased cardiomyocyte apoptosis during the transition to heart failure in the spontaneously hypertensive rat. Am J Physiol 1997;272:H2313–H2319.
33. Leri A, Liu Y, Malhotra A, et al. Pacing-induced heart failure in dogs enhances the expression of p53 and p53-dependent genes in ventricular myocytes. Circulation 1998;97:194–203.
34. Sharov VG, Sabbah HN, Shimoyama H, et al. Evidence of cardiocyte apoptosis in myocardium of dog with chronic heart failure. Am J Pathol 1996;148:141–149.
35. Anversa P, Cheng W, Liu Y, et al. Apoptosis and myocardial infarction. Basic Res Cardiol 1998;93(Suppl 3):8–12.
36. Condorelli G, Morisco C, Stassi G, et al. Increased cardiomyocyte apoptosis and changes in proapoptotic and antiapoptotic genes bax and bcl-2 during left ventricular adaptations to chronic pressure overload in the rat. Circulation 1999;99:3071–3078.
37. Narula J, Haider N, Virmani R, et al. Apoptosis in myocytes in end-stage heart failure. N Engl J Med 1996;335:1224–1226.
38. Olivetti G, Abbi R, Quaini F, et al. Apoptosis in the failing human heart. N Engl J Med 1997;336:1131–1141.
39. Ino T, Nishimoto K, Okubo M, et al. Apoptosis as a possible cause of wall thinning in end-stage hypertrophic cardiomyopathy. Am J Cardiol 1997;79:1137–1141.
40. Saraste A, Pulkki K, Kallajoki M, et al. Cardiomyocyte apoptosis and progression of heart failure to transplantation. Eur J Clin Invest 1999;29:380–386.
41. Narula J, Pandey P, Arbustini E, et al. Apoptosis in heart failure: release of cytochrome c from mitochondria and activation of caspase-3 in human cardiomyopathy. Proc Natl Acad Sci USA 1999;96:8144–8149.

42. Bartling B, Milting H, Schumann H, et al. Myocardial gene expression of regulators of myocyte apoptosis and myocyte calcium homeostasis during hemodynamic unloading by ventricular assist devices in patients with end-stage heart failure. Circulation 1999;100 (Suppl II):II216–II223.
43. Schaper J, Elsässer A, Kostin S. The role of cell death in heart failure. Circ Res 1999;85:867–869.
44. Oskarsson HJ, Coppey L, Weiss RM, et al. Antioxidants attenuate myocyte apoptosis in the remote non-infarcted myocardium following large myocardial infarction. Cardiovasc Res 2000;45:679–687.
45. Sabbah HN, Sharov VG, Goussev A, et al. Evidence for ongoing loss of cardiomyocytes in dogs with progressive left ventricular dysfunction and failure. Circulation 1997;96 (Suppl I):I-754.
46. Frustaci A, Chimenti C, Setoguchi M, et al. Cell death in acromegalic cardiomyopathy. Circulation 1999;99:1426–1434.
47. Goussev A, Sharov VG, Shimoyama H, et al. Effects of ACE inhibition on cardiomyocyte apoptosis in dogs with heart failure. Am J Physiol 1998;275: H626–H631.
48. Wencker D, Nguyen KT, Khine CC, et al. Myocyte apoptosis is sufficient to cause dilated cardiomyopathy. Circulation 1999;100(Suppl I):I-17.
49. Williams RS: Apoptosis and heart failure. N Engl J Med 1999;341:759–760.
50. Hirota H, Chen J, Betz UA, et al. Loss of a gp 130 cardiac muscle cell survival pathway is a critical event in the onset of heart failure during biomechanical stress. Cell 1999;97:189–198.
51. Asai K, Yang GP, Geng YJ, et al. β-adrenergic receptor blockade arrests myocyte damage and preserves cardiac function in the transgenic $G_{s\alpha}$ mouse. J Clin Invest 1999;104:551–558.
52. Adams JW, Sakata Y, Davis MG, et al. Enhanced Gαq signaling: a common pathway mediates cardiac hypertrophy and apoptotic heart failure. Proc Natl Acad Sci USA 1998;95:10140–10145.
53. Feuerstein GZ, Young PR. Apoptosis in cardiac diseases: stress- and mitogen-activated signaling pathways. Cardiovasc Res 2000;45:560–569.
54. Hansdorf RV, Li PF, Dietz R. Signaling pathways in reactive oxygen species-induced cardiomyocyte apoptosis. Circulation 1999;99:2934–2941.
55. Cook SA, Sugden PH, Clerk A. Regulation of bcl-2 family proteins during development and in response to oxidative stress in cardiac myocytes: association with changes in mitochondrial membrane potential. Circ Res 1999;85: 940–949.
56. Cheng W, Li B, Kajstura J, et al. Stretch-induced programmed myocyte cell death. J Clin Invest 1995;96:2247–2259.
57. Sawyer DB, Fukazawa R, Arstall MA, et al. Daunorubicin-induced apoptosis in rat cardiac myocytes is inhibited by dexrazoxane. Circ Res 1999;84:257–265.
58. Ing DJ, Zang J, Dzau VJ, et al. Modulation of cytokine-induced cardiac myocyte apoptosis by nitric oxide, Bak and Bcl-x. Circ Res 1999;84:21–33.
59. Yue TL, Ma XL, Wang X, et al. Possible involvement of stress-activated protein kinase signaling pathway and Fas receptor expression in prevention of ischemia/reperfusion-induced cardiomyocyte apoptosis by carvedilol. Circ Res 1998;82:166–174.
60. Qin FZ, Rounds NK, Mao WK, et al. Antioxidant vitamins prevent cardiomyocyte apoptosis produced by norepinephrine infusion in ferrets. Cardiovasc Res 2001;51:736–748.
61. Frei B. Reactive oxygen species and antioxidant vitamins: mechanisms of action. Am J Med 1994;97(Suppl 3A):5S–13S; discussion 22S–28S.

280 · Oxidative Stress and Cardiac Failure

62. Padayatty SJ, Levine M. Vitamin C and myocardial infarction: the heart of the matter. Am J Clin Nutr 2000;71:1027–1028.
63. Scarpa M, Rigo A, Maiorino M, et al. Formation of α-tocopherol radical and recycling of α-tocopherol by ascorbate during peroxidation of phosphatidylcholine liposomes: an electron paramagnetic resonance study. Biochim Biophys Acta 1984;801:215–219.
64. Patterson C, Madamanchi NR, Runge MS. The oxidative paradox: another piece in the puzzle. Circ Res 2000;87:1074–1076.
65. Diaz MN, Frei B, Vita JA, et al. Antioxidants and atherosclerotic heart disease. N Engl J Med 1997;337:408–416.
66. Carr AC, Zhu BZ, Frei B. Potential antiatherogenic mechanisms of ascorbate (vitamin C) and α-tocopherol (vitamin E). Circ Res 2000;87:349–354.
67. Meydani M. Effect of functional food ingredients: vitamin E modulation of cardiovascular diseases and immune status in the elderly. Am J Clin Nutr 2000;71(6 Suppl):1665S–1668S; discussion 1674S–1675S.
68. Coombes JS, Powers SK, Hamilton KL, et al. Improved cardiac performance after ischemia in aged rats supplemented with vitamin E and α-lipid acid. Am J Physiol Regul Integr Comp Physiol 2000;279:R2149–R2155.
69. Dhalla AK, Hill MF, Singal PK. Role of oxidative stress in transition of hypertrophy to heart failure. J Am Coll Cardiol 1996;28:506–514.
70. Pryor W. Vitamin E and heart disease: basic science to clinical intervention trials. Free Radic Biol Med 2000;28:141–164.
71. Ito K, Akita H, Kanazawa K, et al. Comparison of effects of ascorbic acid on endothelium-dependent vasodilation in patients with chronic congestive heart failure secondary to idiopathic dilated cardiomyopathy versus patients with effort angina pectoris secondary to coronary artery disease. Am J Cardiol 1998; 82:762–767.
72. Hornig B, Arakawa N, Kohler C, et al. Vitamin C improves endothelial function of conduit arteries in patients with chronic heart failure. Circulation 1998;97:363–368.
73. Watanabe H, Kakihana M, Ohtsuka S, et al. Randomized, double-blind, placebo-controlled study of ascorbate on the preventive effect of nitrate tolerance in patients with congestive heart failure. Circulation 1998;97:886–891.
74. Kumar D, Kirshenbaum L, Li T, et al. Apoptosis in isolated adult cardiomyocytes exposed to Adriamycin. Ann NY Acad Sci 1999;874:156–168.
75. Molenaar I, Hulstaert CE, Hardonk MJ. Role in function and ultrastructure of cellular membranes. In: Machlin LH, ed. Vitamin E: A Comprehensive Treatise. New York: Marcel Dekker. 1980;327–389.
76. Dimmeler S, Haendeler J, Galle J, et al. Oxidized low-density lipoprotein induces apoptosis of human endothelial cells by activation of CPP32-like proteases: a mechanistic clue to the 'response to injury' hypothesis. Circulation 1997;95:1760–1763.
77. Haendeler J, Zeiher AM, Dimmeler S. Vitamin C and E prevent lipopolysaccharide-induced apoptosis in human endothelial cells by modulation of Bcl-2 and Bax. Eur J Pharmacol 1996;317:407–411.
78. Siow RCM, Richards JP, Pedley KC, et al. Vitamin C protects human vascular smooth muscle cells against apoptosis induced by moderately oxidized LDL containing high levels of lipid hydroperoxides. Arterioscler Thromb Vasc Biol 1999;19:2387–2394.
79. Manev H, Cagnoli CM, Atabay C, et al. Neuronal apoptosis in an in vitro model of photochemically induced oxidative stress. Exp Neurol 1995;133:198–206.
80. Tagami M, Ikeda K, Yamagata K, et al. Vitamin E prevents apoptosis in hip-

pocampal neurons caused by cerebral ischemia and reperfusion in stroke-prone spontaneously hypertensive rats. Lab Invest 1999;79:609–615.

81. Nakamura M, Wang NP, Zhao ZQ, et al. Preconditioning decreases Bax expression, PMN accumulation and apoptosis in reperfused rat heart. Cardiovasc Res 2000;45:661–670.

82. Kirshenbaum LA, Moissac DD. The bcl-2 gene product prevents programmed cell death of ventricular myocytes. Circulation 1997;96:1580–1585.

83. Hockenbery DM, Oltvai ZN, Yin XM, et al. Bcl-2 functions in an antioxidant pathway to prevent apoptosis. Cell 1993;75:241–251.

84. Zaugg M, Xu W, Lucchinetti E, et al. β-Adrenergic receptor subtypes differentially affect apoptosis in adult rat ventricular myocytes. Circulation 2000; 102:344–350.

85. Ma XL, Kumar S, Gao F, et al. Inhibition of p38 mitogen-activated protein kinase decreases cardiomyocyte apoptosis and improves cardiac function after myocardial ischemia and reperfusion. Circulation 1999;99:1685–1691.

86. Yue TL, Wang C, Gu JL, et al. Inhibition of extracellular signal-regulated kinase enhances ischemia/reoxygenation-induced apoptosis in cultured cardiac myocytes and exaggerates reperfusion injury in isolated perfused heart. Circ Res 2000;86:692–699.

87. Turner NA, Xia F, Azhar G, et al. Oxidative stress induces DNA fragmentation and caspase activation via the c-Jun NH2-terminal kinase pathway in H9c2 cardiac muscle cells. J Mol Cell Cardiol 1998;30:1789–1801.

88. Aikawa R, Komuro I, Yamazaki T, et al. Oxidative stress activates extracellular signal-regulated kinase through Src and Ras in cultured cardiac myocytes of neonatal rats. J Clin Invest 1997;100:1813–1821.

89. Clerk A, Fuller SJ, Micheal A, et al. Stimulation of "stress-regulated" mitogen-activated protein kinases (stress-activated protein kinase/c-Jun N-terminal kinases and p38 mitogen-activated protein kinases) in perfused rat hearts by oxidative and other stresses. J Biol Chem 1998;273:7228–7234.

90. Qin FZ, Shite J, Fan BA, Liang C-S. Antioxidant vitamins attenuate c-jun N-terminal protein kinase activation and apoptosis in heart failure: association with improvement of cardiac function. Circulation 2001;104(Suppl):II-247.

91. Cook SA, Sugden PH, Clerk A. Activation of c-Jun N-terminal kinases and p38-mitogen-activated protein kinases in human heart failure secondary to ischaemic heart disease. J Mol Cell Cardiol 1999;31:1429–1434.

92. Li WG, Zaheer A, Coppey L, et al. Activation of JNK in the remote myocardium after large myocardial infarction in rats. Biochem Biophys Res Commun 1998;246:816–820.

93. Choi WS, Yoon SY, Chang II, et al. Correlation between structure of Bcl-2 and its inhibitory function of JNK and caspase activity in dopaminergic neuronal apoptosis. J Neurochem 2000;74:1621–1626.

94. Park DS, Stefanis L, Yan CYI, et al. Ordering the cell death pathway: differential effects of Bcl-2, an interleukin-1-converting enzyme family protease inhibitor, and other survival agents on JNK activation in serum/nerve growth factor-derived PC12 cells. J Biol Chem 1996;271:21898–21905.

95. Luo YQ, Umegaki H, Wang XT, et al. Dopamine induces apoptosis through an oxidation-involved SAPK/JNK activation pathway. J Biol Chem 1998;273: 3756–3764.

96. Kang CD, Jang JH, Kim KW, et al. Activation of c-jun N-terminal kinase / stress-activated protein kinase and the decreased ratio of Bcl-2 to Bax are associated with the auto-oxidized dopamine-induced apoptosis in PC12 cells. Neurosci Lett 1998;256:37–40.

97. Cook SA, Poole-Wilson PA. Cardiac myocyte apoptosis. Eur Heart J 1999;20: 1619–1629.
98. Sabbah HN. Apoptotic cell death in heart failure. Cardiovasc Res 2000;45: 704–712.
99. Depre C, Taegtmeyer H. Metabolic aspects of programmed cell survival and cell death in the heart. Cardiovasc Res 2000;45:538–548.
100. Haunstetter A, Izumo S. Future perspectives and potential implications of cardiac myocyte apoptosis. Cardiovasc Res 2000;45:795–801.
101. Yaoita H, Ogawa K, Maehara K, et al. Apoptosis in relevant clinical situations: contribution of apoptosis in myocardial infarction. Cardiovasc Res 2000;45:630–641.
102. Lizard G, Miguet C, Bésséde G, et al. Impairment with various antioxidants of the loss of mitochondrial transmembrane potential and of the cytosolic release of cytochrome c occurring during 7-ketocholesterol-induced apoptosis. Free Radic Biol Med 2000;28:743–753.
103. Bagchi M, Balmoori J, Bagchi D, et al. Smokeless tobacco, oxidative stress, apoptosis, and antioxidants in human oral keratinocytes. Free Radic Biol Med 1999;26:992–1000.
104. Qin FZ, Shite J, Liang CS. Reduction of oxidative stress by trolox and superoxide dismutase abolishes norepinephrine-induced myocyte apoptosis and β-adrenergic receptor downregulation in ferrets. J Am Coll Cardiol 2000;35(Suppl):168A.

Index

Familial dilated cardiomyopathy, 22
Females/women, prevalence of diastolic heart failure, 17
Fe^{2+}-N-methyl-D-glucamine dithiocarbamate (Fe-MGD), 83
Fenton Reaction, 134–135, 139–140
Free radicals
 in biological systems, 68–87
 endothelial dysfunction, and thrombosis, 102
 worsening myocardial function, 99
 sites and mechanisms of generation in disease, 72–83

Gene expression, changes in myocardial, 51
Glutathione peroxidase (GPx), 137, 138, 157, 178
Glycoprotein IIb/IIIa inhibitor therapy, 225–227

Heart failure, natural history of
 age, risk factor of, 20–21
 and anemia, 31
 asymptomatic left ventricular dysfunction (ALVD), 7–8
 clinical presentation, 5
 clinical scoring systems, 5, 6
 clinical trial databases, 11–12
 comorbidities in heart failure, 22–31
 defining heart failure, 4–8
 demographic risk factors, 20–22
 diabetes mellitus and glucose intolerance, 27–29
 diastolic heart failure, 7, 17, 20
 disease burden of heart failure, 3–4

disease progression and prognosis, 31–34
epidemiology of heart failure, 12–17
familial dilated cardiomyopathy, 22
family history, risk factor of, 22
gender and ethnicity, risk factors of, 21–22
heart failure exacerbations and relapses, 31–32
hypertension and left ventricular hypertrophy, 26–27
increase in hospitalizations for, 3–4
left ventricular modeling as primary "lesion," 5
neuroendocrine activation, 7
and noncardiac vascular disorders, 31
and nutritional disorders, 31
and poor renal function, 30–31
population-based studies, 8–11
precipitating factors of heart failure, 32
prognosis of heart failure, 32–34
referral-based studies, 11
reverse remodeling, 32
reversibility of ventricular dysfunction, 32
and rhythm disturbances, 29–30
risk profiles and defining epidemiology, 8–22
serum brain natriuretic peptide (BNP), 7
and sleep disorders, 31
and thyroid disorders, 31
and valvular diseases, 29
ventricular dysfunction, 5–8, 17–20
Hemochromatosis, primary and secondary 131–133